The Medical in Mental Health

The Medical Model in Mental Health
An Explanation and Evaluation

Ahmed Samei Huda
Consultant Psychiatrist
Pennine Care NHS Foundation Trust
Ashton-under-Lyne
Lancashire, UK

OXFORD
UNIVERSITY PRESS

OXFORD
UNIVERSITY PRESS

Great Clarendon Street, Oxford, OX2 6DP,
United Kingdom

Oxford University Press is a department of the University of Oxford. It furthers the University's objective of excellence in research, scholarship, and education by publishing worldwide. Oxford is a registered trade mark of Oxford University Press in the UK and in certain other countries

First Edition published in 2019

Impression: 1

Published in the United States of America by Oxford University Press
198 Madison Avenue, New York, NY 10016, United States of America

British Library Cataloguing in Publication Data

Data available

Library of Congress Control Number: 2019932856

ISBN 978–0–19–880725–4

Printed in Great Britain by
Ashford Colour Press Ltd, Gosport, Hampshire

Preface

I wrote this book in order to explain the medical model and to evaluate its usefulness in mental health. The inspiration was twofold. Having read many critical comments about the medical model in mental health, it struck me that many of these criticisms seem based on a lack of knowledge or misunderstanding of the medical model, not just in psychiatry but also in general medicine.

There seemed to be an assumption that doctors in general medicine and general practice and other specialties treated diseases with known pathologies and that they offered very effective treatments that 'cured' diseases. Psychiatrists, in contrast, treated 'non-existent' diseases with ineffective and very toxic drugs. This set of assumptions did not seem to accord with either the research evidence or my own experience in clinical practice.

The second inspiration came when I was reading a textbook on general medicine—*Davidson's Principles and Practice of Medicine* (22nd Edition) by Walker and colleagues (2014)—as part of my continuing professional development. I took notes whilst revising and realized that many of the concerns about psychiatric diagnostic constructs and the effectiveness of treatments also occurred in general medicine. These notes form an important part of the later section of this book where I discuss how psychiatry compares to general medicine.

The apparent contrast between a pristine and scientific general medicine with its miraculous cures and a discredited psychiatry with its 'snake-oil' poisons was a mirage. To come to a more accurate conclusion it seemed that the best method was to define what the medical model was and then to discover the best criteria and standard for determining the effectiveness of its diagnostic constructs and treatments. The best standard for judging the criteria is to compare psychiatry with general medicine.

I have not found any recent book that addresses this issue so I decided to write my own. The classic books on the subject of psychiatry's concepts include a posthumous second edition of a book published in 1980 (Clare, 2011), the text by McHugh and Slavney (1998), and a more recent example by Ghamei (2007); none explain the medical model from the basics or make as detailed a comparison with general medicine. I wanted my book to be accessible to a wide group of people, not just doctors. This wider group included other people who work in mental health—psychologists, social workers, nurses—and their students. I also wanted patients and their families and academics/professionals who are interested in mental health such as sociologists, journalists, and philosophers to be able to read and understand this book. This means that I have assumed no medical knowledge in the reader, which has a drawback in increasing the length of the book as I explain everything.

The question then arises as to my suitability to perform this exercise. My qualification rests mostly on my years of clinical experience and, in the absence of anybody else stepping up to the plate, I have tried to write something from the point of view of the clinical psychiatrist rather than an academic. I have worked as a consultant psychiatrist since August 2002 (including about one year in Australia). I am not an academic psychiatrist—someone whose primary role is doing research—but I do try to look at broader issues and keep up to date with current research developments as much as possible. I spend all my time doing clinical work including sometimes working a full day, seeing patients in the middle of the night, getting up in the morning and doing a full day's work again. I only have 15 minutes to see patients for review outpatient appointments. This gives me a perspective on the importance of practical clinical usefulness that may escape my more academic colleagues. This has resulted in much of the book not being written in an 'academic style', which means I tend not to give references for statements that seem obvious or self-explanatory based on my experience. The earlier, more explanatory chapters tend to be less thick with references than the later chapters, which discuss the results of research. The simplest and most honest credential is that nobody else has done it recently, so I volunteered myself.

I have tried to be as accurate as possible and include the best-quality evidence throughout the book. I lay no claim to world-leading expertise in any of the subjects covered, so inevitably there will be shortcomings in both the evidence and analysis presented. What I am is interested in the field and I try to answer the questions as best as I can and to account for my intrinsic bias. I attempt to present the information fairly. It has been said that a high-level academic expert is more likely to be biased when they review the evidence on a subject (Chapter 9, Greenhalgh, 2010). Perhaps academia requires adopting 'strong' positions that lead to them ignoring evidence that contradicts the position they adopt and only talking about evidence that strengthens their point of view. I have seen books that are, frankly, biased and misleading about mental health but which try to spin this bias as a positive, by claiming to be 'balancing' the views with which they disagree.

This book is divided into three parts. The first five chapters explain the medical model and related issues and provide the background information. Chapters 6 and 7 are the 'hinge' of the book, where I review criticism of psychiatric diagnosis and treatment, respectively, and work out what are the relevant questions to ask to compare psychiatry with general medicine. In Chapters 8 to 16, I examine the usefulness of the medical model in mental health by discussing the evidence to settle the questions of how psychiatry compares to general medicine.

The amount of information and breadth of topics that I can cover means that a lot is left out and what is covered is done so very briefly. Important subjects that have been omitted include the effects of social factors on biology and a chapter on psychological factors in the aetiology of mental health problems. The latter was omitted as it was not one of the key questions to be addressed, but it is obvious to everyone the key role psychological factors have in psychological health issues (as well as in general medicine, but to a lesser degree). The tyranny of space allowed me has meant I sometimes use abbreviations. For example, I use the term 'psychobiological' not in reference to a Meyerian concept but as an abbreviation for 'psychological and biological'.

When referring to doctors, except when referring to specific individuals, I will try to use female pronouns as most doctors are female.

Any mistakes in this book are my sole responsibility.

Finally, I hope the reader finds this book informative and useful.

Acknowledgements

I would like to thank my wife, Aman Sharma, for putting up with me spending so much time on this book, to my parents who were always keen to see me in print, and to the Pennine Care Knowledge Management Team who assiduously tracked down hundreds of papers for me cheerfully and promptly. To all the people all over the world who encouraged me and offered useful feedback for this book, a big thank-you. I would like to mention in particular Professor Keith Laws, David Spindle, and Amir Sariaslan for their suggested alterations and encouragement. I would also like to thank the reviewers of my book proposal for their useful feedback. I owe a great deal of thanks to my editor, Peter Stevenson, for his endless support and encouragement and for agreeing to publish this book, and his assistant, Lauren Tiley, for her hard work, and Janet Walker performed a sterling job as copy editor.

Contents

Chapter 1

Explanation of basic concepts of medical terminology

A useful analogy can be drawn from John Steinbeck's novella *The Pearl*. A poor pearl diver finds a large and seemingly flawless pearl. The diver takes the pearl to a buyer to get it valued. The buyer shows the surface of the pearl magnified by a lens to the diver. What seems flawless is, under closer inspection, revealed to be rough and pitted. The buyer then offers a price far under the true price of the pearl, arguing that it is marred and therefore is not as valuable as it seems. If the buyer can pay a price far below the true value, then it serves to increase the profit made.

The diver suffers in this situation from 'information asymmetry disadvantage'. He lacks the knowledge that all pearls, when seen under a magnifying glass, are pitted and rough. The buyer knows this information and tries to exploit the diver by only showing the rough surface and not revealing this vital 'comparative information' (i.e. that all pearls look like this under the magnifying lens) to allow the diver to make a proper comparative judgement about the value of the pearl.

When people write about the faults in psychiatric practice and concepts, they often do so by comparing it to the rest of medicine. However, this omits the important comparative information. This may be because, like the diver, they lack knowledge of this comparative information and make assumptions about how scientific and effective the rest of medicine is. An example of this is to draw instances from general medicine of excellence in terms of practices and outcomes or depth of knowledge in the genuine belief that these are representative of all general medicine, and that, therefore, psychiatry appears worthless in comparison.

On other occasions, critics of psychiatry (like the buyer) are aware that their comparisons are flawed but they hope that the person they are addressing has an 'information asymmetry disadvantage' that they can exploit. They point out psychiatry's limitations without providing the information as to how it compares to medicine. A variant of this ploy is to cherry-pick examples of excellence from general medicine and claim they are a fair representation of the difference between general medicine and psychiatry.

The teaching of medicine focuses on practices and facts and not on their conceptual foundations. Often doctors know *what* to do, not *why* or what the *nature* of what they are doing is. Doctors are taught to be reflective about their practice nowadays, but this usually focuses on their actions (or sometimes their feelings) and not on underlying concepts. There is an absence of understanding of concepts in the medical curriculum (see the General Medical Council (GMC) and the United States Medical Licensing

Examination (USMLE) websites for the UK and US medical student curriculum, respectively). Thus, they may have stereotyped and limited views of what a diagnosis is, or the fact that illness and disease are always objective entities clearly demarcated from health. In their writings on medical matters doctors may use these unrealistic concepts, and readers without medical training may accept these unrealistic concepts about medicine as the truth. Doctors may be aware that they are sometimes guilty of over-simplification and they occasionally state this explicitly, but generally, most writing on diagnosis assumes that the reader is aware of this reductionism. Thus begins a chain of misinformation that spreads to people who have no medical training and who accept these medical concepts as the 'whole truth'. Therefore, they have an 'information deficit' and do not realize this, having, in good faith, read and accepted what doctors have written. They may then use these flawed medical concepts to write about medicine for people of similar professional backgrounds to themselves. This chain of misinformation then spreads like a virus.

The aim of this book is try and reduce 'information deficit' so that the reader can make up her or his own mind about the medical model in mental health. I will endeavour to be as fair as possible in describing and interpreting the evidence whilst recognizing that I cannot be perfectly neutral. Let me start by describing some essential concepts that are necessary to understand before progressing with the rest of the book.

This chapter will discuss the 'consultation' between a doctor and her patient. The doctor is said to have authority based on her knowledge, her professional behaviour, and her ability to influence the patient. The doctor's authority requires a framework of how to assess the patient and make clinical decisions. The medical model is one such framework: the doctor assesses the patient, recognizes a problem with associated knowledge, and then suggests a course of action based on this knowledge.

There is then a discussion of concepts such as 'illness', 'disease', and 'health'. Is it possible to make an easy, comprehensive, and reliable definition of these states? How do we apply these concepts to mental health? Finally, there is a discussion of how the medical model is one way of helping people but often other perspectives are needed.

The consultation

The encounter between a doctor and her patient can be described as a 'consultation' and is 'the central act in medicine' (Chapter 1 in Pendleton et al., 1984). In this consultation, both the patient and the doctor have agendas. These agendas may be similar or may differ to various degrees. The 'classic' agenda is where a patient has a problem for which they think may need medical attention: they want the nature of the problem identified, what is likely to happen, what caused the problem, and what the doctor recommends as treatment. Other agendas may be present. A patient may need to get an episode of sickness certified so that work won't punish them for taking sick leave. Another example is where a patient is detained against her will in a psychiatric ward and wants to convince the doctor that she does not need to be detained any longer. A doctor may want to ask a patient to take part in a research study. An unscrupulous doctor may wish to persuade a patient to accept unnecessary treatment in order to exploit her financially.

The doctor in this consultation is said to have three different forms of 'authority'—by which is meant 'the right to be heard' rather than 'the right to do what one wishes'—'sapiental', 'moral', 'charismatic' (Chapter 1 in Pendleton et al., 1984). This translates into roles or functions (see Figure 1.1). 'Sapiental' authority is the authority that a doctor derives from her knowledge, skills, experience, and expertise; the consequent role or function would be her knowledge of medical conditions and how to recognize and treat them. 'Moral' authority refers to the authority doctors receive from society due to their adherence to a code of ethics placing the patient's interests and care above all other interests as well as a 'professional' set of behaviours—such as being respectful, attentive, willingness to attend patients at all hours, and so forth.

I prefer the term 'professional' authority as doctors are not necessarily more 'moral' than others but are given authority by society because of the set of behaviours and attitudes that are characteristic of their profession. It may also derive, at least in part, from the doctor's knowledge and claim to expertise in a specific situation. The result is that society permits doctors to perform certain roles and grants them certain permissions such as being allowed to ask patients about intimate bodily functions or personal matters, to touch the patient during physical examinations, or to make decisions on health in the patient's best interests if they are incapacitated, or conduct evaluations on patients such as whether to allow access to healthcare, welfare benefits, or avoidance of punishment by the courts.

'Charismatic' authority is harder to define but refers to the ability of the doctor to persuade the patient to place their trust in her and believe that the doctor's decisions and actions will benefit them. This can increase the chances of the success of the doctor's proposed treatment, or at least the chances of the patient saying the treatment is successful. The doctor may derive this authority from their own self-confidence (which could be entirely misplaced) or from some other aspect of their personality. Sometimes it can flow from other forms of authority; if a doctor is clearly highly 'moral', exhibits a great deal of professionalism, or has a high degree of 'sapiental' authority by being renowned for being knowledgeable or highly skilled.

The obverse of 'charismatic' authority can see a doctor seeking and displaying power in order to satisfy her own needs as well as to impress patients. This type of authority tends to be allowed greater 'leeway' in terms of behaviour and medical interventions so long as the results are positive. Another role may be that of 'iconoclast' (i.e. shaking up a previously established way of organizing or delivering medical care if it can be shown that the method they use is superior to the orthodoxy). Great care must be taken that doctors don't confuse the authority bestowed upon them with licence to do what they want against the patient's or others' interests.

Other factors can influence doctors' agendas such as society, culture, and context; for example, a patient may need a sickness certification as part of the requirements of the society they live in, others may not. An involuntarily detained patient may seek to persuade the doctor that they were well enough to be released from detention and sent home. Other factors may be the health beliefs of the patient; for example, if they demand an antibiotic to help them with an upper respiratory tract infection

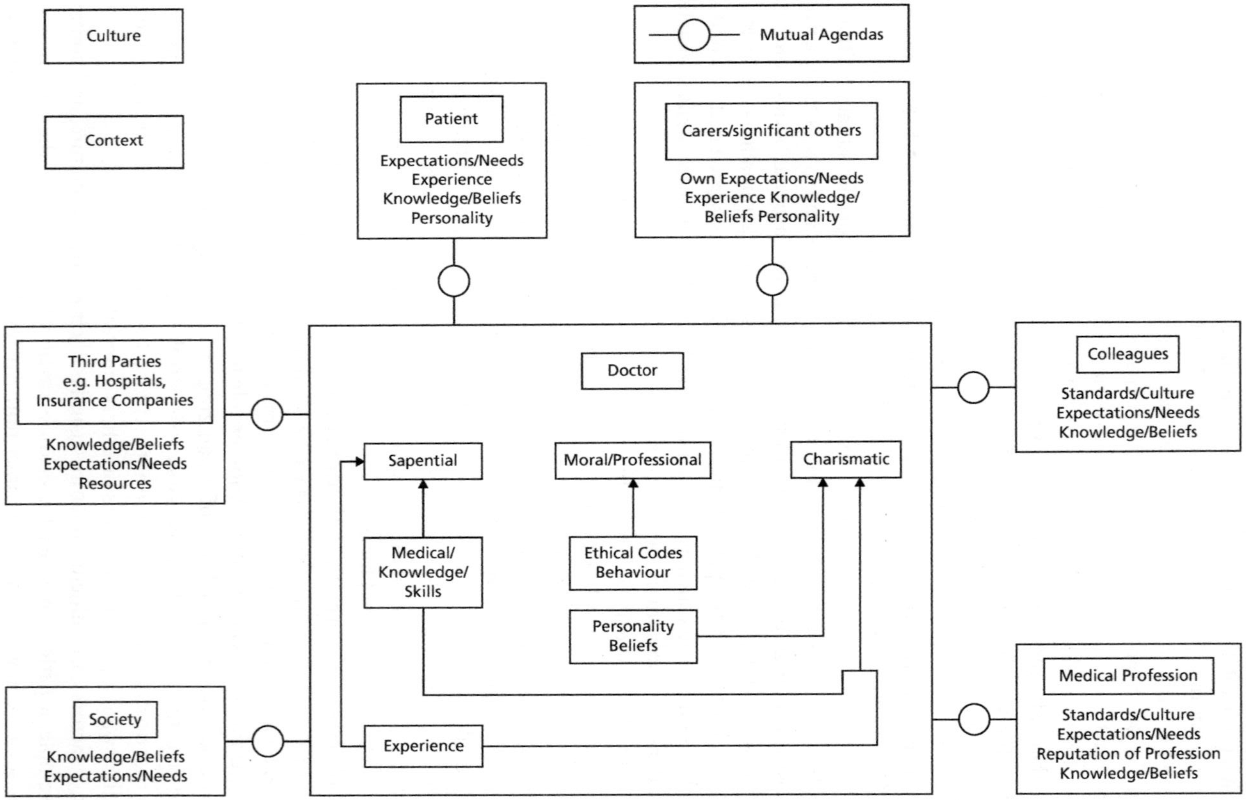

Figure 1.1 The consultation.

even if it is likely to be a viral infection and therefore an antibiotic is not an indicated treatment. The patient may have researched the possibilities of what could be causing their problem and might be seeking confirmation of what is wrong from the doctor or believes an investigation should be ordered. An unscrupulous doctor may try to exploit the patient. Personality, beliefs, and knowledge can affect all parties' agendas, not just the patient's. The start of the consultation should involve the doctor talking to the patient in order to discover what they want and then try and address their needs as best as possible.

Other parties are also involved in the consultation and have their own agendas. Often healthcare is paid for by a third party such as a health insurance scheme or a hospital or a government body. General practitioners (GPs) in the United Kingdom are usually self-employed but are paid by the National Health Service (NHS) for providing a primary care health service. These third parties have their own agenda in a consultation; they want effective health care to be provided but they also have an interest in cost-effective care and sometimes outright cost containment. Their definition of what is good quality health care and cost-effectiveness is influenced by their knowledge and beliefs and external constraints (such as budgets, directives, and guidelines on health care for certain conditions such as the National Institute for Health and Care Excellence (NICE) Clinical Guidelines). Medical care is very expensive so third parties are likely to want doctors to justify this expense. The third party expects the doctor to focus on providing healthcare based on their medical knowledge, skills, and experience in a professional manner. Given the expense, third parties expect doctors to see as large a number of patients as possible in as little time as possible.

Another example of third party involvement is when a doctor is asked for their medical opinion about a patient for a specific purpose. Examples include the courts (who may want to know whether a person is fit to stand trial), welfare agencies (whether a person is fit to work or how much care they need), or occupational health (if there are any health impediments to somebody carrying out a job). In these cases, these third parties are relying on the sapiental authority of the doctor to give an accurate knowledge-based answer and the professional authority of the doctor to give an impartial answer.

Society has input into the consultation, too. It has expectations of what it wants from doctors (for instance, to be knowledgeable, caring, professional, and honest) but also what patients can demand and get help for from their doctors. It was doctors' professional authority (i.e. their ability to be held to account by relevant authorities, their ethical codes of behaviour, and their ability to be administrators) rather than sapiental authority (i.e. knowledge of mental health problems and effective treatments) that led to them being put in charge of asylums in the nineteenth century (Chapter 2 in Burns, 2006). If psychologists or social workers existed as highly developed professions with professional authority during the Victorian era, then perhaps they would have become asylum superintendents instead of doctors.

Patients' carers, significant others, and relatives also have an agenda regarding the consultation. They (usually) have the patient's best interests at heart and want to see them get better. Sometimes variations in the agenda between patients and their significant others exist: perhaps a patient regards an aspect of their presenting problem as not too troublesome but their spouse finds it highly bothersome.

Doctors' colleagues such as nurses or other professionals also have agendas for the consultation. Perhaps they seek the knowledge of the doctor to resolve a query about the patient's clinical condition or deal with a clinical emergency, their sapiental role. These colleagues have their own knowledge bases and professional codes of ethics so only need from doctors what they cannot provide using their own sources of authority. They may need the doctor to confirm queries about health-related issues such as ability to walk a certain distance, capacity to make decisions, or to complete forms related to welfare benefits or other societal requirements.

The medical profession also has an agenda for consultations between doctors and patients. It derives societal authority and benefits from its good reputation. It therefore has an interest in making sure that consultation between doctors and patients does not bring the profession into disrepute. If the medical profession can reduce the frequency of inadequate or harmful practices by doctors and maintain a high level of good performance, then it can continue to justify doctors' high prestige and salaries. For this reason, the medical profession is suspicious of 'charismatic' practices as they can often cause unintended harm.

I have been discussing the different agendas parties to consultations bring to that engagement between doctor and patient. Moving now to standards, there must be a balance struck between standardizing good clinical practice and stifling innovation that may lead to improvement. The medical profession tries to maintain sapiental authority by education and training; encouraging continuous professional development; taking part in medical research and publishing the results in the medical scientific literature in order to update the knowledge base of other doctors. Doctors maintain professional authority by devising and teaching codes of ethics and professional guidelines as well as having established professional bodies responsible for disciplining doctors for breaches of professional ethics, such as the GMC in the United Kingdom.

The sapiental role/authority also requires a system which organizes and uses medical knowledge (such as what types of problems patients present with, the likely course of these problems, how to detect and identify them, what interventions help, etc.), skills, expertise, and experience. It requires a framework to systematize how this knowledge is acquired, how it is improved through research, how it is recalled and used in consultations and other clinical situations to make decisions that benefit patients. This framework can be regarded as a 'model' (model in this case refers to a system that tries to represent a field of interest for a specific purpose).

The medical model

The medical model as described in this book refers specifically to a system that a doctor would use to help in clinical or research practice to help identify clinical problems, make predictions as to outcomes and responses to treatment of these clinical problems, and an underpinning, understanding, or explanation for these predictions that could also form the basis of research.

Throughout the ages, doctors have used a variety of medical models such as imbalances of bodily fluids (the 'humoural model') or disturbances of energy flows in the body. Even in the same era (such as ours), different doctors will use different models. In fact, the same doctor may use different models, depending on which clinical problem or condition he/she is dealing with at the time. Although they are closely intertwined, we should separate the medical model as a description of a model of practice of how doctors interact with patients—in terms of methods of assessment, classification of their problems, and how they 'manage' their patients' health problems—from the various explanatory models that doctors used to explain their patients' health problems to themselves and their patients.

People often refer to the 'biomedical model' and sometimes understand this incorrectly to mean a model that focuses exclusively on a person's biology and biological interventions. The biomedical model also integrates the effects of culture, social factors, personal circumstances and beliefs, diet, upbringing, and so forth on health and illness. It can even accommodate the notion that psychological or social factors may be more important in the causation of certain conditions than biological factors and that the best intervention is not necessarily biological (e.g. medication) and often involves interventions based on psychological or social factors (Chapters 2, 3, and 4 in Guze, 1992). However, the biomedical model tends to view non-biological factors' effect on health as due to their effect on an intermediate biological factor. Doctors increasingly prefer a biopsychosocial model of explanation of health problems (which has ancient roots in medicine such as in the writings of Hippocrates) and that recognizes the importance of psychological and social factors in their own right as important for explaining health problems (Engel, 1981). It is important to recognize that this model does not mean biological, psychological, and social factors carry equal weight as causes for every condition and in every individual, and it can easily lead to 'trite' and 'sterile' statements (Chapter 1 in Ghaemi, 2007).

In this book, I discuss specifically a model of medical care that involves assessing a patient, then making decisions and interventions based on this assessment, followed by monitoring the response to these interventions by further assessments which may lead to changes in decisions and interventions, and so on in a cycle of assessments/interventions/assessment of effect of interventions and changes in severity (see Chapter 5). These assessments are undertaken principally by talking to patients in order to acquire a medical history but also by performing a clinical examination, ordering any relevant tests, and seeking additional details such as information from relatives and/or carers.

The doctor then uses this information to make a diagnosis (or more than one diagnosis). They also incorporate other important information into a 'diagnostic formulation' (see Chapter 2), and decide on a management plan that incorporates discussing with the patient the likely range of outcomes and the choice of recommended treatments and further investigations. A simpler definition of the medical model has been proposed in which doctors advise on, coordinate, or deliver interventions for health improvement based on the best possible evidence and that it is more important to know that a treatment is effective than its mechanism of action (Shah and Mountain, 2007).

The medical model is sometimes described as a 'disease-based model'. This is based on a misunderstanding that a diagnosis always refers to a disease that is clearly separate from other diseases and from optimal health, and that management of patients uses diagnoses focused on biological processes ignoring psychosocial factors In fact, as we shall see later, the medical model is a pattern recognition model: the clinical features of the patient are 'matched' to the clinical features of conditions that have been described in an existing body of medical knowledge (see Chapter 2).

To try to improve communication between themselves, doctors use standardized terminology which is often based on classical Greek. This is because of both the influence Ancient Greece has on Western culture as well as the specific influences of Hippocrates (and his 'School') and Galen, the pre-eminent Greek physician in Ancient Rome, on the development of modern medicine (Chapter 1 in Bynum, 2008).

'Patient' is the most commonly used term for the person being seen by the doctor (or consulting the doctor). Some prefer 'client', 'consumer', or 'service user': these imply a less deferential role and a more symmetrical power relationship with the doctor than the term patient. Even the very word 'patient' implies that the patient should be waiting at least in part for the convenience of the doctor. There are, however, disadvantages with being a patient in terms of an asymmetrical power relationship with the doctor, but there are advantages too.

Being a patient signifies that the person so designated is entitled to the protections and benefits offered by the doctor's professional code (often based on the Hippocratic Oath) as well as those of professionals allied to medicine. Given that doctors are amongst the most trusted professionals (as are the professionals allied to medicine such as nurses, occupational therapists, physiotherapists, etc.), these benefits may be highly regarded.

Surveys of people with mental health and physical health problems found that 75–80% preferred the term 'patient' (McGuire-Snieckus et al., 2003; Deber et al., 2005). Interestingly, there is a more even split between this and other terms, such as 'client', in cases where the individuals concerned are seeing other professionals, such as social workers. This suggests that people are aware of the different nature of the interactions they have with health and social care professionals and the different implications of the various terms.

When dealing with an individual, a doctor should use the term that the individual prefers. For the purposes of describing a group of people who are being seen by doctors in their professional capacities, I will use the word 'patient' throughout this book. There are good reasons why other terms are preferable but 'patient' seems an acceptable term to many people seeing a doctor.

'Symptom' refers to what a patient tells you about what they are experiencing. This is often 'grouped' or 'translated' into a medical term that is used as an umbrella term for similar descriptions of experiences by other patients (Chapter 1 in Brush, 2015). Sometimes this is expressed in plain English; other times a standardized medical term is used. For example, a patient may say 'I can't lie flat as I get breathless', which the doctor may record 'breathlessness on lying flat' or 'orthopnoea'.

The 'medical history' is a record of the information that the patient relays to the doctor. Apart from symptoms, other important information is sought such as age, gender, marital status, employment, family history of medical problems, past medical history, medications allergies, etc. Patients are questioned further to allow a more exact classification of their symptoms (e.g. timing, triggering, exacerbating, and relieving factors, and so on).

There is a systematic process drummed into medical students as to how to ask these questions, how to order them, and then how to record them. The aphorism is that 90% of the time a diagnosis can be made from the patient's history alone. A study looked at referrals to consultants in general medicine from their GP (Hampton et al., 1975). Most of the patients had already received a diagnosis from their GP. In 66 out of 80 patients, based on the history alone (i.e. just over 80%) and reading the referral letter from the GP, the consultant was fairly confident in their diagnosis. A further seven patients required a physical examination to be confident of the diagnosis whilst seven patients required physical investigations to make the diagnosis.

'Signs' are features of the patient that are detected by the clinician though observation and examination. They may include a wide variety of possibilities from rate of breathing, rashes on the skin, lumps, movement and speech abnormalities, unusual facial expressions, and so on. They may also include an *absence* of a feature or a reduction in a normal attribute or behaviour that would one expect to find, for example a missing finger or a silent chest with reduced or absent breath sounds. The more *reliable* the sign, the more likely different clinicians are to agree on the presence or nature of the sign. Something can be both a symptom and a sign (such as a patient complaining about a fever). The different signs are again 'grouped', based on similarities to signs observed in other patients (e.g. shallow breathing, different types of rashes, abscesses, and so forth).

For thousands of years, the patient's description of what has happened to them, their symptoms and signs, along with the timings of fluctuation of the severity of these symptoms and signs were the mainstay of the information that the doctor could acquire about the patient, apart from some simple bedside tests such as tasting the urine in patients with profuse urinary outputs to see if it was sweet like honey (with the patient diagnosed with diabetes mellitus) or very weak-tasting (the diagnosis being diabetes insipidus).

This information would be collated to form a 'clinical picture'. Both symptoms and signs would be translated into standardized terminology (even if the patient's own words were used in conversation with them). This was to facilitate communication between colleagues who would be discussing the same phenomenon. This standardized terminology was also used in textbooks, meaning that doctors had to translate how the patient described their health experiences into this standardized terminology in order to match it to what was learned from textbooks. The clinical picture would not just comprise symptoms, signs, fluctuations, and the results of any tests but also the description of what has happened to the patient and their personal details. Demographic data such as age, gender, what job the patient had, what effects their environment had on their health, what illnesses were commonly found in the patient's family, and other information that was felt to be clinically relevant were included in this overall picture. Hippocrates is reputed to have said 'it is more important to know what sort of person has a disease than to know what sort of disease a person has'.

This wider viewpoint of what is important to know about patients, not just their type of illness, has been claimed as inspiring many complementary traditions. It is, however, the direct forefather of the biopsychosocial medical model, which looks at the multiple influences on the person that influence health and what is perceived as good health. This model is more clearly seen in psychiatry but it is there, lurking in the background of all medical specialties to a greater or lesser degree. Traditionally, when doctors present cases to each other it usually begins with a brief demographic statement about the patient, ‘This 62-year-old businessman presents with a typical history of . . .’. It can also be seen as the root of many psychosocial models of distress, even if they eschew this distress being seen as a ‘health’, let alone an ‘illness’ issue.

Health, illness, and disease

The definitions of illness, health, and disease are the subject of extensive debate amongst philosophers of medicine. It is particularly relevant in mental health for reasons we shall discuss later in this chapter. This subject could occupy the rest of this book. If the reader is interested there are many books on this topic. I recommend *Psychiatry and Philosophy of Science* (Cooper, 2007) and *Concepts of Psychiatry* (Ghaemi, 2007). A good website that discusses how concepts of health and illness are based on objective criteria and the influence of social values can be found at <http://plato.stanford.edu/entries/health-disease/>.

Doctors are seen as primarily interested in illness and disease as opposed to health (although as we shall see later, doctors are involved with situations that are not regarded as illnesses). ‘Illness’ is a tricky term to define precisely. It is generally thought of as an often unpleasant state that is more than just the presence of disease (even if a disease can be identified) but also incorporates features specific to the individual such as their particular experience and personality (Chapter 1 in Pendleton et al., 1984). Patients with illness present to their doctor who may then try to discover if an underlying *disease* is present causing the illness (see Chapters 3, 4, and 5). Most of the discussion that follows uses the term ‘disease’ rather than ‘illness’ as ‘disease’ is the term that tends to be used in relevant philosophical discussions.

It is easier to describe (and recognize) examples of disease than to give a watertight definition that encompasses all states and conditions commonly (and uncommonly) regarded as diseases that also demarcate them neatly from states regarded as ‘healthy’ using purely objective measurements and terms. In other words, somewhere along the line we must include more subjective measures such as judgement of a professional. This professional in the case of diseases is usually, but not always, a doctor.

Trying to define disease in terms of subjective distress caused by the state so labelled would exclude some types of disease in which the patient doesn’t recognize an obvious deficit of functioning due to a brain problem—such as a stroke—causing anosognosia (an inability to recognize a disease or illness present). Other states that would be excluded from this definition include asymptomatic carriers of infectious disease—such as ‘Typhoid Mary’—although in cases like this, a test can be used to identify the presence of an infectious agent, but this relies on the presence of a capability to perform such a test. Examples such as high blood pressure are often asymptomatic but they are associated with increased risk of diseases like heart attacks or strokes. Of course, they have an objective element—the measured blood pressure—but this criterion of objective difference and increased risk of definite disease would also classify pregnancy as disease, which would be wrong (leaving aside the problem of demarcating neatly what blood pressure figures should be regarded as healthy and which should be regarded as disease).

Definitions that rely on abnormal functioning or harm flounder on defining exactly, without confounding examples, how such abnormal functioning or harm is to be demonstrated. Often what is decided as abnormal functioning or harm involves subjective judgement by a doctor. This can be regarded as a normative judgement. By this I mean a professional healthcare worker, in this case a doctor, makes a decision as to whether something is 'normal' or 'not-normal', in this case specifically a disease. The professional should make this judgement based on their professional knowledge and judgement. People, including doctors, disagree on whether specific states are diseases (Tikkinen et al., 2012).

Historically, these judgements were made before an accurate knowledge of the scientific basis of causation of these states. Doctors, and other professionals, made a judgement of a state being a disease often founded on a belief that this state differed from health, based on stress or harm caused to people or the risk of harm to self or others ('Typhoid Mary' had no symptoms but was regarded as having a health problem due to the risk she posed to others), and further that this state was *appropriately* regarded as a disease or at least a state suitable for medical attention by the society in which the doctor lived (Ereshefsky, 2009). Hippocrates stated that epilepsy, regarded as a sacred illness bestowed by the gods, could also be regarded as an illness for doctors to treat. He did this in the absence of the knowledge that it was caused by unusual electrical activity in the brain (or any way of proving this); the explanation used by ancient doctors was that it was caused by an imbalance of humours (bodily fluids) (Chapter 1 in Bynum, 2008).

What was regarded as disease will also vary, depending on the society the patient inhabited. Clare quotes the example of a South American tribe who regarded coloured skin spots caused by dyschromic spirechotosis (due to a treponemal infection) as a precondition for getting married and the absence of such skin spots as a sign of abnormality (Dubros, 1965; Chapter 1 in Clare, 2011). This is an example of how social values and their role influence and, in some cases, decide what 'disease' is. Of course, there are many examples of obvious disease that most or even all cultures would accept as such. People coughing up blood would be regarded by most people as being self-evidently diseased. However, there are also examples—as described above—where different societies or social groups (such as professionals) or different individuals will disagree about whether a condition constitutes a disease or not.

There is also the question of what measurements used to demonstrate demarcations between health and disease are truly 'objective', by which I mean that the results of such measurements and demarcations are completely unaffected by subjective judgement at some point and/or whomever observes and interprets these measurements. At some point in the creation of these measurements, the conception of these measurements, and the observation of these measurements, there is an element of subjectivity. Certainly, in the assigning of measurements to 'disease' or 'health' most research starts from the basis of a judgement as to what is 'health' or 'disease', then identifying what range of measurements are associated with either state. We then come to the issue of how people observe and finally interpret these measurements (assuming the measurements are observed by a completely perfect process). Even when examining clinical signs, there is often a degree of interpretation by the observer, often seeking a verbal confirmation from the patient ('does it hurt if I do this?') (van Praag, 1992). It seems that true objectivity is hard to demonstrate and, not for the first or last time, there is a 'dimension' of objectivity/subjectivity. Some methods or demarcations are 'more objective', others 'more subjective'.

Disease seems objective in that it suggests a demonstrated abnormality of structure or function, it seems to represent a state independent of the observer but there are elements of subjective judgement involved. This abnormality is clearly demonstrated using tests or investigations such as X-rays, microscopic examination for bacteria, or even more subjective tests such as an extreme score on questionnaire measuring psychological phenomena. This difference is supposed to be clearly seen between states of health and between different examples of disease.

Unfortunately, the concept of disease is also subjective in several respects. First, the process of demonstrating a disease process involves an initial step of labelling a condition or state as a type of illness and *then* performing research to see what differences in structure and/or functioning is associated with this type of illness, which is called disease (see Chapters 3 and 4).

Second, when interpreting the findings of any investigations there is often a point at which subjective judgement by a professional is involved (even if this is an informed judgement). For example, when examining a microscope slide for cells displaying signs of transforming into cancerous cells, there is a gradient or dimension of increasing signs of being a cancer cell. The pathologist must interpret where on this dimension the cell lies and to give a judgement as to which category the cell is best allocated. What is more, another pathologist looking at the same slide may disagree as to the most appropriate category. Even when bacteria are present in the body there is still an element of judgement regarding whether it is a pathogen causing disease (Casadevall and Pirofsky, 1999).

Third, in order to demonstrate what is abnormal, you have to be confident you have the capability to measure abnormality as well as being able to measure and demonstrate normal functioning. Unfortunately, for certain bodily functions and systems, our knowledge of how to measure and demonstrate even 'normal functioning' is beyond us. The most obvious example is higher brain functions such as thinking, emotions, and memory. If you cannot accurately and reliably measure and demonstrate 'normal' functioning (assuming you can satisfactorily establish what is 'normal') then you cannot demonstrate and prove 'abnormal' functioning. Thus, rules or definitions of how to define abnormalities of structure or function reliably run into difficulties and perhaps a messy solution is best (see Chapter 3 in Cooper, 2007).

Fourth, the very concept of what a disease is has varied with culture and history (Wulff, 1999).

In summary:

- It is easier to give examples of disease and to recognize clear examples of disease (i.e. they are prototype concepts—see Chapter 3) than to create a comprehensive water-tight definition of disease that clearly demarcates it from health and applies for every type of health state that is regarded as a disease.
- Disease is usually labelled as such based on whether it involves harm (such as distress, discomfort, impaired functioning, or damage to bodily functions or structures) or elevated risk of causing a more clearly recognized illness in the patient or others.
- The judgement by the professional as to whether a condition should be regarded as disease can be more or less/not contentious depending on the nature of the condition.
- Decisions as to whether a state of a patient's health is to be regarded as a disease will always involve elements of subjective decision-making: the health professional's judgement (a normative judgement) and the views and values of the patient's society help to decide what changes constitute illness or disease.

Disease and illness, if thought to be dependent on presence of disease, are concepts involving *subjectivity*. Concepts of disease involve 'biological, sociological, political, philosophical, and many other considerations' (Chapter 4 in Schoenbach and Rosamond, 2000). Health is also tricky to define clearly and reliably and separately from illness or disease (Chapter 3 in Pendleton et al., 1984). The World Health Organization, in its Constitution of 1946, famously defined health as 'a complete state of physical, mental and social well-being, and not merely the absence of disease or infirmity'.

Sir Aubrey Lewis, the Australian psychiatrist, said of this definition that nothing could be more 'comprehensive than that, or more meaningless' (Lewis, 1953).

How many people's 'health' would meet this definition? If it does not meet this definition does this mean people are unhealthy, ill, or even diseased? Who decides if somebody has 'well-being'? Health proves to be another tricky concept to define reliably and satisfactorily. Health, like illness and disease, is easier to recognize but much harder to define in a value-free way that reliably identifies people who are healthy from people who are not, and in a manner with which everyone will agree.

Disease and illness are terms that imply that the states thus labelled are definitely medical problems and appropriate for doctors to assess and to treat. There are many examples of cases where this would not be contested, and most would agree that it is appropriate for medical attention be directed towards these. The issue becomes more contestable in more marginal examples. 'Disorder' has been suggested as a substitute term for disease, using the criteria of presence of harmful dysfunction, involving both scientific and social value judgements (Wakefield, 1992). I will use the term 'condition' instead. Although this term has medical connotations, these are not as strong as they are for disease and illness and it sounds less harsh or judgmental than 'disorder'. By 'condition' I mean a description of a state in a person that may come to the attention of health services (Ereshefsky, 2009) but does not mean that this state is definitely an illness or disease, or even a state that should be regarded as a primarily a health problem (instead of, for example, a social problem). Some conditions should not be regarded as an illness or disease at all, although they may be regarded as suitable for medical attention, like pregnancy.

Given the element of subjectivity and the role of professionals in deciding which conditions constitute illnesses or diseases, is it the case that conditions labelled as illnesses or diseases should *only* be viewed with the medical model? Emphatically, no! Many conditions can and should be viewed using multiple models. For example, the social model of disability is far more useful for planning adaptations to the environment, allowing maximal participation by everyone in society. This model identifies what the barriers are to participation by people in society: an obvious example is stairs, with no ramps, as a route of access to a building.

The medical model can thus be viewed as follows:

- One way of conceptualizing and helping a condition and not necessarily the *only* way.
- Not automatically the *best* way of helping to achieve all or indeed any desired outcomes.
- A model that is willing work in conjunction with other models, in a multi-model, multidisciplinary way (i.e. with others such as carers, other professionals), each contributing a part to achieve desired outcomes.
- A model that at times may be unhelpful or even harmful for certain conditions.

Hippocrates illustrates this with his views on epilepsy, the so-called sacred illness. Although he was of the view that epilepsy had natural causes, this did not mean it was not *also* a sacred illness, in the sense that it had a spiritual dimension. This is an example of what has been described as 'promiscuous realism' (Dupre, 1996), the theory that there are often multiple ways of viewing the same subject. Each different view or way of viewing or representing the subject illuminates a different aspect, the implication being that amalgamating these different views gives you a better glimpse of the whole subject. The model that you use in a situation depends on how useful it is for you to achieve the goals that you seek; for example, trying to reduce the chances of a harmful outcome in a patient or reducing symptoms.

A parable illustrating this view is the story of the blind Indian men encountering an elephant. One felt the trunk and pronounced it was a snake, another felt the flank and said it was a wall, and so forth. They are only describing what they are experiencing from their perspective. One can argue that they are making the mistake of assuming that what they experience is the sum of what should be said of the subject and that they do not realize it is only a fragment of the whole. If they discuss their own conclusions with each other they can put all this information together and come up with a complete picture of an elephant rather than the individual parts they each feel.

We have discussed the influence of subjectivity on deciding what is illness and disease. In *The Myth of Mental Illness* Szasz was concerned that deviant, albeit ordinary, human behaviours and problems were being 'pathologized' for the purpose of social control (Szasz, 1960). His contention was that 'medicalizing' a particular condition/behaviour was justified only if an objective disease—defined as either a structural or functional abnormality of an organ—could be demonstrated.

There are several problems with Szasz's view, but the most relevant one for this book is that it is too prescriptive to be of any use in an applied science such as medicine.

Generally speaking, conditions are 'medicalized' before causal understanding is obtained. This is especially the case in psychiatry, since our understanding of the mind–brain functioning is still unfolding.

We are unable to demonstrate the biological processes creating, for example, thoughts. Since we are unable to demonstrate the processes of 'normal' mental functions of the brain, it follows that we may be unable to demonstrate 'abnormal' mental functions unless they are caused by obvious structural abnormalities (such as brain tumours causing mental symptoms), or obvious functional abnormalities (such as the dysregulated electrical activities in epilepsy), or they are the same pathological processes found in the rest of the body (such as autoimmune diseases causing behavioural abnormalities). This set of problems has been referred to as 'the mind–brain problem' (Chapter 1 in McHugh and Slavney, 1998). It is possible that we will never properly understand the physical underpinnings and functions of the mind (Chapter 6 in Guze, 1992).

Hence, if we have an imperfect knowledge of bodily systems, as we do for the higher functions of the brain, we cannot tell if abnormality of function or structure *precedes* or *causes* the behaviour labelled as an illness. Szasz argued that we should only label states or conditions as illness if we can definitely demonstrate disease. In a debate with Szasz, Clare pointed out that this meant, for example, that tuberculosis could not have been regarded as an illness until the causative bacteria was discovered by Koch in the late nineteenth century; the millions of people dying of 'consumption' or tuberculosis, as we now call it, were purportedly dying of a purely social construction until that moment. This was a definitive argument that Szasz was unable to counter (Chapter 8 in Clare, 2011). We should remain cautious of applying the label of illness to conditions when we do not have an objective confirmation of a disease process validating this label.

Tuberculosis is an example of diagnosis with clinical benefits ('utility'), in this case recognizing the risk of death, the need for medical intervention, and an explanation for the symptoms and signs of the patient, before the discovery of adequate scientific knowledge explaining the cause of the diagnosis ('validity') and ultimately leading to the discovery of more effective treatments. Doctors are clinicians who use science in order to benefit their clients. Before they had adequate scientific knowledge they still offered benefits to their patients—such as placebo benefits from treatments they prescribed—and developed clinical concepts and practices that were found to be useful. If doctors had discovered that magic or witchcraft was superior to science, they would have abandoned science and embraced eye of newt and toe of frog!

Our knowledge of both the normal and abnormal functioning and structure of the body is incomplete. The immune system, for example, contains much that we still don't understand but of all bodily organs, the brain remains the greatest mystery.

Conclusion

Doctors embody three types of authority that transform into roles or functions: sapiental (e.g. knowledge), professional (e.g. ethical codes of behaviour), and charismatic (the ability to persuade the patient to obey the doctor and have faith that they will benefit). Fulfilling the sapiental role requires doctors to have a framework to work in or model to learn, and to use their knowledge. Not all interactions between a doctor and patient will make use of this model.

The medical model refers to both how a doctor assesses a patient and manages her health problem, as well as an explanatory model used by doctors to illuminate the health problem at hand. Doctors prefer a biopsychosocial model that takes into account biological, psychological, and social factors as an explanation of health problems. It is easier to give examples of disease (we can use the broader term 'illness') than to create water-tight definitions of disease. There is often a medical professional's normative judgement that the patient is presenting with a disease. 'Disease' implies a demonstrated abnormality in the patient of structure or process that explains the health problem (though even this often involves normative judgement). 'Condition' refers to a state that is associated with distress or harm or risk of harm to the patient or others. Some conditions thought suitable for medical attention are not illnesses or diseases, such as pregnancy.

People have argued that for an illness to be present there must be demonstrated disease, but, amongst other reasons, this is a false argument as this assumes a current perfect state of knowledge as to what, precisely, constitutes a disease. This definition of demonstrated disease is particularly difficult to apply in mental health as we know little about the normal functioning of the brain, let alone abnormal functioning.

The medical model, as a way of working to help people with health problems, is one way of helping people, a model of practice. There is also a medical model of viewing and explaining these problems, a model of explanation. 'Promiscuous realism' and practical experience suggests there are multiple models of viewing people's problems, and multiple ways of helping people with these problems. The medical model is not necessarily the best way to view or help a problem. Doctors work with other professionals who use other useful explanatory models and/or ways of working with people.

Chapter 2

The role of diagnosis in medical practice and society

This chapter discusses how doctors organize the information they learn and how they apply this knowledge in clinical practice. Doctors accumulate a tremendous amount of information, both semantic knowledge (e.g. facts about health and illness) and procedural knowledge (e.g. how to examine a patient and perform medical procedures). This information is structured to aid learning and utilization. This information is split into two types of knowledge, clinical and medical. 'Clinical knowledge' refers to the type of knowledge that the doctor uses when they are with the patient (e.g. how to talk to a patient, how to observe them and examine them, and what the correct modes of behaviour are). 'Medical knowledge' refers to semantic knowledge such as anatomy, physiology, pathological changes in disease, what medications to use in certain situations, and so on. Some practical examples of clinical and medical knowledge are shown in Table 2.1.

This is exemplified by the textbooks medical students read for the general medicine (called internal medicine in North America) part of the curriculum. Two types of textbooks are often recommended: *Macleod's Clinical Examination*, and either *Davidson's Principles and Practices of Medicine* or *Kumar and Clark's Clinical Medicine*. The first textbook (*Macleod's*) focuses on history-taking and clinical examination (i.e. clinical knowledge). The second pair of books cover the variety of conditions seen in general medicine (including mental health conditions) (i.e. medical knowledge). North American medical students may use *Bates' Guide to Physical Examination and History-Taking* for clinical knowledge and *Harrison's Principles of Internal Medicine* for medical knowledge. These types of knowledge are not completely separate; both clinical and medical knowledge textbooks will include information on symptoms and signs.

The role of diagnosis in organizing and accessing information

One of medicine's challenges is how to translate the knowledge of diseases and other conditions from medical knowledge into clinical decision-making that benefits the patient in front of the doctor. This is accomplished by matching the patient's presenting problem to the best fit for conditions known to the doctor. There are over 10,000 known medical conditions (Muth and Glasziou, 2015) and whilst we can't expect a doctor to know or to have even heard about all of them, we do expect the doctor to

Table 2.1 Clinical and medical knowledge.

Clinical knowledge examples	Medical knowledge examples
How to take a history of medical problems from a patient and enquire about symptoms	Functioning and structure of 'normal' or healthy functioning of the human body, mind (psychology), and society (sociology)
How to observe and examine a patient for signs of illness How to behave with patients: acting respectfully and caringly	Illnesses and associated information such as common pathological processes (e.g. inflammation or infection), diagnostic investigations, and medical treatments
Appropriate ethical behaviour	Injuries and likely complications
	Drugs and effects on human body and side effects

know something about a large proportion of them, particularly common conditions. This is an information and performance logistics problem: the acquisition of a body of useful knowledge during training and then the ability to recall relevant parts of that knowledge whilst seeing patients. The doctor often finds herself under multiple pressures when performing clinical assessments:

- *Time pressure*: such as only 10 minutes allowed per GP consultation or a queue of patients waiting to be seen in the emergency department.
- *Large number of potential presenting problems*: the patient can present with a large number of problems or collection of problems (sometimes these problems may not need or be appropriate for medical attention). These problems can present in a variety of manifestations and combinations.
- *Matching patients' problems to learnt knowledge*: the doctor must sort through a large volume of information stored in her mind about the range of problems she has learned in order to recognize what the current presenting problems are. She must then decide what the appropriate course of action is.
- *Physiological pressures*: the patient may be in pain or experiencing distress that affects their ability to communicate with their doctor. Sometimes the patient has impaired consciousness or is unconscious, making it difficult or impossible for the patient to communicate with the doctor. The doctor may be seeing the patients at 3 a.m. or fatigued for another reason, may be hungry or even unwell herself.
- *Expectations*: the doctor is aware that she has a duty to perform her medical tasks to a minimum standard expected of someone with her experience and extensive training. These expectations come from herself, her patient, her colleagues, especially fellow doctors (who, apart from concern for the patient, do not want the reputation of their profession to be damaged by sub-standard practice), her employers, and society (which expects doctors to perform to high standards as part of its social contract with doctors, which includes paying them well and regarding them in high esteem).

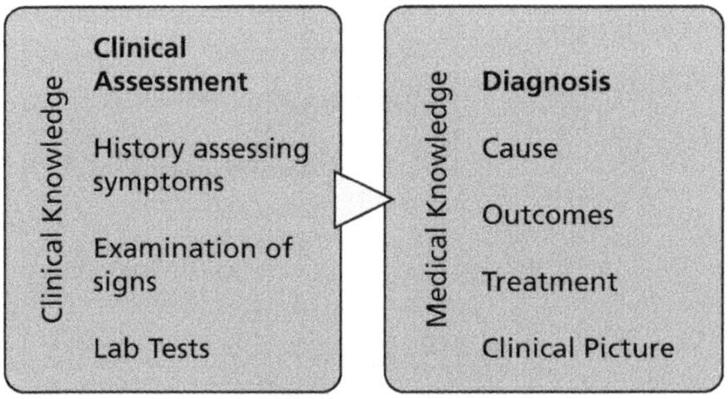

Figure 2.1 Diagnosis as a bridge between medical and clinical knowledge.

- *Consequences of decisions and actions*: she is also aware that the consequences of her getting something wrong could involve serious, adverse consequences for the patient such as pain, disability, continued distress, or even death.

The system medicine has developed has been 'battle-tested' over thousands of years of practice under these exacting conditions. However, in the particulars of their specific job, doctors may find it fruitful to learn about systems of working other than adhering to the classical medical model; for example, doctors who practice psychotherapy or doctors in general practice (Chapter 1 in Pendleton et al., 1984).

Doctors use the information gained from clinical knowledge (i.e. being able to ask the patient relevant questions as well as knowing how to observe and examine the patient). This information then needs to be linked to knowledge of conditions in medicine. Diagnosis is used as a bridge between these two types of knowledge, semantic and procedural, as well as a means of organizing substantial areas of both types, and has been used to organize information about a range of conditions of medical interest for thousands of years (Chapter 1 in Bynum, 2008).

For each diagnosis, the doctor will learn important information such as cause, outcome, treatment, and, crucially, how to recognize a given condition by the 'clinical picture' offered by the description of what has happened to the patient (which may include information on triggers or causes of the problem), the symptoms, signs, and lab tests associated with the diagnosis. This information is based on research and experience of people with a similar clinical problem (Chapter 1 in Sackett et al., 1991). Furthermore, diagnosis acts as the link between clinical knowledge and medical knowledge (see Figure 2.1).

The different conditions given a diagnostic label are organized into categories based on 'systems' aligned to specialties (e.g. cardiovascular system/cardiology, nervous system/neurology). This allows a 'meta-structure' of conditions based on a system's organization; for example, see the chapter headings in *Davidson's Textbook of Medicine* (Walker et al., 2014). This is a way of organizing medical knowledge: each system is a 'branch', with separate conditions acting as 'leaves'; see Figure 2.2.

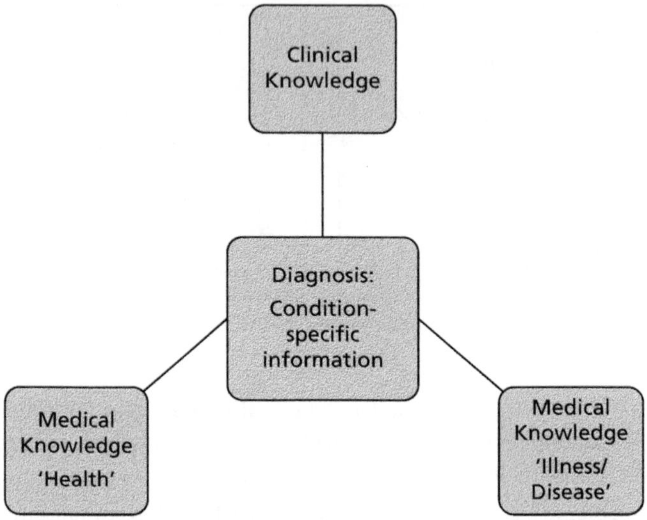

Figure 2.2 Structure of how doctors integrate different types of knowledge with individual patient.

Diagnosis in clinical practice

Patients can present with a nearly infinite potential combination of symptoms and signs that need to be interpreted (Schwartz and Wiggins, 1987a). General practitioners might encounter a patient with almost any potential medical condition and only have about 10 minutes to identify the problem and devise a treatment plan before doing the same again, and again, for consecutive patients for several hours. An inexperienced doctor in hospital can see a severely ill person at 3 a.m. and must recognize and initiate life-saving action whilst knowing that there are several other similarly sick patients still waiting to be seen. There are multiple pressures acting on the doctor, as described earlier, as well as the problem of the doctor possessing incomplete information about the patient or the condition.

Rules of thumb (or 'heuristics') that can be memorized through repetition and constant use are helpful (Croskerry, 2002; Chapter 5 in Brush, 2015), but they also possess the potential drawback of being over-relied on or may lead to cognitive errors (Croskerry, 2003; Berner et al., 2008). Heuristics are used as they save time, cost, and cognitive effort (Graber et al., 2002) and are particularly useful when the doctor is under pressure (Croskerry, 2009). Heuristics may take the form of learning of small lists and rules, for example, for:

- Different conditions associated with a variety of clinical signs or symptoms.
- Procedures to perform in certain situations.
- Common or dangerous problems and how to investigate, treat, and manage them.

These heuristic methods rapidly identify useful information. This has been referred to as 'system 1' cognitive processing style, which is fast, intuitive, and effortless (Bate et al., 2012). This is based on the theory that there are two types of cognitive processing systems used in decision-making, a faster 'system 1' and a slower 'system 2' (Croskerry, 2009).

System 1 is generally preferred due to its greater economy of use of time and cognitive resources. The conclusions are often 'plugged in' to a network of information to guide the doctor's actions and recommendations, often in the form of 'mindlines'. These are 'collectively reinforced, internalised tacit guidelines' that act as 'socially constructed knowledge in practice' (Gabbey and May, 2004), used by doctors and created via contact with local opinion-leaders as well as more formal guidelines.

The most pragmatic and common way for experienced doctors to recall clinically relevant information is to perform 'pattern recognition' of resemblance to a 'prototype' clinical picture associated with a particular diagnosis (Chapter 1 in Sackett et al., 1991; Croskerry, 2009; Bate et al., 2012; Preface in Brush, 2015). This process is rapid (see, for instance, Cooper, 1983, and Chapter 5 in Brush, 2015) and the doctor may not be aware of doing this. It has been compared to a skill that improves with practice and occurs below the level of consciousness (Schwartz and Higgins, 1987b). This may be supplemented by awareness of conditions important not to miss as they may cause serious harm to the patient (Croskerry, 2002). The features of the clinical picture that allow the doctor to identify the diagnostic construct (the diagnostic criteria) are not necessarily the same as the whole or substantive nature of what is represented by the diagnostic construct and may not describe all the features of the clinical picture associated with the diagnostic construct (Kendler, 2017). For example, myocardial infarction may be recognized by raised serum enzyme levels or ECG changes but the myocardial infarction itself involves obstruction to the heart's blood supply leading to death of cardiac muscle; depression encompasses a greater degree of experiences than those listed in its diagnostic criteria.

Using clinical knowledge to gain information that creates a clinical picture, doctors rapidly form multiple hypotheses about several diagnoses that may be present (based on their medical knowledge) (Barrows et al., 1982). They then select the most likely diagnosis based on how well the 'clinical picture' fits the 'prototype' of one of a large number of potential diagnoses in their medical knowledge (Shedler et al., 2010). They will then 'run' with this hypothesis until contradictory information arises that disproves this hypothesis (Schwartz and Higgins, 1987b). Then they must look for another diagnosis that fits the current clinical picture in a better way.

Although this seems a straightforward process of two sequential stages (identify elements of clinical picture then match to nearest diagnosis as in Figure 2.3), it is usually an interaction rather than a sequence; ideas of possible diagnosis plus concepts of typical examples of these diagnoses influence how and which symptoms/signs are assessed or recognized (Berrios and Chen, 1993). This interaction of what the doctors expect to see based on rapid hypotheses about likely diagnoses influences what information the doctor searches for and how they interpret it.

An 'exhaustive' version of reaching a decision on a diagnosis is to collect all the clinical information first and *then* fit it to the best matching diagnosis (Chapter 1 in Sackett et al., 1991; Graber et al., 2002). Research studies that use diagnosis often adopt this 'exhaustive' technique to try to improve the reliability of this diagnosis. This may be combined with standardized ways of interviewing and examining the patient and standardized ways of performing clinical tests to further improve reliability.

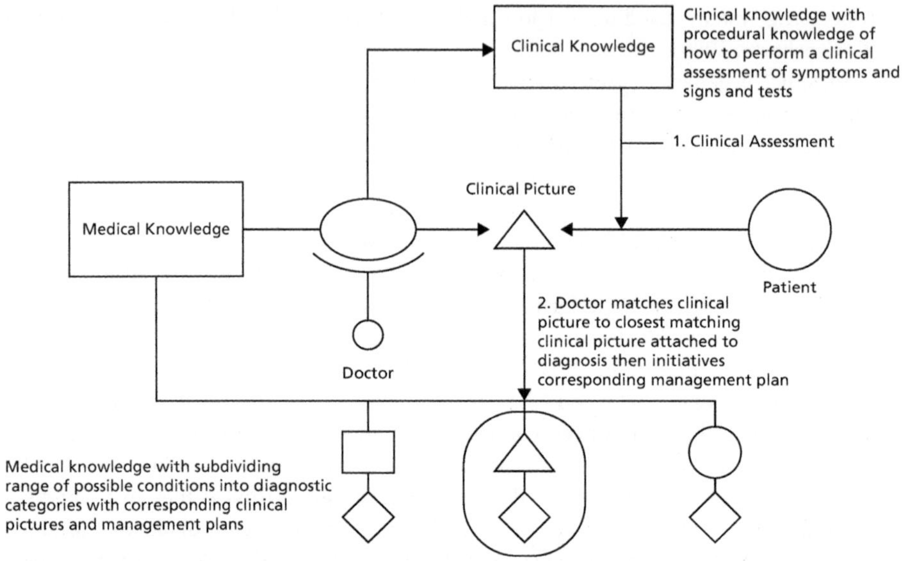

Figure 2.3 How doctors incorporate clinical and medical knowledge using diagnosis in deciding management plan.*
Step 1 Clinical assessment of patient by doctor utilizing clinical knowledge produces clinical picture.
Step 2. Doctor matches clinical picture to closest matching clinical picture and its corresponding diagnosis, then initiates management plan associated with that diagnosis.
*Additional useful information acquired from clinical assessment is omitted to simplify diagram. Unidirectional arrow used to depict relationship between clinical picture and matching diagnosis but is actually a two-way process.

This 'exhaustive' technique is not as common in clinical practice because it involves increased costs, time, and effort.

Four different diagnostic techniques have been described, all based on identifying previously described conditions with relevant clinical information attached (i.e. a diagnosis) (Chapter 1 in Sackett et al., 1991).

1. The pattern recognition technique described earlier.
2. 'Multiple branching' (i.e. a decision tree, informing clinicians which assessments to take and what the results mean in terms of a diagnosis or further assessments required). Although Sackett and colleagues (1991) suggest this is often used by other professionals using the medical model or in 'triage' situations, it is often used by doctors for 'broad clinical problems' (see Chapter 3) until a more definitive diagnosis is made.
3. The exhaustive approach, described earlier, of completing the history and examination and other investigations before deciding the likely diagnosis.
4. The hypothetico-deductive strategy. Doctors (and medical students) very quickly—within seconds or minutes (Chapter 1 in Sackett et al., 1991)—form a list of diagnoses likely to explain the patient's situation. They then look for confirming

information (and information that disproves the likely diagnosis, but note that doctors are less good at noticing this). This meshes well with the pattern recognition technique as doctors look to identify if the suspected diagnosis is present.

An alternative to these techniques is to build a bottom-up view of what features the doctor can detect in the form of symptoms and signs, and then try and work out, using their medical knowledge of how the body is supposed to work normally, what is the underlying abnormality present. Looking at the clinical signs and symptoms present, they can deduct from physiological and anatomical principles what may have gone wrong and thus deduce a chain of pathological events. This method—of identifying the condition by cross-matching what has been observed to have gone wrong in the patient with what is known that can go wrong in a system, then using deduction to identify the diagnosis—is commonly practiced in neurology.

There is still an element of 'pattern recognition' in this method but there is a greater element of deduction. This type of deductive/analytic approach has been referred to as the 'system 2' cognitive processing style (Bate et al., 2012). It is slower than system 1, with rational deliberations based on careful evaluation of the known information. System 1 is preferred but if it fails to come up with an answer that satisfactorily explains the clinical situation then the doctor will use the system 2 cognitive style. Although described as two different systems, they may really be opposite ends of a spectrum of cognitive processes (Croskerry, 2009).

To stereotype these two approaches: Dr Quick and Dr Slow both see the same patient. The patient is in his 60s, sitting up in bed with many pillows, leaning forward with marked respiratory effort and tinge of blue around the lips. Both legs are swollen and if pressure is applied to any swollen areas such as on top of the feet or the ankle, an indentation is formed in the skin that very slowly returns to normal. Dr Quick is already thinking is the patient is presenting with congestive cardiac failure. Dr Quick looks for information in the history and examination and what tests to order to confirm the diagnosis, and brings to mind a memorized treatment plan for congestive cardiac failure. The mental processes involved in how the doctor sorts through the information to select the initial diagnosis rapidly are still unknown to some extent (Chapter 14 in Cooper and Sartorius, 2013).

Dr Slow is performing a comprehensive history and examination of every possible symptom and every possible clinical examination. Dr Slow has noticed the signs of increased fluid in the extremities, particularly in the gravity-dependent regions of the lower legs. Both doctors further note the raised jugular venous pressure and other physical signs such as the 'crepitations'. Dr Slow knows about physiology and anatomy. By a gradual process of deduction, Dr Slow works out all the possible causes of the observed symptoms and signs using her knowledge of basic medical sciences.

Dr Slow may order tests and then try to interpret the results using her knowledge of medical sciences. Dr Slow gradually deduces that the problem may be due to a problem with insufficient cardiac functioning, then she must try to deduce what interventions may be useful. This process relies on Dr Slow avoiding deductive errors in trying to determine what is happening.

This deductive process takes a lot longer (Chapter 2 in Brush, 2015) than performing a clinical assessment of the patient to identify relevant information followed by recognizing a prototypical picture of a diagnosis (Scadding, 1967), which then triggers information-seeking that confirms the diagnosis and what interventions should take place to identify causes and alleviate the condition. Dr Quick has most likely started treatment whilst Dr Slow is ploughing through her first set of deductions. This example is clearly loaded in favour of Dr Quick. Dr Slow is entitled to point out that often patients do not present with a typical clinical picture, or the clinical picture is misinterpreted and the wrong diagnosis is chosen (Croskerry, 2002; Berner et al., 2008), leading to Dr Quick at best wasting time, at worst using interventions that decrease the chance of a positive outcome. Sometimes the clinical picture is very complex—due to co-occurring conditions or presence of other factors—and requires some element of deduction to understand the situation in full and choose the correct interventions.

Dr Slow's method results in a treatment plan which is devised based on detailed findings related to that specific patient and how the condition manifests itself in that particular individual. She could quite rightly argue that Dr Quick's method rests on assumptions, generalized inferences drawn from the study of other patients with the same diagnosis who may be different in varying degrees to the patient being seen. Nevertheless, the ability to recognize conditions that are similar in important respects to those that have been seen and studied before gives Dr Quick's approach two distinct advantages over Dr Slow's: speed of decision-making and the ability to base decisions on evidence gathered from the study of patients with similar problems.

Dr Quick points out that Dr Slow relies on accurate knowledge of both the normal functioning of the affected bodily systems as well as what could go wrong with the functioning of these systems. This knowledge, where it exists, arose relatively recently in the history of medicine, which goes back thousands of years, some of it from the eighteenth century, much of it more recently, most of it is incomplete. Many systems of the body are still only partially understood, the immune system and basic brain functions such as control of movement, for example. The mind and its functions (e.g. thinking and memory) are even more poorly understood. Given this imperfect knowledge there will be many cases where deduction alone is insufficient, even today. In these cases of a knowledge gap making deduction difficult or even impossible, what is the doctor to do? Can she tell the patient to 'come back when we know more (might take thousands of years)', and send the patient away?

Long before doctors possessed accurate and useful knowledge of the science of human illness, they were still able to make diagnoses that provided useful information on the expected range of outcomes as well as sometimes guiding what treatment to offer. This was based on careful observation of groups of patients with the same diagnosis (see Chapter 5). This was possible even if doctors had inaccurate models of illness such as the 'humoural theory' (Chapter 1 in Bynum et al., 2008). In medicine, a diagnosis could have *utility* (usefulness such as knowing the broad range of outcomes and sometimes different treatments associated with the illness) without *validity* (in this case defined as knowing the pathological processes causing the diagnosis).

Diagnosis was not historically a 'scientific' classification system based on accurate knowledge of the causes of what was being classified but instead a 'clinical' descriptive classification system based on what was useful to the doctor at the bedside in recognizing conditions with implications for prognosis and, sometimes, treatment.

Throughout history, doctors gave the impression (and often believed themselves) that they had an accurate scientific understanding of the body and its illnesses. Historically, even if the knowledge of a given conditions' causation is poor, diagnostic constructs could still offer some utility from information gained by careful observation.

Diagnosis at the hub of clinical decision-making

In clinical practice, a mixture of the two types of thinking—fast, intuitive, system 1 and rational, deliberative system 2—are used to identify a diagnosis and its implications as well as to deduce further information about what is happening in the body in terms of knowledge of functioning and anatomy (Croskerry, 2009). The doctor will often form a quick impression as to the type of the condition they are presented with (usually in the form of a diagnosis) but will often have to use deductions to make sense of other clinical information they detect and to aid decision-making. If they are unable to come to a diagnosis quickly or their initial diagnosis does not fit with the clinical information, then the doctor uses a more deliberate analysis of the clinical data to deduce a new diagnosis. This is a hypothetical-deductive style of clinical thinking.

The diagnosis is used as the hub of clinical decision-making (Kendell and Jablensky, 2003; First et al., 2004; Gale, 2006):

- It links the clinical knowledge of identifying symptoms and signs to the medical knowledge of conditions of medical interest and their causes, outcomes, and treatments.
- It forms an important part of the information seeking that a doctor performs in order to recognize a clinical picture linked to a diagnosis through pattern recognition.
- Once a diagnosis is arrived at it then drives a further process of clinical decision-making and information-seeking.

A diagnosis is not the same as certainty and not the sum total of information required about a patient (Chapter 1 in Ghaemi, 2007). Attached to a diagnosis is useful information which guides the clinical management plan (Chapter 1, Sackett et al., 1991; Chapter 3 in Guze, 1992) and triggers further enquiries, not the least of these being is the diagnosis correct and should it be changed, what types of further tests and examinations the healthcare team should perform and when, and what additional information should be sought by the clinical team (see Figure 2.4). The information attached to a diagnosis often takes the form of probabilities.

- *What types of clinical picture does this diagnosis present?* The range of probabilities of how the diagnosis will present in terms of symptoms, signs, lab tests, or other important clinical features. This will tell the doctor how to recognize the condition, what information to seek, and how to find it. It will guide the doctor regarding what questions to ask, how to interpret the answers, what tests to run, and what pattern of results to look for, often as part of a pattern recognition exercise.
- *What if the diagnosis is wrong?* The possibility that the diagnosis is correct (its reliability) according to some external criteria—usually for most medical specialties a test (such as biochemical test, pathology of diseased organ, imaging test) but it could also be another expert doctor's opinion. This possibility of the diagnosis

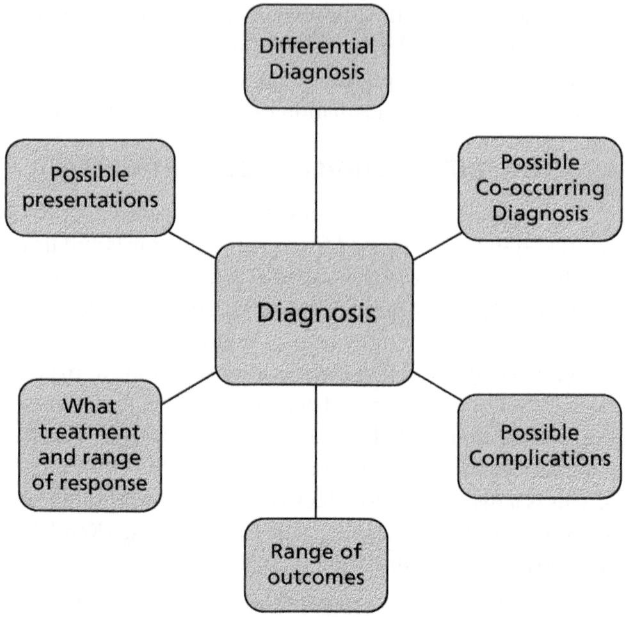

Figure 2.4 Diagnosis at the hub of linked information and information seeking.

being incorrect means the doctor should continue to be vigilant and search for information that suggests the diagnosis is incorrect. If such information is unearthed then the doctor should revise (change) the diagnosis to one that fits the information better, including the 'null option' of 'no diagnosis'. The doctor should keep a differential diagnosis (or many differential diagnoses, or even the 'null option' of no diagnosis/no illness) in mind, ready to adopt if it fits the available information better.

- *What other conditions could be present?* The presence of more than one condition is known as co-morbidity or co-occurrence. One condition may increase the chances of developing another condition. Some conditions may have similar underlying causes, thus increasing the probability of more than one conditions being present or that different conditions are actually different aspects of a broader underlying condition (see Chapter 3). This alerts the doctor to look for signs or symptoms or to run tests or investigations for these other potential diagnoses.
- *What complications should I look out for?* There can be a risk of additional problems or features being present, or developing subsequently, that are known to be associated with the diagnosis. This triggers the doctor to look for these other potential problems by asking the patient for symptoms indicating another problem is present, examining the patient to look for these problems, and running further tests to identify these problems. Even if the problems are not present at the initial assessment, they can develop later. Armed with this knowledge, the doctor can be alert for them occurring.

- *What treatment should I offer*? The range of possibilities of treatment and the range of responses to treatment—what are the different alternative treatments (not just medication)/help available? How likely will the diagnosed condition respond to treatment? How long will this treatment take to improve the condition? What are the signs of this improvement taking place? What side effects may occur with treatment and how do I identify these? Patient-specific information may also affect treatment outcome (e.g. if they are allergic to the medication; if they have any biochemical features that affect the drug such as rapidly metabolizing it; whether they are on any other medication that affects the proposed treatment; whether there are any features of the specific illness in the patient that will affect the treatment outcome such as severity, etc.).
- *What do I expect to happen in people with this diagnosis*? The range of possibilities of outcomes seen with this diagnosis. Most illnesses don't have a fixed outcome but have a range of probable outcomes. This permits the doctor to discuss these details with the patient. The range of factors that are associated with better and worse outcomes are also linked with the doctor's knowledge about the diagnosis and allow the doctor to look for their presence and modify them if possible.

Diagnosis is provisional and is always open to review as more information comes to light. A reluctance to change the diagnosis in light of contradictory information is a type of medical decision-making error (Croskerry, 2003). Diagnosis is the hub of linked information that the doctor has learned about a condition that guides the doctor's management plan. It is not a comprehensive statement of all that is needed to make clinical decisions. Deciding on the diagnosis is just the start, not the finish, of clinical decision-making.

Diagnosis can be thought of as a *quantum reflexive hyperlinked seed*. 'Quantum' reflects the uncertainties regarding whether the diagnosis is right, the probabilities of outcome, treatment, and so on. It is 'reflexive' in that the information associated with the diagnosis includes procedures to monitor whether it is accurate or should be replaced by a new diagnosis. It is 'hyperlinked' in that the diagnosis is a hub that links multiple domains of information about the condition as well as what additional information needs to be acquired that is specific to the patient, not to the diagnosis. The 'seed' describes the compact nature of a simple term like diagnosis which is jam-packed with the information and procedures needed to develop a management plan to help the patient by a doctor with the ability to respond and act on the information given to her by the patient. Diagnosis is a short-hand method of incorporating relevant clinical information and using it, and it evolves as knowledge improves (Chapter 3 in Guze, 1992).

Who benefits from making the diagnosis? Surprisingly it is the doctor who is the *direct* beneficiary. She has gone from a situation of great uncertainty—the patient presenting with a near-infinite diversity of problems and their manifestations—to one of greatly reduced uncertainty. She has reduced the great uncertainty to a better idea of the range of probabilities of complications, outcomes, what other conditions could be present, treatments and their effects, and so forth. The patient is the *indirect* beneficiary. The doctor is now better equipped to give the patient important information about their condition such as a prognosis or available treatments to help both, doctor and patient, jointly make a management plan.

Another way that the patient benefits is that the problem for which they are seeking medical attention has been given a name. This naming has several implications, the first being that this type of problem has been seen before by the medical profession and has been incorporated into medical knowledge. Second, as noted earlier, the medical knowledge associated with this name should increase the doctor's ability to offer help with the problem such as offering the patient some idea of the likely outcome or, better still, identifying an effective treatment. Third, it gives a sense of validation: this problem offers the patient legitimacy in claiming the role of a 'sick' individual (see later) and seeking help from others, not just health professionals. Fourth, it can provide an explanation for what the patient is experiencing even if the explanation is 'that we tend to see *x* in cases of *y*'—a better explanation is possible if we understand the aetiology of a diagnosis and the mechanisms by which its associated problems are produced.

At times, the diagnosis is not welcomed or it may even be contested by the patient, who may feel that the diagnosis is wrong and should be different. They may feel that their situation should not be given a diagnosis at all. They may object to a negative aspect of the diagnosis such as a poor prognosis or stigma attached to the diagnosis.

The value of an individual diagnosis relies on the accuracy and depth of information (such as range of likely outcomes and responses to treatments) attached to that diagnosis and the usefulness of associated procedures (such as which tests to run to look for important additional information). If the diagnosis itself is associated with poor quality information or even misleading information, then it is not of much use. There may be problems with certain diagnostic constructs but that does not mean there is a problem with the system of using diagnostic constructs, which guides treatment and management, as a whole.

Factors other than diagnosis are used in guiding clinical decision-making. Within a diagnosis there may be individual features associated with a diagnosis that guide treatment. There may be factors associated with the individual that guide clinical decision-making (e.g. smoking may affect outcome or individual drug allergies that mean certain treatments are avoided). There may be economic, cultural, geographic, or other factors beyond the individual that guide clinical decision-making.

For example, different countries and regions offer different advice as to what antibiotics to use, depending on local bacterial antibiotic sensitivities. Different resources available may drive what types of investigations and treatments are offered. An example of cultural factors includes male-dominated societies where decisions about whether to perform a caesarean section may legally need to wait for permission by the father to proceed, even if the mother's and/or baby's life is in danger.

The patient's clinical problems may also be formulated as a problem list, with a plan for each item of the list. Often diagnosis is integrated into this problem list where appropriate. If the problem is 'breathlessness', then clearly the diagnosis explaining breathlessness is relevant. Sometimes the problem is one of poor functioning of an aspect of the body (e.g. poor urinary output) and the solution will involve both deduction and knowledge associated with the diagnosis. Sometimes the problem list incorporates items for which the diagnosis is of no help at all. For example, if the problem is homelessness (i.e. a socioeconomic problem), then the diagnosis may be of little use (although a diagnosis of a medical problem that may improve an individual's eligibility for housing may be of enormous importance; see later in this chapter).

Often the diagnosis is incorporated into a 'diagnostic formulation',. Doctors take 'histories' from patients. The vital clinical information about the patient is often compressed into a brief summary. This will include important clinical findings and other information as well as important negatives (what has been shown to be absent), and includes the likely diagnosis as well as relevant differential diagnosis. This is moving from a general summary of information from the diagnosis alone to a more individually specific summary of the clinically relevant information than the information gained from the diagnosis alone (Schwartz and Higgins, 1987a). This summary is then exchanged between doctors when one 'presents' the case to the other—often a more junior doctor to a more senior doctor. This summary attempts to explain why this particular person is presenting with this particular problem (and, further, why they still have the problem and indicating what we should be doing about it).

The doctor is not just focusing on the diagnosis but also taking in the wider realm of relevant clinical information; that is, the typical medical model does not *exclusively* focus on the diagnosis or disease but instead on a more comprehensive assessment of the patient, of which diagnosis is but a part.

In order to fulfil its role in clinical decision-making, the diagnostic system has several qualities.

- Aids *communication and consistency between professionals.* When two health professionals are discussing the same diagnosis they need to know that they are referring to the same condition. If doctors mean different things by the same diagnostic label, then the information attached to the diagnosis becomes unreliable and even contradictory or dangerous (Stengel, 1959; Chapter 2 in Cooper and Sartorius, 2013).
- It *improves the consistency of medical practice to an established standard.* Diagnosis often forms the basis of guidelines or recommendations issued by professional or governmental bodies. This reflects its role as a tool of communication. A good example in the United Kingdom is NICE which publishes guidelines on good clinical practice for different conditions using a diagnostic label so that individual clinicians can identify to which patients the guidelines apply.
- It acts as an *organizing function of medical knowledge.* As described earlier, diagnosis is used to organize medical knowledge.
- It is the basis of *research.* A condition with a diagnostic label can be used as a basis of research for causative factors, disease process, and effective treatments. Diagnostic categories are useful in forming the basis of and ordering contemporary research, which in turn is based on the careful observations conducted by medical predecessors such as Hippocrates, Galen, Avicenna, or Ibn Sina (Bynum offers a brief history of medicine including descriptions of these medical giants and their ideas; Bynum, 2008).

- It forms a *barrier against idiosyncratic concepts or the abuse of medicine.* Medicine can be abused by the powerful to justify social oppression. Medical authority can also be used to exploit vulnerable people who are desperate for help with a condition by giving this predicament a diagnostic label and offering to help—for a fee, of course. By creating a standardized terminology of diagnostic labels, doctors can try to minimize the spurious authorities of a 'wild diagnosis'. An example is the former Soviet Union where political dissidents where diagnosed with 'sluggish schizophrenia'. The absence of this diagnosis from the official diagnostic classification of the World Health Organization in itself could not stop this abuse but it highlighted the fact that it *was* an abuse of medical authority in the name of the state (Chapter 2 in Cooper and Sartorius, 2013).

It is not a necessary characteristic for diagnostic constructs to be scientifically validated entities, clearly separated from health and from other entities. Different types of conditions described by diagnostic labels are discussed in Chapters 3 and 4.

Other functions of diagnosis

Medicine and its practice have a powerful impact on society. Doctors and their ways of how they think about illness dominate how people think about health and illness. Doctors determine, to a large extent, the *discourse* society employs about these matters. A diagnosis doesn't just have an effect on how doctors think about their patients and their clinical management of them, it also has powerful social effects on how society interacts with patients. Diagnosis enacts a strong influence on the administration of healthcare, access to benefits and the collection of statistics. Nikolas Rose, Professor of Sociology at the Department of Social Science, Health and Medicine at King's College London outlined ten of these additional functions or *implications* of a diagnosis (Rose, 2013):

1. Access to treatment
2. Payment for treatment or ability to claim payment of treatment from health insurance
3. Permitted absence from work or reduced other social expectations
4. Eligibility for social welfare benefits
5. Administration of healthcare, including recording activity and claiming payment for said activity and organizing services
6. A reason for involuntary detention and/or treatment (in conjunction with other factors)
7. Eligibility for special educational support
8. Collection of health statistics such as incidence and prevalence of conditions
9. Health statistics used to plan health service provision
10. Eligibility for research funding and for charities to be organized around a diagnostic construct

Let us look at these points in detail. The first, and related second, points are that to gain help for a problem from the healthcare system, the individual must have a problem that is recognized by medicine as being a *legitimate* medical problem with a diagnostic label confirming its place in the body of known medical conditions. These healthcare services require a diagnostic code to justify providing the service they offer. Without this code, they may not be able to provide the service: if publicly funded, the said service may be restricted to those with a diagnostic code of some kind—the taxpayer may not want health services to deal with problems that are not deemed to be appropriate for the health service to be treating. If funded by a third party payer such as an insurance company, then the service provider may need a diagnostic code in order to claim payment so that the insurance company can be sure it is funding legitimate claims. The diagnosis therefore provides an 'authorization key' to justify access to and use of a service.

The third point is about diagnosis granting access to welfare payments; society wants some means by which authority for service provision is granted in order to justify welfare payments to an individual (to avoid paying out money unnecessarily). A diagnosis that is known to be associated with an impairment of functioning that gives a health reason for someone being eligible for a particular welfare payment is one such justification. It should be noted that health reasons are powerful motivators to society for *perceived eligibility of need* for additional support including welfare payments. As part of their professional responsibilities to society, doctors are expected to provide accurate diagnoses of conditions, providing a legitimate health-based reason for accessing these welfare payments.

Parsons' concept of the 'sick role' is useful in this context (Parsons, 1951). Parsons was an influential sociologist who postulated that to be described as 'sick' was to enter a state of 'deviance' from social norms. This state had certain rights or exemptions but also certain responsibilities.

- The person was exempt from normal social responsibilities (e.g. not having to turn up to work whilst unwell, or seek work if their illness prevented them from working.).
- The person was not to be blamed for this state or held responsible for their condition.
- The person was expected to try to get well and not exaggerate their infirmity in order to avoid tasks.
- The person was expected to seek help from socially sanctioned healing professionals and follow their recommendations.

This is a great simplification and plenty of exceptions to it can be found. Diagnosis of a 'legitimate' medical condition (i.e. a condition known to medicine and which is regarded as serious enough to justify granting the benefits of the sick role for the situation) may need to be combined with evaluations of degree of impairment of functioning before being accepted as a key to validating the eligibility of an individual to welfare.

Even dimensional concepts of illness need a categorical statement of someone being 'sick enough' to justify being granted the benefits and exemptions of the 'sick role'. Sometimes the 'sick role' is used to justify the imposition of responsibilities on the 'sick' person. Sometimes this includes restriction of liberty or imposition of treatments, as we shall discuss later (Chapter 13).

Being given a diagnosis may, and often does lead to people treating the person diagnosed differently. Often people are identified with their illness (Chapter 11 in Cooper and Sartorius, 2013); think, for instance, of 'diabetic', 'epileptic', 'schizophrenic', 'leper'. Apart from other people treating the diagnosed individual differently, the diagnosed and labelled person may regard themselves differently. This identification of a person with their illness can have many ill-effects, including stigma—from society, from healthcare professionals, and about themselves.

Rose's point 6 is an example of how being given a diagnosis means people may treat you differently than others in an unpleasant or detrimental way. Being given a diagnosis may mean that certain legal rights such as liberty may be allowed to be waived. For example, 'Typhoid Mary' was detained initially for a period of years and then later until she died because she was a carrier of typhoid and had been linked to several deaths. People with mental health conditions who refuse to be admitted to hospital may be detained involuntarily (although other conditions such as concerns for the person's health, safety, or other people's health may apply). A diagnosis may have unwelcome consequences for people, including stigma or loss of liberty.

Rose's Point 10 concerns how a diagnosis can act as a 'rallying point' around which a cause can coalesce and can also be used to justify research funding. Identifying a diagnosed condition and attaching information to that label such as impairments, consequences, and complications that can be expected helps justify fundraising or access to existing research funds to help identify a cause, treatments, and support for people with the condition. People being approached to give money trust that the cause is legitimate because of the diagnostic label.

Points 5, 8, and 9 represent two opposite ends of the same process. In most situations, a third party pays for some/all the costs of healthcare. This is usually a government, insurance company, or a charity. (Some services are still paid directly by the patient.) These third parties need a system of procedures to manage costs, plan services, and ensure they aren't being exploited by healthcare providers (such as doctors, other health professionals, or larger groups such as clinics or hospitals).

Diagnosis provides an important piece of information in verifying that the charges made to the third party are reasonable. There is inevitable variation of costs for conditions with the same diagnosis, but an insurance company is likely to smell a rat if billed $500,000 for a case of ingrown toenail but more understanding if the same charge was levied for a case of severe pancreatitis requiring a prolonged stay in an intensive care unit and several urgent operations.

Professor Mary Boyle, strongly opposed to the use of diagnosis in mental health, admitted that it is a convenient system for social functions of diagnosis such as administration and eligibility for services (Boyle, 2007).

A healthcare provider which relies on funding from third parties such as governments or insurance funds will require an administrative coding system of healthcare needs, such as a diagnosis, to justify expenditure on providing healthcare and charging third parties. The alternative would be a system where the patient has to pay for all the costs themselves to the healthcare provider out of their own pocket. Diagnostic codes are often used as the basis of collecting information—as well as procedures—on activity by healthcare providers and then provided to the third parties.

Governments collect and publish health statistics. They also submit these health statistics to the Global Health Observatory of the World Health Organization. To allow comparisons within and between countries, the statistics need to be cited using common terminology to summarize health information such as a standardized diagnostic coding system.

These statistics also allow identification of worrying trends that demand action. Epidemiologists collect data on the *prevalence* (the number of people with a specific condition over a period of time) and *incidence* (the number of new cases of condition over a period of time). Apart from managerial and financial concerns outlined earlier, this type of information provides vital intelligence. For example, if higher rates of an infectious disease than are usual are detected, this alerts the relevant authorities that there is the risk of an epidemic developing and to take the relevant preventative actions (such as vaccinating people at risk). This is why certain diseases are 'notifiable', such as measles or poliomyelitis, and must be reported centrally if cases are diagnosed by the clinician. Another instance is where unusual illnesses are noticed to be more frequent than expected. It was an upsurge of unusual infections in the United States that led to the identification of AIDS and its causative agent, HIV (Chapter 4 in Schoenberg and Rosamond, 2000).

Conclusion

Doctors needed a way of organizing the large amount of knowledge learnt about conditions of medical interest. This system of organization helps them learn this information and then access it when seeing their patients. The system used was a way of categorizing illness and other conditions under a diagnostic label. Doctors learn clinical knowledge about how to assess patients and this produces a clinical picture. This clinical picture is then matched to the closest resembling prototype of a clinical picture attached to a matching diagnosis. This allows them to access medical knowledge attached to the diagnosis, such as the range of likely complications, co morbid/co-occurring conditions, outcomes, and treatment responses to expect. This forms the hub of clinical decision-making. However, every diagnosis is *provisional* and can always be discarded if subsequent information suggests another diagnosis (or no diagnosis) fits the available information better.

Diagnosis of a condition needs to be reliably agreed between clinicians in order to fulfil its additional roles of communication between professionals as well as a classification system for research. A universally agreed diagnostic system can also act to highlight idiosyncratic or even oppressive practices by individual clinicians or even entire countries.

Medical concepts have a powerful effect on how society views health. As a result, medical diagnosis has many social effects as well as having an important role in the measurement of health by statistics; the administration and management of healthcare as well as access to healthcare; how health problems are researched; and how welfare benefits are tied to health status. Some of the social effects resultant on being given a medical diagnosis may be beneficial, such as reduced expectations of the person to fulfil a social role such as work. Some of the social effects are less benign, such as loss of liberty or stigma.

Chapter 3

The nature of diagnostic constructs

A diagnosis is a construct used by doctors for certain purposes. It is a classification of conditions of interest to doctors and other healthcare professionals. This chapter will review why and how classification is used before discussing the different types of conditions classified using diagnostic constructs.

Classification

Classification refers to both the action of classifying and the end result of this process. Classifying involves grouping phenomena (whether real or conceptual) according to similarities. This is a process that is common to the most primitive organisms as necessary for survival (Sokal, 1974) and forms the basis of human cognition (Parnas, 2015). Classifying our experience of the world is both necessary and universal amongst living organisms.

The result of this process is a 'classification' which is a schema of objects or concepts (often referred to as a 'taxon'). The next step is identification: recognition of which category in the classification a newly encountered example should be allocated to (Sokal, 1974). In medicine, for example, when seeing a new patient there is an 'identification' of which diagnosis the patient's clinical picture fits best (see Chapter 2).

One purpose of classification is 'economy of memory'; saying someone is a native French speaker avoids having to list the millions of words, grammatical and sentence structures that they can be expected to know and use. 'Without this ability to summarize information and attach a convenient label to it we would be unable to communicate' (Sokal, 1974).

This ability to communicate allows transmission of knowledge between individuals. Classification facilitates the acquisition of knowledge in research by allowing grouping of objects or individuals on the basis of similarity in a quality (such as gender, weight, or presence of an illness). This ability to summarize information allows people to learn and memorize many concepts or constructs rather than learn about a few concepts in massive detail.

Sokal notes that classification tries to describe relationships between classified concepts or objects (Sokal, 1974). This may attempt to describe an underlying principle reflecting the natural world or some artificially imposed constraints such as a maximum number of categories, or, in medicine's case, an easily recalled way of recognizing previously described states with attached useful clinical information in the patient that the doctor is clinically assessing. Trying to classify biological entities into neat categories clearly separated from each other is much harder than classifying entities in physics or chemistry (Dupre, 2001).

In medicine, we could choose to avoid classifying problems that patients present with for two reasons: the first is that there is no need for classification because the important features of the problem are essentially the same in everyone; the second is that there is no classification possible due to the uniqueness of the individual's problems.

Every patient has three types of attributes (Kendell, 1983):

1. Attributes shared by all patients.
2. Attributes shared with some patients.
3. Attributes unique to that patient.

If the first approach is taken by focusing on the attributes shared by all patients, then several problematic implications result (Keeley, 2015): that everyone has the same outcome, the same causes, and they should all have the same treatment or intervention. People with lung cancer clearly have a different prognosis and receive different treatments than people with colds. Of course, there should be common elements of treatment such as kindness, respect, listening, and compassion. Nevertheless, it is important to differentiate conditions in order to gain important clinical information such as differing range of outcomes, treatments, or complications.

The second approach, focusing on the unique attributes, is seductive as it appeals to individualism: everyone is unique and therefore the conditions they present to doctors are unique and so should not classified. It is a common saying that 'labels are for jam jars, not people' and 'you shouldn't put people in a box'. First, it is not the people themselves that should be labelled or put in a box but the problems that they present (APA, 1994). Categorizing people's personalities comes close to classifying all a person's nature but doctors are, in theory, only classifying those aspects of a person that have brought them to medical attention, not the person in entirety, but this distinction is often hard to establish or, in the case of the patient, *felt*. Second, not everything *should* be given a medical classification. Nevertheless, concluding that people are unique and that their presenting problems are *completely* unique, therefore making it impossible to classify their problems, leads to major problems. Using this logic, information gleaned from one patient cannot be applied to other patients. If everyone's presenting condition is so unique there are no similarities between them, there is no point observing, analysing, or researching a given person's health problem as it will only apply to that individual (Hill, 1952). Doctors will be 'flying blind' every time they see patients.

That this is argument presents an 'appalling vista' does not make it wrong, but a cursory experience of medicine suggests that similarities do exist between people with the same diagnosed condition. People with a cold have more similarities in their symptoms and their likely outcomes with others suffering the same condition than with people diagnosed with lung cancer. In other words, it is important to classify a person's problem but this does not mean we should equate the person with that diagnostic label. Patients present with unique combinations of several factors but some of these factors may be in shared with other people. We can learn about these common factors in patients in order to help us gain useful information the next time we encounter these common factors in future patients. These factors could be demographic issues such as gender or wealth or ethnicity. They may be better viewed as dimensional constructs (like height or weight) or as 'non-medical', for example, psychological factors like self-esteem. There is thus a need to recognize similarities between patients in the form of a classification to learn useful information and then apply it when we see patients. This does not mean that all these factors should be classified under a categorical diagnostic system.

A third argument is that classification of medical problems causes more harm than good. We discussed in Chapter 2 the malign effects of stigma and other undesirable outcomes due to a person being 'labelled' with a medical diagnosis. Given the importance of classification to medical practice to inform clinical decision-making it is difficult to accept this argument as valid without severely impairing medical practice healthcare. There may be specific situations where it does apply, particularly where the harms caused by giving a diagnosis outweigh any benefits.

For example, the Soviet Union's labelling legitimate political protest as 'sluggish schizophrenia' carried no benefits for the patient as there are no medical treatments for this fictitious condition and plenty of harm done to the patient via involuntary incarceration and unnecessary treatments. The argument that classification does more harm than good is an argument for avoiding *inappropriate* medical classification, not against medical classification as a whole. It can also be used as an argument for a properly constituted medical classification that excludes situations that are inappropriate for medical attention (Chapter 1 in Cooper and Sartorius, 2013).

Some form of classification of the conditions that people present with is necessary in order to acquire useful information about them (e.g. range of outcomes, complications, or what treatment to use). Medicine has reduced uncertainty by using diagnostic constructs to guide clinical decision-making, in research as well as these constructs having other social and administrative functions (see Chapter 2).

There are two types of concepts commonly used in classification. The first is defined by a set of criteria that are said to be individually necessary and jointly sufficient (Ramsey, 1992). They are individually necessary in that each criterion must be met before a proposed example of the concept can be regarded as a true example. Jointly sufficient in the sense that if all these criteria are met then the proposed example is a true example of the concept.

To identify a shape as a square we may use the following criteria:

- Four sides equal in length
- Four straight sides
- Sides join at angle of 90 degrees only

To identify a shape as a square we go through these individual criteria and if all are fulfilled then the shape is a square. The problem with this type of classification is that it is often overly rigid and does not describe all examples of a member of a class (Dupre, 2001). For example, if a dog is defined as having an essential criterion of having four legs, how does that account for three-legged dogs?

Humans do not tend to classify what they encounter by exhaustively ensuring a list of criteria is fully met before identifying the correct category. Instead, people often try to identify key features and match what they encounter to prototypes of likely categories (Rosch and Mervis, 1975; Ramsey, 1992; Keeley, 2015). The closer an example is to the prototype the quicker it is identified as a member of that class (Rosch and Mervis, 1975). For instance, a more typical bird such as a sparrow is more quickly recognized as a bird then an atypical bird such as a penguin. These key features can also vary by context or circumstance (Ramsey, 1992), resulting in a flexible construct reactive to circumstances.

This makes good evolutionary sense. Imagine trying to identify a potential predator. Waiting until the potential predator fulfilled *all* the criteria that defines the particular predator might leave us in dangerous proximity to it. A better method is to look for key features that might help us distinguish crocodiles from floating logs. Piecing together an identification of a potential predator from an incomplete picture has survival value. We may trigger false alarms but as long as these false calls are not overly frequent, distressing, or preoccupying, the trade-off in terms of increased survival potential is worth it.

The central prototype of the construct is a 'prime example of a given category' with 'overlapping borders with neighboring prototypes'. A sparrow is a better example of a prototypical bird than a penguin. Prototypical concepts condense information including how to recognize the concept, what other 'neighbouring' concepts are similar to it, and how to distinguish between the two, despite overlaps in distinguishing features (Parnas, 2015). Members of a construct may have familial resemblances to each other (Rosch and Mervis, 1975). A prototypical construct is therefore ideal for medical diagnosis, especially when there are no clear boundaries between diagnostic constructs (see later in this chapter).

Prototypical concepts have four types of qualities (Hampton, 2006):

- *Vagueness*: lack of clear rules that apply in every case means that some examples of a concept are unclear.
- *Typicality*: different examples of concepts differ in their degree of 'typical' nature of the concept.
- *Generic nature*: people can construct generic rules for deciding membership of a conceptual class but these do not apply in each and every example.
- *Opacity*: this refers to the difficulty in defining clear rules of what constitutes membership of the conceptual class.

Doctors use both prototypical concepts and concepts defined by criteria to create diagnostic constructs. Prototypical concepts fit better with type 1 processing whilst concepts defined by criteria, although not necessarily individually necessary and jointly sufficient, are a better match for type 2 processing (see Chapter 2). Doctors look for key features to match a prototypical profile of the condition that matches the closest clinical picture and differentiates it from similar prototypes. They then complete further history-taking, examination, and laboratory tests to confirm that the necessary and sufficient features are present to confirm the diagnosis based on meeting specific criteria (which can be accompanied by prototypical descriptions) (Parnas, 2015).

The features that doctors use to classify conditions are divided into two broad categories (Chapter 4 in Schoenberg and Rosamond, 2000; Scadding, 1967):

- Manifestations or 'external features' of the condition such as symptoms, signs, the course of the condition, laboratory test results, and how the condition responds to treatment. Diagnoses based on these manifestations alone can be said to be 'nominalist' (Chapter 4 in Schoenberg and Rosamond, 2000; Zachar and Kendler, 2007) in that they 'label' conditions because clinical practice can benefit from useful information attached to that label (see Chapter 2). Nominalist categories offer labels for specific states, and are very useful. They may or may not correspond with an underlying structure in nature which is independent of humans (i.e. they have utility without validity; Kendell and Jablensky, 2003). Most diagnoses in history were based on these manifestation criteria as our knowledge of the causation or mechanisms of illness was usually poor until recently.
- Causal or 'internal features' of the condition such as identified causes or mechanisms—changes in process or structure of the body or identified abnormalities such as presence of micro-organisms defined as pathological. Sometimes the causal factor may be an event such as injury or a traumatic life event. Causality will be discussed in Chapter 4. These types of diagnostic constructs are often 'essentialist' as they are describing an underlying nature producing the clinical picture (Chapter 4 in Schoenberg and Rosamond, 2000: Zachar and Kendler, 2007) and are said to have validity (Kendell and Jablensky, 2003). Essentialism, as applied to medical diagnostic categories, would state that each member of a category is defined by something they have in common with each other (their underlying essential nature) and this separates them from members of other categories. These diagnostic categories represent some underlying structure in the world independent of humans (Zachar and Kendler, 2007). The ability to understand and demonstrate causes or mechanisms implies greater utility as it opens the door to further research into reducing the effect of the cause or mechanism, or reversing it, or even preventing further cases (e.g. immunization).

The different types of problems or conditions that are classified with a diagnosis are listed below (see Chapters 9 and 11 for the data providing the basis for diseases/syndromes and spectrums):

- A broad category of clinical problems for which a specific condition has not been identified yet, such as 'acute abdominal pain', or of persisting clinical problems despite an identified diagnosis.
- A classic disease or syndrome clearly demarcated from good health and each other in the form of syndromes.
- A spectrum between health and illness with an unclear demarcation, or boundary, set between the two;
- A spectrum of illness or condition with an unclear demarcation set between these illnesses or conditions.
- Spectrums of illnesses or conditions with frequent co-occurrence.
- Injuries.
- Other conditions that are felt to be of interest to healthcare professionals but that are not illnesses, such as pregnancy.

Similar divisions of diagnostic constructs in mental health have been suggested before, including by Karl Jaspers (see Maj, 2005, 2013) and by the John Hopkins Department of Psychiatry (McHugh and Slavney, 1998).

Broad categories of clinical problems

Broad categories are used when patients present with problems where a specific condition has not yet been identified. For example, a patient presents with an 'acute abdomen'; they may have, for example, abdominal pain, vomiting, or tender abdomen. The doctor has not yet identified a condition (e.g. acute pancreatitis). A diagnostic label is helpful for this 'interim' position.

The value of an 'interim' diagnosis is twofold. First, it acknowledges this state of uncertainty. Second, these 'interim' diagnoses are associated with valuable information in themselves: likely conditions associated with this problem; how to identify the specific condition (what differentiating features of the differing clinical pictures to be aware of to make the differential diagnosis); what investigations to perform to identify likely conditions; what important complications to look out for; what treatments can be offered or avoided if the condition is unclear.

Medical students are taught these broad categories of problems with lists of differential diagnosis, what clinical pictures to be aware of to aid diagnosis, what tests to perform, treatments to use and avoid (see Figure 3.1). Examples of these broad categories include 'acute abdomen', 'chest pain', 'unconsciousness', and so on.

Another example of a broad category includes notable clinical problems not covered by the diagnosis alone. This is to highlight to the healthcare professional that these important clinical problems still need to be dealt with or at least she should remain aware

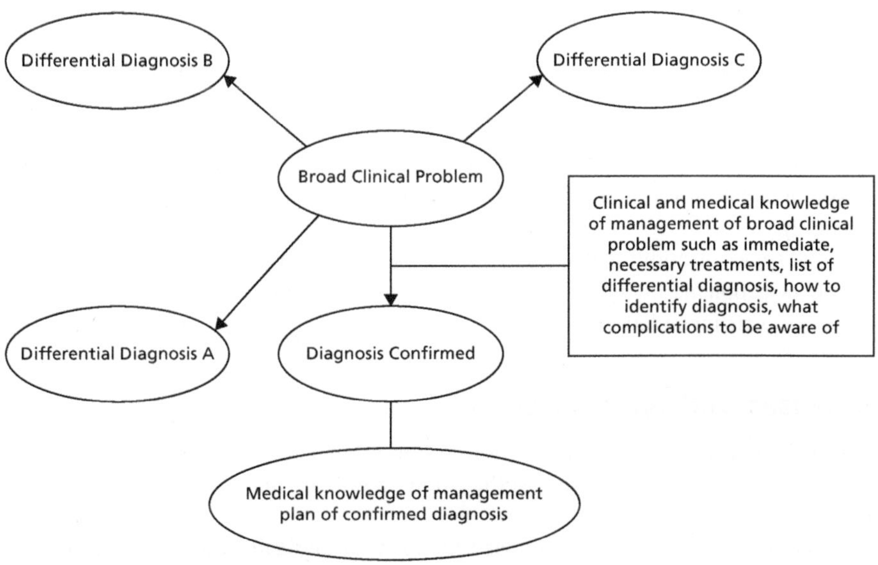

Figure 3.1 Broad clinical problems.

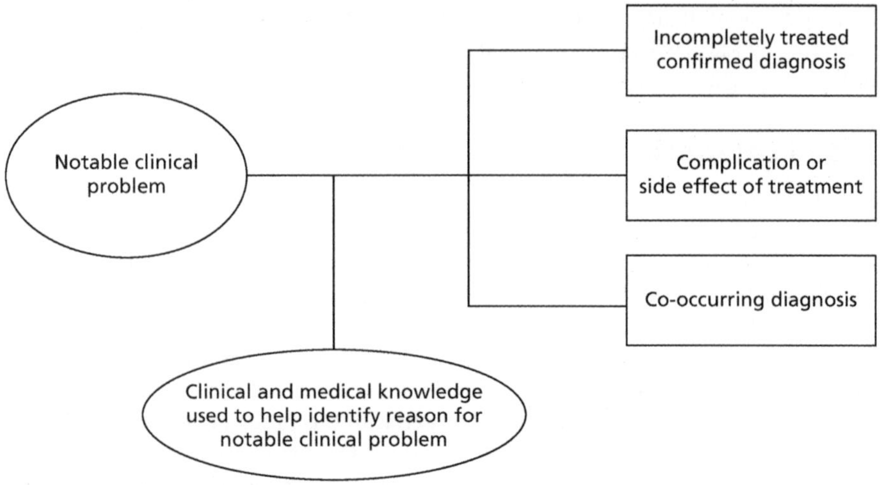

Figure 3.2 Notable clinical problems.

of them. Examples include critically low blood pressure, hypoxia (shortage of oxygen), and high risk of suicide. A diagnosis may have been identified and action taken to treat this diagnosed condition, but the use of this additional term signals that the identified diagnosed condition has been incompletely treated or that extra measures need to put in place to take account of a persistent problem. It also highlights that another condition may be present, (a co-occurring condition), and to look for signs of this too, especially if this additional problem is not a noted complication of the primary diagnosis.

Finally, it also makes the clinician aware that complications of medical treatments, including drug side effects, may be the cause of this notable clinical problems and the treatment may need reviewed. For example, antidepressant drugs can cause suicidal thoughts as side effects. If a doctor prescribes an antidepressant for depression and the patient subsequently reports suicidal thoughts, the doctor needs to be aware that this could be because of the medication they prescribed, not a direct result of the depression. The doctor needs to use their medical knowledge to distinguish between the two possibilities because if it is a side effect then the antidepressant needs to be stopped promptly.

These types of additional clinical problems (see Figure 3.2) may be referred to simply as 'problems' on a list that is recorded in conjunction with a diagnosis (as part of a diagnostic formulation).

Diseases and syndromes

The term 'syndrome' refers to a situation where certain clinical features such as particular symptoms and signs occur together more frequently than chance ('cohere'). This results in distinctive clinical pictures.

In the seventeenth century, Thomas Sydenham promulgated the theory of 'species' (i.e. 'syndromes') of medical illnesses, that particular causes of illness created a unique

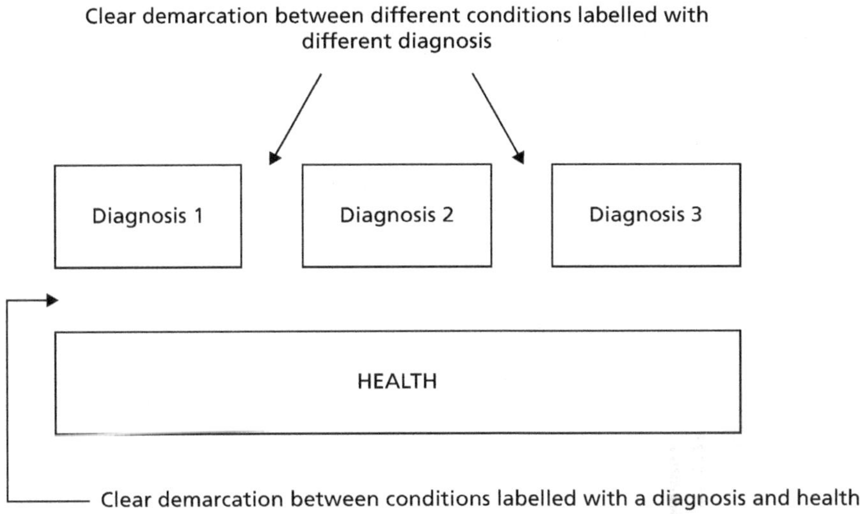

Figure 3.3 Diseases or clear-cut syndromes.

clinical picture that could be differentiated from other causes of illness with different clinical pictures. Careful history-taking and observation and examination allowed doctors to distinguish these 'species', and further work could then identify their causes (Chapter 4 in McHugh and Slavney, 1998). Sydenham believed that diseases processes produced the same symptoms in different people (Chapter 2 in Bynum, 2008).

A cause or disease process would lead to a distinctive, uniform clinical picture that would be separate from health as well as from other illnesses (as in Figure 3.3). Sometimes the distinctive clinical picture would be a response to a treatment even though the reason for this would be unknown at the time (Chapter 2 in Bynum, 2008). For example, the response of malarial fevers—or 'quartain ague', as Sydenham called it—to 'Peruvian bark' proved the value of differentiating it from other fevers. The effective ingredient of 'Peruvian bark'—quinine—was unknown to Sydenham, as were the effects of quinine on the causative micro-organism of malaria, or even that malaria was caused by a micro-organism. This ignorance of mechanism of action did not invalidate the benefit of making the diagnosis and offering effective treatment. This clinical syndrome was believed to be associated with a distinctive change in structure (anatomy) or processes (physiology) (Chapter 13 in Ghaemi, 2007).

This became the dominant model of illness in medicine (Kincaid, 2008; Huklenbroich, 2014), and especially folk ideas about medical illnesses. Illnesses were caused by diseases and were relatively uniform in their symptoms, signs, course, and responses to treatment. The presence of distincitve feautures that cohered was not enough to signify an illness. There also had to be some distress or risk of adverse event or loss of functioning present (Wakefield, 1992; Huklenbroich, 2014).

The process of advancement of medical science became clear (see Figure 3.4): identify a distinctive syndrome, clearly different from the healthy state and from other syndromes, through observation and careful recording of the clinical picture, then see

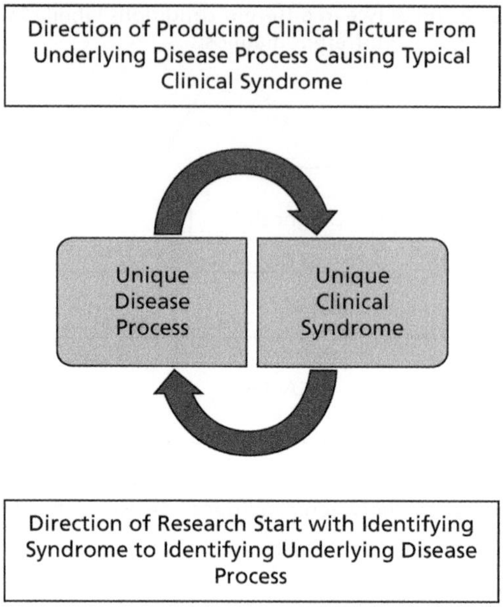

Figure 3.4 Relationship between disease and clinical picture and its effects on clinical practice and research.

if other cases of this sydrome could be identified. Once there was agreement that a true syndrome was identified, then work could begin on further identifying cases and gathering information such as prognosis, likely responses to treatments, complications, and causes. Importantly, it also meant that work could begin on identifying the underlying disease process. The identification of a clear abnormality of structure or function in the body causing the diagnosed condition means it becomes possible to devise tests to demonstrate this abnormality. This allows doctors to identify cases of this diagnosis using more objective methods of laboratory or imaging tests rather than relying purely on symptoms or signs, and helps demonstrate the scientific validty of the diagnosis. If the disease process can be identified then that leads to further research on reducing the effect of the disease, reversing the disease, or preventing it.

Research led to discoveries of gross anatomical or biochemical or microscopic evidence of differences between both healthy people and people with the syndrome, and between people with different syndromes (Chapter 3 in Bynum, 2008) (see Figure 3.5). Further advances led to further differentiation of disease processes and causes between people with superficially similar clinical syndromes. This could have implications for outcomes, co-occuring conditions, complications, or appropriate treatments.

Medical research often proceeds on the assumption that a disease mechanism is present, even if it has not been identified. This is especially so when there seems to be clear-cut differences between a recognizably 'healthy' state and an 'ill' state, as described by the clinical picture such as clear differences in symptoms or signs. This asssumption, often wrong, is based on historical experience; disease mechanisms have

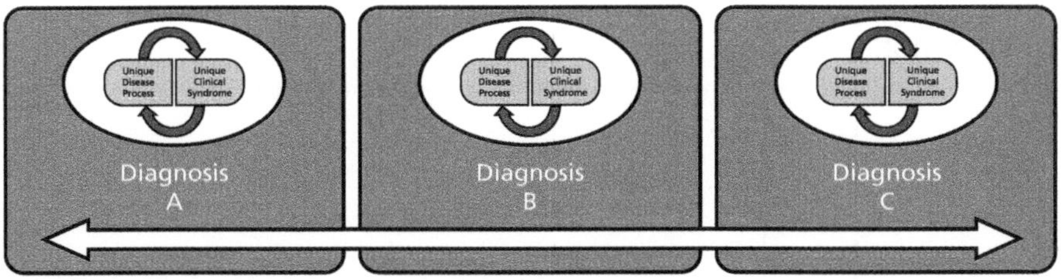

Figure 3.5 Separate diseases producing distinctive clinical pictures.

been discovered before for previous syndromes and we expect to find them for currently idiopathic (or 'unknown cause') syndromes.

It is not always necessary for a clear-cut, essentialist disease to cause a clear-cut syndrome. For mental health conditions, the causes could be psychosocial, generating a clinical syndrome in response. People in response to acute psychological trauma may display features of 'psychological shock', often diagnosed as 'acute stress reaction' (or similar term). Psychosocial causes are important in medicine as a whole, not just mental health, even if they act via biological factors. For example, 'deprivation dwarfism' is a syndrome of physical and psychological abnormalities characterized by the triad of extreme short stature, voracious appetite, and marked delay in sexual maturation. The condition has been noted in children who have experienced nutritonal, emotional, and psychological deprivation (Silver and Finkelstein, 1967). The causative deprivation is usually severe and the treatment ultimately is psychosocial, placing the child in a more nurturing environment providing their basic social needs of food, shelter, and care.

If an underlying disease process leads to a distinctive clinical picture then the diagnostic label often names the disease process (e.g. urinary tract infection describes the pathological presence of bacteria in the urinary tract). If the syndrome can be clearly separated from health and from other illnesses then this fits an essentialist model (Zachar and Kendler, 2007). These types of diagnostic constructs are defined by something they have in common, a disease process at best or a clinical picture at least, that distinguishes people with the diagnosis from healthy people and people with other diagnoses. It is important to recognize that these types of diagnostic constructs are not always caused by a disease process.

Spectrums of health

One of the most commonly used diagnostic constructs is for conditions that lie on a spectrum of health (see Figure 3.6); examples include high blood pressure or type 2 diabetes. The spectrum represents a range of values given to an attribute or variable. These attributes are often biological in nature, such as blood pressure or plasma glucose levels, but not always *primarily* biological. In mental health, attributes such as depression or anxiety may have a biological component (such as activity in brain neurones when having sad or anxious thoughts), but these biological phenomena are an aspect of a whole, including psychological and social factors, but not necessarily a

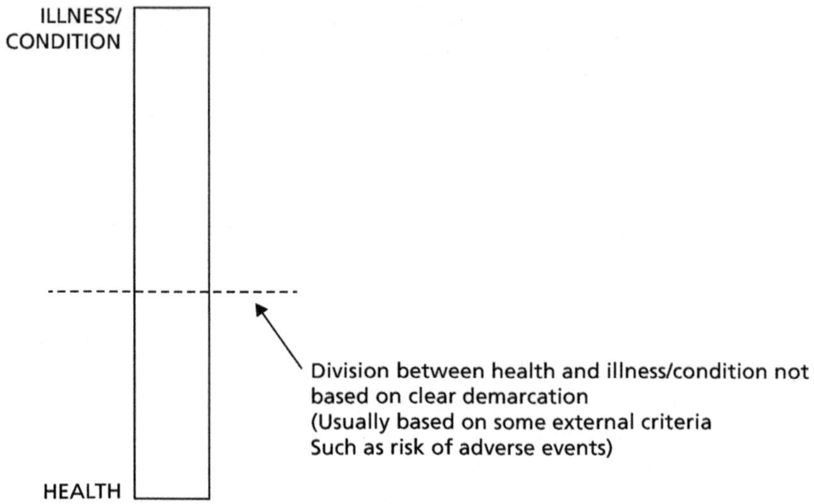

Figure 3.6 Spectrums of health.

cause of this attribute. These biological phenomena may just be a *consequence* of these psychological and social phenomena. They can still be viewed as a spectrum of distress distributed in the population at large with larger amounts of anxiety or depressive symptoms meeting a threshold for diagnosis *if* help from healthcare professionals is helpful. In variables that show a 'normal' distribution, extreme values are only possessed by a small percentage of the population.

Cultural factors also effect diagnostic constructs based on primarily biological thresholds. At medical school, I was told that German physicians recognize a condition called 'low blood pressure' (without an obvious cause such as major blood loss or other causes of haemodynamic shock) which they treat with salt tablets.

Thresholds are a pragmatic solution to the need to make binary decisions in clinical practice (e.g. a cut-off that indicates sufficient level of a clinical problem to justify or indicate benefit from medical treatment). A similar process is used in criminal law courts when the threshold of 'beyond reasonable doubt' is applied to the evidence to decide a verdict of guilty or not guilty (a lower threshold is used for verdicts in civil cases of 'on the balance of probabilities'). Thresholds are drawn based on levels of distress and/or impaired functioning or a risk of adverse health outcomes (such as strokes or heart attacks for high blood pressure) to make decisions about whether to recognize the situation as a health problem that may benefit from treatment. This is a nominalist construct; we are giving the name of a diagnosis to parts on this spectrum because there are benefits in doing so (Zachar and Kendler, 2007). Another reason may be to identify cases to allow counting and thus estimation of clinical need for epidemiological reasons or for planning purposes (Chapter 4 in Schoenberg and Rosamond, 2000).

Once we *reduce* a dimensional concept into categories we *lose* information. For example, we may describe someone as tall but this is not as informative as giving their height (6 feet 4 inches). Putting information into categories can make it easier to store and recall in memory. Some decisions may need information to be in categories in order to use it. Doctors are used to categories for clear-cut syndromes and diseases so they extend this to 'collapsing' a dimension into a category by applying a threshold (Keeley, 2015).

In medicine, categorical decisions are often required (admit to hospital or not admit, use treatment A or treatment B). This becomes easier to research (by defining groups meeting and not meeting criteria for a condition, then gathering information on differences between the two groups) and to learn this information, then recall it and use it in clinical practice.

Once a threshold has been decided upon and a category defined for research then information from this research can then be utilized. Identifying examples of this category can be determined by assessing if people cross this threshold, and the information from research can be used to benefit the person who has been identified as a case.

NICE has produced a set of guidelines for hypertension (NICE, 2011). It first sets a threshold of systolic blood pressure (140) and diastolic blood pressure (90). If people meet this threshold for systolic blood pressure or diastolic blood pressure—as well some other rules concerning accurate measurement—then they are diagnosed with hypertension. Advice is then given as to how confirm the diagnosis, what investigations to perform, what complications to be aware of and how to detect them, what treatments to offer, and how to monitor response to treatment.

There are few absolute (or even relative) differences in risks for people who are only just on either side of this threshold (e.g. people with a blood pressure of 134/84 compared to people with a blood pressure of 140/90). For other conditions diagnosed based on distress caused or functional impairments, there is little absolute difference in terms of distress or functional impairments between people above the threshold and people just below the threshold ('subthreshold' cases).

Setting the threshold too low may dramatically increase the number of people given the diagnosis, thus increasing healthcare costs, increased side effects caused by medications or interventions with little benefit (benefits may be greater at more extreme points on the spectrum than in the middle), not to mention people suffering malign social effects of being given a diagnosis without concomitant clinical benefit. Set the threshold too high and some people who could benefit from treatment, in the form of reduced distress, improved functioning, or reduced risk of adverse events, will miss out because they will not meet the criteria for the diagnosis and so may be denied access to potentially beneficial healthcare. These thresholds may be particularly hard to set if less objective criteria such anxiety or depressive symptoms are used to set a threshold (see Maj, 2012 on the difficulties for setting a threshold for depression).

For pragmatic reasons, a threshold needs to be drawn. For many illnesses like hypertension, type 2 diabetes, or mental health conditions, these are often done by committees of experts. These experts debate amongst themselves, using the research evidence as well as their eloquence, to set the thresholds for defining the condition of interest. These experts are not disinterested guardians of wisdom, they often have their own pet theories and wish to see them prevail. They often have been shown to have financial conflicts of interests in terms of some form of connection to drug companies (Chapter 3 in Taylor, 2013), even if it is in the form of research grants rather than direct payments . Another important flaw is the frequent lack of input from patients in the process. Despite these flaws, a threshold needs set for the reasons outlined above.

Many of the attributes that lie on a spectrum have complex multiple reasons for the actual value in an individual. Height, for example, is distributed on a spectrum which ranges from very short people to very tall. The height of a person is often determined by genetics but more importantly diet, socioeconomic status, lifestyle, etc. Extreme values of these multifactorial attributes are, therefore, often due to a complex combination of factors rather than a simple disease process.

Conditions that are on a spectrum of health can be associated with pathology and disease as a consequence of these conditions. Hypertension, as an example, is associated with pathological changes such as damaged arteries leading to diseases such as heart disease or strokes.

Care must also be taken that what seems like a condition on a spectrum of health is not actually a disease or syndrome. If all that is measured about an individual is height, it may be assumed that an individual at either end of the spectrum may be there due to the usual factors that affect height in everyone. However, diseases or syndromes may be the cause of extremes of height such as excess or lack of growth hormone, Marfan syndrome (a disorder of connective tissue often leading to increased height), or genetic conditions linked to restricted growth. By taking into account other factors than just a single variable, we may be able to detect separate syndromes other than spectrums of health. Sometimes we are unable to measure accurately other variables that would demonstrate these clear-cut differences, particularly in mental health. This can mean that conditions that appear on a spectrum of health due to our currently limited forms of measuring and assessing mental health variables may actually be syndromes, if only our ability to assess and measure all relevant variables were better.

Spectrums of conditions

This describes two kinds of situations that are not mutually exclusive. The first is where it can be hard to separate conditions from other conditions with different diagnostic labels. Examples include some autoimmune diseases and the division between dementia of Lewy body disease and Parkinson's disease. When I was at medical school we used to talk about differentiating chronic bronchitis from emphysema, but now they are usually combined together into 'chronic obstructive pulmonary disease' (COPD). It was recognized that features of both conditions were often found in the same patient. The difficulty and limited usefulness of separating chronic bronchitis from emphysema when both were frequently present to some degree in patients led to preferred use of a combined diagnostic category.

For other diagnoses, there is felt to be some clinical utility to give separate diagnostic labels even when these conditions cannot be clearly separated on the basis of clinical manifestations (symptoms, signs, course, response to treatment, lab tests) or mechanisms or causes. Some people, for example, suggest that psychotic illnesses, like schizophrenia or bipolar disorder, are on a single spectrum. Some have argued that the separation of diabetes into 'type 1' and 'type 2' is a pragmatic (or nominalist)

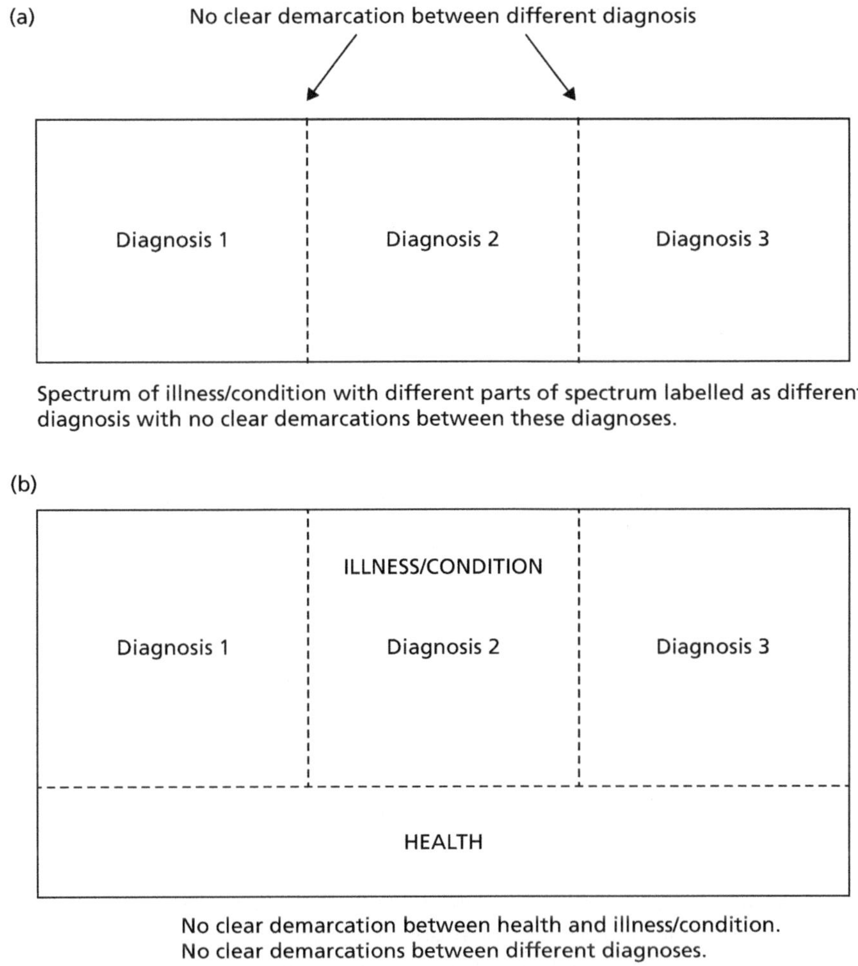

Figure 3.7 (a) Spectrums of illness/condition with clear boundary with health. (b) Spectrums of illness/condition with no clear boundary with health.

construct identifiying two extreme ends of a continuum, and these are not truly seprate categories (Gale, 2006).

These concepts (see Figure 3.7(a) and Figure 3.7(b)) —are examples of nominalist diagnostic constructs (Zachar and Kendler, 2007).

The second type of situation (see Figure 3.8) is where there is a high degree of co-occurence between conditions given different diagnostic labels but where, in fact, they are most likely to be different aspects of an underlying condition. An example is metabolic syndrome where high blood pressure, obesity, hypercholesterolaemia, type 2 diabetes, and other conditions can occur in different combinations in different people. This is probably due to a mulitfactorial combination of diet, lifestyle, genetics, and so forth combining to give several different effects. Although some of the treatments

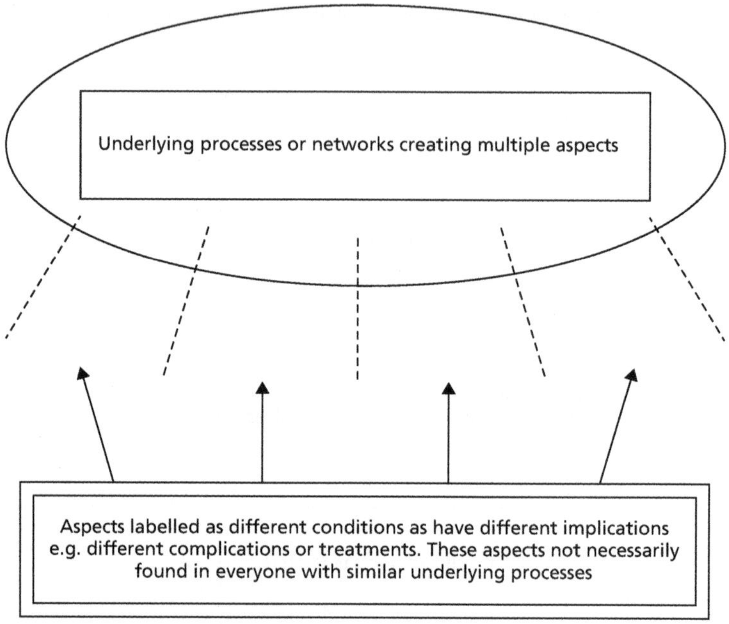

Figure 3.8 Spectrums of conditions.

are common for these 'different' conditions (changes in diet or increased exercise), some of the treatments and complications are different for these separately labelled conditions. Many mental health conditions have similar causes too—such as childhood trauma or psychosocial adversity or distressing life events—so unsuprisingly, more than one mental health condition may be present. Like the metabolic syndrome, more than one feature of mental health problems is often present, and because of differing complications, prognosis, or treatments it may be worthwhile identifying these different aspects separately as opposed to using a super-category of 'distressed'.

The analogy of colours in the rainbow can help explain the first type of spectrum (of illness/condition). A rainbow is a spectrum of colours. Western and Japanese cultures recognize seven main colours in the rainbow; other cultures recognize fewer numbers, as few as two. When tested, (non-colour blind) people from all cultures can reliably recognize differences in tone/colour. (This means clearly distinct, different colours can be reliably recognized even if there is no word in the person's culture for that colour).

Differences between colours are not absolute (e.g. orange eventually becomes yellow, but the border between the two is indistinct). Differences between neighbouring colours are more difficult (e.g. orange/yellow or indigo/violet) than differences between clearly different colours (e.g. orange/violet).

This is a spectrum phenomenon (but with an external validated criterion of light frequency/wavelength) that we categorize into separate colours, not by this external criterion but how it appears to us (so a colour is subjectively decided upon and then the corresponding wavelength scientifically discovered). The number of categories is culturally determined and we can reliably differentiate between colours/tones if they are on clearly different points of the spectrum, but less reliably if they are close together on the same spectrum.

We categorize colours because it is useful for various purposes (e.g. description). We categorize based on prototypes (e.g. of typical green) that are not clearly separated; the archetype is of the 'greenest' green. There is no assumption of 'clustering' (i.e. that in nature, light frequencies/wavelengths encountered will be more common for each named archetype/category, or that the prevalence of light frequencies will be more common in the centre of the archetype/categories' light frequency value).

There are multiple uses for colour (e.g. decorative purposes, signalling, to help identify objects in nature, etc.) and a necessity for communication about colour (e.g. between designers and manufacturers, to check consistency of colour production). Pantone™ is a system which enables consistency of colour and communication about it, with names and codes for different standardized colours. To improve reliability, Pantone's™ colour guides should be used for 12 months, otherwise colours may vary too much from each other, due to fading. The user of the Pantone™ code identifies a particular colour and specifies that that specific colour be used by the recipient of the communication. This is similar to a diagnosis identifying a prototype that is recognizable to the person receiving the communication.

There may not be valid and clear boundaries between conditions that are points on a spectrum given different diagnostic labels. However, there may be some clinical utility in identifying different points of the spectrum. There may be differences in the clinical manifestations of symptoms/signs or in a likely range of outcomes or complications. The treatments and responses to them may vary. Classification using separate diagnostic labels therefore may have clinical utility without there being valid clearly demarcated entities.

The second type of spectrum (of illnesses/conditions) can be thought of in terms of naming different aspects of a complex state. In metabolic syndrome, we may be noting the presence of whether there is elevated blood pressure or high levels of serum cholesterol. We discuss each aspect as *if* it was separate, given the different types of information attached to each aspect (e.g. complications, responses to treatment). We may give advice or offer interventions that benefit *all* aspects (such as improved diet, more exercise, or less alcohol), as well as interventions that are specific to particular aspects (antihypertensives for high blood pressure, statins for high serum cholesterol). Although given different diagnostic labels, these aspects are not independent of each other. Unfortunately, a lot of the research information we have, such as responses to treatment, do not take into account the high degree of co-occurrence found in these types of conditions (Muth and Glasziou, 2015). This means our medical management has a higher degree of uncertainty than we wish. Nevertheless, the benefits of recognizing these different aspects is often felt worthwhile due to differences in complications or treatments. Clinical utility is used as a justification for the use of the diagnostic construct in the absence of clear valid differences between these related diagnoses.

The purpose of classification in clinical practice is clinical usefulness. If it is impossible to delineate clearly separate categories, either because they do not exist because the condition is a spectrum or because we lack the capability to demonstrate the boundaries between conditions, then the next best option is to use a clinically useful classification based on identifying points on a spectrum. As long as people are aware that they aren't necessarily describing clearly separate categories—either from states considered healthy or from other conditions—then, if a diagnosis can be reliably distinguished from other diagnoses and carries clinically useful discriminatory information (such as likely range of outcomes or different responses to treatment), it is a 'worthwhile' diagnosis.

Injuries

There is an almost unlimited number of ways a person can be injured. The clinical implications of an injury depend on both the *cause* and *nature* of the injury and the *characteristics* of the injured region. There are some similarities in effects of injuries such as bleeding, pain, or possible infection, as well as response to injuries such as inflammation, healing, or clotting. Injuries (external entities to the body affecting the body) are not diseases (which are found in the body, including its' surface or contents) and so should be regarded as a separate type of diagnostic construct. The phrase 'depression isn't like a broken leg' is sometimes used to emphasize the difference between mental and physical health, but this fails to take into account that hypertension is not similar to broken legs either.

The use of this type of diagnostic construct is that it allows information to be gleaned about similar injuries grouped together into a diagnostic label—information about likely causes, clinical picture, likely complications, likely range of outcomes (e.g. the usual time for a fracture to heal), and the best treatments. Injuries can directly cause mental health problems such as changes to personality after frontal lobe of the brain injuries. Some people conceptualize some mental health problems as similar to a 'psychological injury' in response to a psychosocial trauma.

Other conditions of interest to healthcare professionals

This is a disparate group of conditions seen by health or related professionals. They are not illnesses, diseases, or injuries, but it is felt that health professionals offer some benefit. It is easier to give examples of broad types than a comprehensive definition.

Some of the conditions are not illnesses but are states associated with an increased risk of illness or health-related adverse events, such as pregnancy, where ante-natal care has been shown to be beneficial in early detection and thus increasingly effective treatment of illnesses associated with pregnancy such as gestational diabetes. Childbirth, a natural process, is also of interest to healthcare professionals even if taking place at home as there are often situations that are threatening to the child and/or mother which require rapid intervention. Either creating diagnostic labels or using existing terms as if they are diagnostic constructs (e.g. 'pregnancy') are of value in denoting a state of interest to healthcare professionals even though they are not diseases or illnesses.

A second, broad type of condition is one to which healthcare professionals can bring useful skills or can offer other benefits. Examples include cosmetic surgical procedures or terminations of pregnancy for which there is neither foetal abnormality nor threat to the pregnant woman's physical health. Terminations are more appropriately and safely carried out by doctors rather than 'backstreet abortionists'. For cosmetic surgery, the diagnostic construct is often a description of the procedure carried out rather an abnormality. Some people seek cosmetic procedures where conditions are a clear example of an illness or disease (such as a 'cleft lip'), or when a body part is too much at one end of a spectrum. At other times, it reflects a personal wish to alter some bodily attribute. It is better that suitably trained health professionals perform the procedure to increase the chances of a successful result and reduce the risk of adverse effects of the procedure.

The third type of broad situation includes problems or difficulties where help is sought from a health or allied professional. In order to get access to help, a diagnostic label may be needed (see Chapter 2). The constructs themselves can be simply a description of a problem such as child behavioural difficulties or marital difficulties. The diagnostic constructs are often very broad and non-specific. The distress or adverse consequences as a result of these difficulties should not be underestimated. Many people regard mental health problems as this type of diagnostic construct—not an illness or disease but a condition where help from professionals may be beneficial.

These diagnostic constructs tend to comprise a broad range of people who are very 'heterogeneous' in terms of the causes and manifestations of their problems. It is still possible to gain information about likely range of outcomes or likely range of responses to interventions or treatments but the degree of uncertainty around the information is higher than diagnostic constructs based on disease processes. Ultimately, accessible information, even with a high degree of uncertainty attached to a diagnostic construct, is better than no information at all.

Another major concern of these types of diagnostic constructs lies in the fact that they can lie beyond the realm of defined illness and yet still be presented as if they are an 'illness' (think, for example, of 'loneliness'). Apart from the financial concerns of third-party funders of healthcare as to whether they should be paying, there are legitimate concerns by society with regard to the 'medicalization' of given situations (Chapter 3 in Sackett et al., 1991). This cannot be just 'left to the professionals', who clearly have a self-interest in extending the range of situations where they can claim it right and proper for them to intervene.

Therefore, there must be a continued negotiation between society and health professionals as to what are 'legitimate' areas in which health professionals may be involved. Health professionals' sole claim to bring these matters into their 'domain' rests on their ability to prove that their skills are necessary to gain maximum benefit or prevent harm, and it is up to society to decide if this claim is sufficient on a case-by-case basis.

Conclusion

Classification is necessary in medicine, indeed it is necessary if we are to make sense of anything that we encounter and to communicate with others. If we avoid classification, then we cannot differentiate outcomes and offer the same intervention to everyone. If we avoid classification on the basis that every case is absolutely unique then we cannot learn useful information from previously seen patients to apply to new patients.

Doctors are humans and so tend to use classification based on prototypical concepts—identifying a diagnosis based on its resemblance to a prototype. This may be confirmed by further information gathering to see if the case meets the full criteria of a criteria-based diagnostic construct. Diagnoses tend to be categories even when they describe points on a dimension or spectrum. This is because categorical decisions are often made by healthcare professionals and this fits better with categorical constructs. Diagnostic constructs comprise several types: a broad clinical problem needing further clarification; the classic disease or clear-cut syndrome; a spectrum with health; a spectrum of illness(es) or condition(s); injuries or situations that are of interest to health professionals.

Diagnostic constructs do not have to be clearly demarcated from healthy states or even each other to be useful. They only have to be identified reliably and carry discriminatory information such as likely range of outcomes, complications, and likely range of responses to treatments. Diagnostic constructs are not just applied to illnesses or diseases but also to situations where health professionals believe they can be of benefit. This may be because they can reduce distress, or there is a higher risk of illness or adverse events, or they can reduce the risk of adverse events or increase the chances of a treatment's success. A diagnostic label may also be necessary to access care from a service. Where diagnostic constructs are used for conditions that are not illnesses, diseases, or injuries then there needs to be scrutiny by Society of health professionals' classification and domains of self-proclaimed expertise to prevent over-medicalization.

Chapter 4

The clinical picture, creating diagnostic constructs, and causation

In this chapter, different models of how the clinical picture is produced by an interaction of biological, interpersonal, and social/cultural factors are discussed before looking at how doctors group similar clinical pictures together into a diagnosis with clinical utility and, hopefully, scientific validity. Different methods of identifying causation of conditions are outlined and how illnesses are often caused by an interaction between causes, characteristics, and contexts.

The production of the clinical picture

The clinical picture is the doctor's interpretation based on what has happened to the patient, and considers symptoms, signs, and results of investigations that are available to her. Psychiatric symptoms and signs have been described as 'hybrid objects' (Berrios, 2013), and this model leaves aside the question of causation. The term 'objects' describes constructs that are used to depict or explain aspects of the world. The generation of psychiatric symptoms as signs are said to be 'hybrid' because they involve combinations of biological and semantic elements—a biological element/kernel is contained within two layers of configurating envelopes.

The cause of the biological element is not depicted in this model. The biological element refers to the brain activity associated with the symptom or sign. This might be, for example, nervous activity that is a corollary of the patient's thoughts or that controls muscular movements or a seizure in the temporal lobe causing an olfactory hallucination.

The two configurating envelopes describe the semantic and contextual elements that act to configure and modify the interpretation and expression of the biological element successively. The first envelope involves individual and sociocultural forces (such as personality traits and culture) whilst the second envelope consists of interactional forces (e.g. between doctor and patient or within a broader social context) (Markova and Berrios, 2015).

A patient's culture and individual experience, such as education, shape how they view and describe their experience, their own personal viewpoints and attitudes that further influence how they perceive and construct their experience, and the words they use. This also has effects on the doctor's viewpoint and the terminology used to describe the patient's verbalized experiences and behaviour. A doctor's training and education influences how they perceive and describe patients' problems; for example, they use the medical model and its standardized terminology such as symptoms and diagnostic constructs because it has been drummed into them via their medical education. The quality of the patient experience, such as the rate of change in their condition (e.g. a rapidly worsening problem is more likely to draw the patient's attention), the context in which their experiences happen (e.g. if voices are heard on a busy bus commenting on the patient's appearance—these voices may be less noticeable than if nobody else is there), and the quality of change (how much it differs from what the patient or doctor expects) will also influence how the patient and the doctor interpret their experiences.

The second type of configurating envelope describes interactions including that between the patient discussing their experiences with somebody else other than the doctor (Berrios, 2013). For example, if a patient is being interviewed by a doctor, it is likely that the clinical interview will be directed by the doctor to see if the patient's experiences match a list of symptoms that the doctor thinks relevant, based on potential likely diagnoses. This line of enquiry may direct the patient's attention to aspects of the experience they had not considered, or may structure the patient's description of their experience so that it matches other patient's similar experiences that the doctor has encountered.

Although the doctor is nominally directing the interview, the nature of human conversation is that interaction between two parties involves give and take. The patient may not wish to discuss certain facts or experiences that would be relevant to the clinical picture. The presence of other experiences that the doctor may regard as symptoms or behaviour that the doctor may regard as signs may also influence how the doctor regards an individual experience as fitting a 'bigger picture'. The patient is not passive during the clinical examination either; for example, they may show evidence of pain if the part of the body being touched is tender. There are also cultural and semantic factors at play in the laboratory tests, although these have less of an effect than on interpretation of signs and symptoms.

This model describes how a biological element interacts with semantic and cultural factors and interpersonal/dialogical factors to produce a psychiatric symptom or sign in the doctor's mind. Two dichotomous examples are given by Berrios (2013). The first is where the contribution of the biological element to the final sense or meaning is far stronger than the semantic and other elements, such as where an epileptic seizure gives rise to hallucinations. The second type is where the semantic element is the biggest contributor; for example, someone in a low mood may describe a negative state directed towards themselves such as guilt or low self-esteem related to a whole cultural system of expectations that they perceive they have not met. In reality, there is not a clean-cut division between these two types; more likely there is a variable contribution of biological and semantic and other elements in the construction of signs, symptoms, and the overall clinical picture.

This type of model can be extrapolated to other medical specialties. For example, someone can have an obvious biological element such as a fever (raised temperature) or rash. This would be understood using the cultural framework of the patient combined with the training and education of the doctor. A physician from Ancient

Rome may view the whole problem in terms of imbalance of humours, and a physician in the classic Chinese tradition would consider the same problem in terms of energy flow imbalances. There are also biological elements to be considered with regard to the doctor, too. They may be tired from being up all night and so miss an important clinical symptom or sign. Other semantic issues can come into play: if a doctor is rude to the patient then the patient may not discuss all their symptoms with them. If the patient's problem is of an intimate nature such as genital problems, seeing a doctor of the opposite sex may cause them to be less forthcoming about their problem.

Another model of how psychiatric symptoms are produced uses a metaphor of light passing through filters and lenses (Chapter 1 in Clare, 2011). The light represents life events and stresses (the more severe the stressor the denser the light) passing through a series of lens/filters of past experience, psychological defences, physiological reaction, coping strategies, illness behaviour resulting in a final dysfunction measured on an Illness Rule. The patient's past experiences act as a polarizing filter altering how they view current stressors. Psychological defence mechanisms may act to reduce or block (or increase) the effect of the stressor. Physiological reactions engendered by the stressors passing through these lenses and filters (such as increased heart rate/blood pressure or increased production of the body's corticosteroids) are described as psychophysiological reactions.

These psychophysiological reactions may increase the subjective experience of being under stress. Coping mechanisms now come into play and may act to reduce the effect of the stress (or maintain or increase them; e.g. if a patient copes with stress by drinking excessive alcohol). Finally, there is the effect of illness behaviour or how the patient behaves in respect with their illness such as seeking or avoiding medical help or taking their medication regularly. The final result is the degree of dysfunction caused by the stressor. This can be placed on a spectrum of Illness rule , a range of possible expressions of dysfunction caused by this stressor.

This model can again be extrapolated to other medical illnesses. A cause of illness undergoes a series of interactions with intermediate factors before we arrive at that individual patient's expression of the illness in terms of signs, symptoms, and lab test results.

A final model of how the clinical picture is produced relies on an interaction of a variety of different factors such as biological, interpersonal/psychological, or cultural/social factors which can operate within the patient, the doctor, and in society. These factors interact with each other and the metaphor of light can be used (see Figure 4.1): diffraction patterns (caused by slits) that could interfere with each other, filters that only allow certain light frequencies through, and lenses that can focus the light onto a smaller or larger area. Note that there is no assumption of a simple causal relationship between these factors for the purposes of this model; they interact with each other. If the doctor's mind is a blank screen, the 'clinical gaze' of the doctor is a light source, and these intermediate factors is a collection of lenses, filters, and slits, then we have a good model of how the final clinical picture is projected into the doctor's mind and is perceived. The light passes through these intermediate factors resulting in a pattern projected onto the screen, the pattern resulting in a clinical picture, including a description of what has happened to the patient and signs, symptoms, and results of any laboratory investigations.

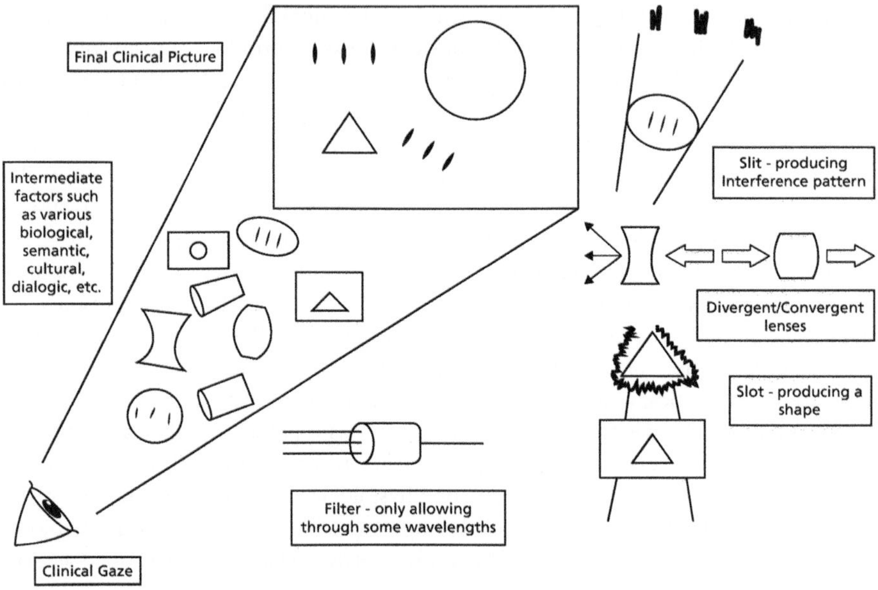

Figure 4.1 Model of production of the clinical picture.

This clinical picture is an interpretation by the doctor of the information gleaned from her assessment. Another doctor may arrive at a different clinical picture when they assess the same patient. Two patients with a similar type of underlying problem may present clinical pictures that are different to varying degrees to the same doctor. Given the large number of variables that can potentially affect this clinical picture and how they interact with each other, the degrees of difference in clinical picture produced may vary greatly or very little, either between doctors with the same patient or between patients with similar underlying problems. We shall now look at how this operates in practice, starting with an instance where the variation of clinical picture is small, followed by an example where the variation is large. It should be remembered that variations in clinical picture exist on a spectrum, with extreme examples at each end of the spectrum being chosen for illustrative purposes.

It should also be noted that the clinical picture is a moving picture in the doctor's mind. There are multiple reasons why the clinical picture changes. The condition itself may evolve; as medical conditions progress they can become more severe or develop fresh complications (e.g. heart attacks can cause cardiac arrhythmias or heart failure). Medical interventions may alter the clinical picture (e.g. intravenous fluids may increase blood pressure). Other intermediate factors may also alter the clinical picture (the patient may begin to trust the doctor more and provide more information about past experiences). More information may become available (investigation results are delivered and this information is added to the clinical picture), confirming or questioning the current diagnosis or warning of complications.

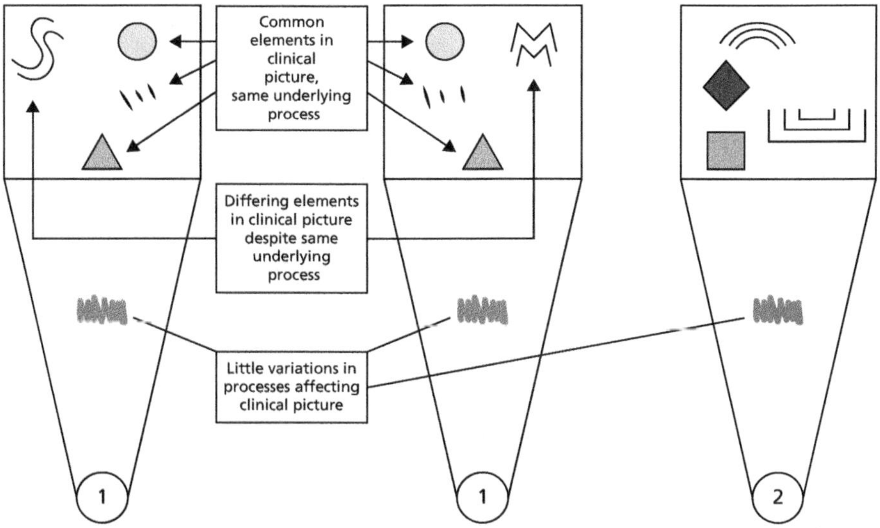

Figure 4.2 Conditions with little variation in clinical picture.

The first example we shall discuss is where there is little variation in the clinical picture (see Figure 4.2). The condition may have a largely biological cause or a largely psychosocial cause. Whatever the causation, the intermediate factors discussed above have little effect in generating much heterogeneity in the clinical picture.

Figure 4.2 shows two people with similar underlying conditions and one person with a different condition. (It could also be said to represent the same person seeing two different doctors with a second person with a different condition seeing one of the doctors, but we shall stick with the first description initially.) Intermediate factors are simplified in the figure for pictorial purposes. The two people with the same condition have many common elements of the clinical picture: they have similar histories, symptoms, signs, and results of investigations. They also have some differing elements. The person with the different condition has a different clinical picture (in this example, there are no common elements for ease of illustration, but this is not often case, with some common elements often found to exist between different conditions). The similarities in clinical pictures allow doctors to recognize that the two patients have the same condition. In the alternative example of the same patient seeing two doctors, the similarity in clinical pictures increases the chance of both doctors agreeing to the same diagnosis.

It should also be noted that people with no condition are omitted from the Figure 4.2. Once subjected to the 'clinical gaze' of a medical assessment, it is common for people to display some features interpreted as symptoms or signs. Even clinical investigations may reveal abnormalities when no condition appears to be present, such people without thyroid problems testing positive for thyroid peroxidase autoantibodies (Chapter 20 in Walker et al., 2014).

The next example illustrates conditions where there is a great effect of the intermediate factors on the final clinical picture (see Figure 4.3). The reason for this may be due to differing levels of severity of causative or maintaining factors (or even different causative or maintaining factors altogether) for people diagnosed with the same condition. There may be a greater impact of other biological, semantic, cultural, or other interpersonal factors on the clinical picture. A patient with a different condition is also included in the example. As in Figure 4.2, Figure 4.3 can also be interpreted as a patient being assessed by two different doctors, with a second patient with another condition being seen by one of the doctors. People with no conditions are excluded for reasons of simplicity.

In Figure 4.3, we can see there are still some common elements of the clinical picture (but fewer than before) and a greater number of differing elements. There are also some common elements with the patient with a different condition. A greater 'interference' effect of intermediate factors leads to a greater 'spread' of possible variations in elements of the clinical picture, resulting in different conditions being more likely to have some elements that resemble each other. Given the bigger quantity of non-common elements between individuals with the same condition (or the same individual assessed by different doctors), there is a higher chance of non-agreement as to the diagnosis. The matching of the clinical picture to the correct diagnosis of the condition is made harder by this larger amount of non-common elements. There is increased 'noise' to the 'diagnostic signal' so that doctors may not agree that these two patients have the same diagnosis, or two doctors may disagree on the diagnosis in the same patient.

In addition, the presence of common elements in patients with a different condition may lead to an incorrect diagnosis by the doctor. If condition 2 has some common elements with condition 1, this may lead the doctor to diagnose wrongly

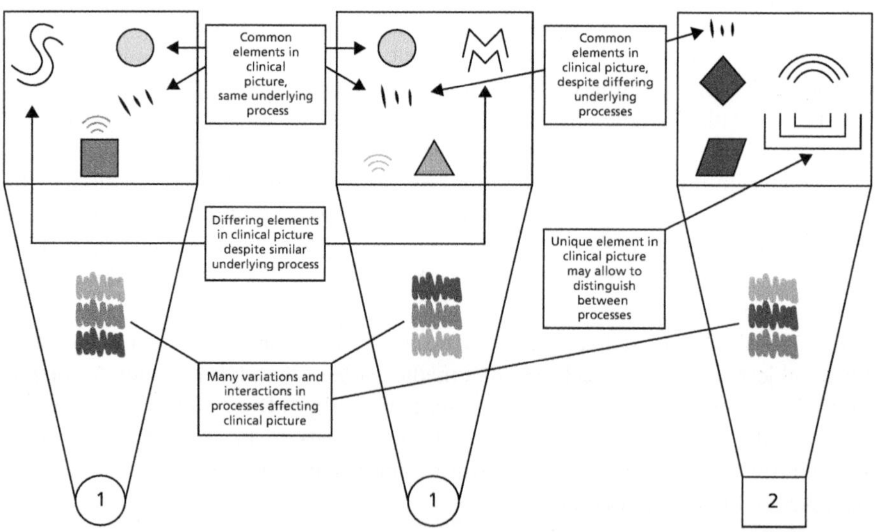

Figure 4.3 Conditions with great variation in clinical picture.

patients with condition 2 as having condition 1. This is more likely if the doctor overlooks elements of the clinical picture that are more associated with condition 2 than condition 1; the doctor may forget or overlook these elements in their diagnostic assessment. Sometimes the doctor may not have the ability to detect these differentiating elements of the clinical picture; for example, they may not yet have access to reliable investigations or tests to tell condition 1 apart from condition 2.

Situations where intermediate factors have a great effect on the clinical picture can thus be seen to affect the reliability of the diagnosis between patients with the same underlying condition and between doctors seeing the same patient, and for other conditions sharing common elements of the clinical picture.

Making a diagnosis is a skill involving recognizing important salient points in a clinical picture. The accuracy in correctly identifying the diagnosis that best matches the information available requires knowledge and decision-making abilities. Like many skills, success in arriving at a correct diagnosis depends on a mixture of factors—the innate skill of the doctor, their level of training and practice, their knowledge, and the difficulty of the diagnostic task. Mental health conditions often involve a greater effect on the final clinical picture by intermediate factors, and this is combined with a lack of effective investigations. This can make diagnosis in mental health cases very challenging.

The next example (see Figure 4.4) illustrates conditions that can be thought of as sitting on a spectrum of good health, such as high blood pressure or depression. It specifically depicts conditions with multiple aspects on a spectrum with each other (and sometimes with health)—such as metabolic syndrome (including conditions such as high blood pressure or obesity) or anxiety/depression. In this example, patients have many common elements in their clinical picture, but these exist on a spectrum. Each element's point on the spectrum depends on the interaction of a variety of intermediate factors. This represents their complex aetiology which is often a mixture of many genes having small individual effects interacting with multiple environmental factors.

In this example, common elements may be present in all or most of the patients. They may differ only as to the extent of their severity or intensity. The classification of these conditions can be undertaken in a variety of different ways. Once an element has reached a particular threshold (such as blood pressure exceeding a certain value) then it can be described as a separate condition such as high blood pressure. The presence of each element is only noted once it has passed a threshold of significance. The information attached to each element or aspect can then be used (such as likely prognosis or complications and what treatments are effective for that element). This is a simple categorical system such as that used in classifying patients with differing severity of aspects of metabolic syndrome such as high blood pressure, type 2 diabetes, or non-alcoholic fatty liver disease. In this example, only aspects that exceed a certain threshold (see Chapter 3) are noted as being present. For each patient, the elements in the clinical picture that do not meet specified thresholds are not classified with a diagnostic label.

Another classification method is to describe the value/state of each individual attribute. Each patient could have their blood pressure, plasma glucose and HBA1c,

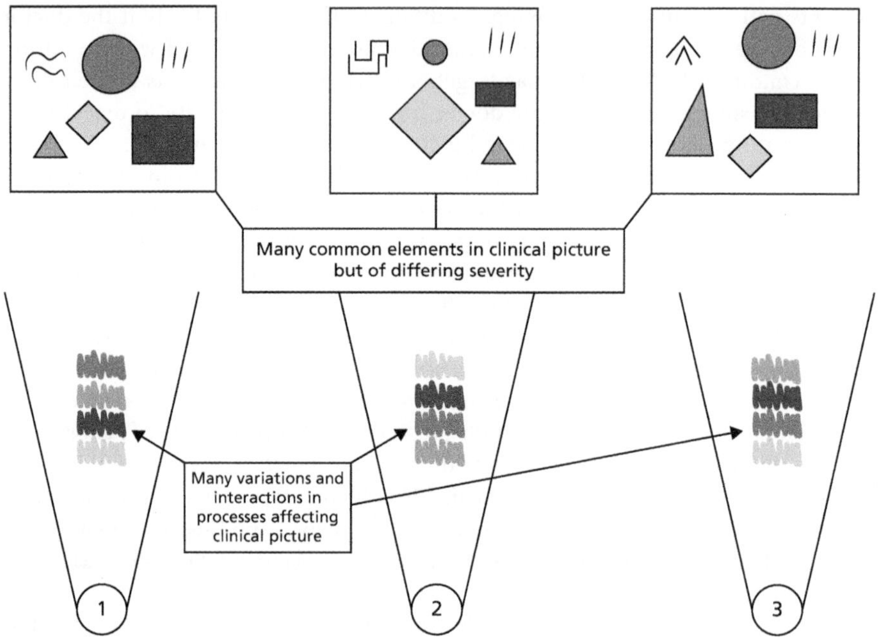

Figure 4.4 Production of clinical picture in spectrum conditions.

serum total cholesterol, body mass index, state of fattiness of liver, and so forth, described. This type of classification is easier to apply in situations where it is limited to a relatively small number of attributes as it is cognitive resource intensive. Professionals whose way of working with people involves spending a lot of time with small numbers of individuals in non-urgent situations can use far more complex classification systems such as these multi-dimensional classifications.

Depending on the amount of time available and/or the purpose for which a classification is intended, a categorical or dimensional classification may be more appropriate. Dimensional classification omits less data than categorical classification, with fewer assumptions than placing combinations in a category. It does involve having to keep in mind a great deal of data, however, and this takes time and considerable cognitive resources. Other implications of using dimensional classification will be described later. Sometimes this dimensional data can be summarized into simpler forms. For example, you can calculate risk of cardiovascular events by combining several different elements of the clinical picture (such as blood pressure, body mass index, cholesterol, and ethnicity) into a percentage chance of experiencing an event over a period of years (see Kannel et al., 1976; Hippisley-Cox et al., 2007).

For classification of conditions, the purposes for which the information is used, as well as the restrictions in which the doctor operates, will determine choosing between categorical or dimensional classifications.

From clinical picture to classification

The first step in classification is describing conditions able to be recognized in clinical practice and used for grouping participants in research, based on perceived similarities in their clinical picture. These diagnostic constructs have utility if they are able to be recognized based on the description of the clinical picture they depict and have attached useful information for clinical decision-making (see Chapter 2). There will have been information gathered about them; historically, doctors would combine expert opinion based on the authority of renowned physicians with observations based on their own experience. More recently, information will have been provided by research on participants identified as having the condition by their clinical picture matching an accepted description.

This type of diagnostic construct is a 'clinical' diagnosis based on the clinical picture (Scadding, 1967; Chapter 4 in Schoenberg and Rosamond, 2000). It is used on the basis of clinical utility. Information can be gathered on prognosis, complications, co-occurring conditions, and responses to treatment even if the reasons for this are not understood. The level of explanation in this type of diagnosis is often basic. 'We tend to see/or have seen before/this complication (or other phenomenon) with this diagnosis'. The 'explanation' is merely a descriptive statement of association with the diagnostic construct.

The next step is to research these clinical diagnostic constructs to identify differences of structure (pathology) and/or functions/processes (usually pathophysiology but also meant broadly to include psychological or social mechanisms) that may be measured by the appropriate techniques such as biomarkers that are associated with the clinical picture. The final step is to identify the causes of these differences in structure/processes, otherwise known as the aetiology (Chapter 4 in McHugh and Slavney, 1998). I shall describe these diagnostic constructs as having 'scientific validity' but there exist multiple definitions of validity (see Chapter 6). The differences in structure/processes may not be strongly caused by a top-down process like a disease but by a network of interactions (although an initial cause may have triggered the network). Some have found modelling mental health symptoms as an interacting network more useful than as a top-down process (Borsboom and Cramer, 2013; Borsboom, 2017).

A scientifically valid diagnosis can exist in two forms, identified differences of structure and/or process (or mechanism) or of causation, and sometimes a 'complete' combination of aetiology/pathology/pathophysiology and clinical picture (Campbell et al., 1979). Once a difference of structure/process is identified, then the gathering of information can be improved upon: investigations can be developed to identify cases of this diagnostic construct and improve the reliability of this expanded clinical picture.

The improved reliability of detecting cases through investigations makes it easier to perform research on causes and treatment. From a patient's point of view, the demonstration of proven differences can protect them from accusations of having an 'invalid' problem. The benefit of increased knowledge of the condition's mechanisms (including psychosocial mechanisms) includes increased explanation and understanding of prognosis, complications, and co-occurrence. It allows us to understand why current treatments benefit as well as opening up new avenues for researching improved treatments. There is additional benefit of explaining the processes behind the development of patient's problems. It can be clearly seen that whilst a clinical utility type of diagnostic construct has its merits that a scientifically valid diagnostic construct is superior.

The best progression for a diagnostic construct is to begin with a clinical utility diagnosis, a descriptive diagnostic construct based on the clinical picture, then progress to scientifically valid diagnostic construct, based on mechanism or understanding the condition's aetiology (Gale, 2006). The pitfalls on this pathway are several.

First, that there is no often no one-to-one relationship between clinical picture and an underlying condition associated with specific differences in structure/process or causes. Tuberculosis can resemble many other diagnoses in its clinical picture (Sievers, 1961), apart from tests that demonstrated the presence of the bacteria causing TB (mycobacterium tuberculosis). If the doctor does not think to order the investigation (or an investigation is not available) then she may not be able to distinguish between TB and these other conditions. Two of the five cases described had misleading laboratory test results which shows that no single type of information is foolproof. The doctor needs to take into account the whole clinical picture and that an initial diagnosis may have to be revised.

Second, as TB illustrates, there is conversely many clinical pictures that can be associated with a single underlying condition; that is, there is no one-to-one relationship between condition and clinical picture.

This results in a situation where a clinical picture, particularly if it lacks important information such as results from investigations that can differentiate different conditions or no such investigations are available, may result from several different mechanisms and/or causes. The resultant diagnostic construct is heterogeneous. They describe people who have similarities of their clinical picture but often different types of causes. These heterogeneous diagnostic constructs tend to carry greater uncertainty over the information attached to them than a homogenous diagnostic construct (describing people with similar mechanisms and/or causes). This greater uncertainty of information is still better than 'no information' if no classification is attempted.

In the past, fevers were classified according to their course over time (an aspect of their clinical picture) into 'acute', 'chronic', 'indolent', and so forth, in a heterogeneous diagnostic construct. As medical knowledge advanced this classification was dropped and fevers are now described with an aetiologically based diagnosis causing the fever, for example, the type of infection or a flare-up of an autoimmune disease. In some cases of fever there is no obvious cause found and the diagnostic construct of 'pyrexia of unknown origin' (PUO) is used. This demonstrates that doctors used a diagnostic classification based on the clinical picture but as soon as they discovered a way to separate a heterogeneous diagnostic construct in a scientifically valid way into more homogenous diagnostic constructs they adopted these superior diagnostic constructs.

A further problem with clinical utility diagnostic constructs is the potential they have to hinder progress towards a more scientifically valid diagnostic construct. I used the word 'perceive' rather than 'notice' in the first stage of a doctor identifying a putative diagnostic construct based on similarities in the clinical picture. By this, I meant that the doctor perceives a pattern, not necessarily that a pattern of a syndrome exists. It may be that they are just describing a point on a spectrum rather than a syndrome.

Once this particular description of a diagnostic construct based on a clinical picture enters the collective consciousness of doctors and becomes used in research and training, it gains utility from information attached to this diagnostic construct. However, the diagnostic criteria used for this clinical utility type of diagnosis may not be the best way to identify the causes or processes underlying the clinical picture; for example, it may be too heterogeneous a construct, making research to establish a scientifically valid diagnosis more difficult than it needed to be.

A superior potential set of diagnostic criteria that are better able to predict outcomes, complications, or responses to treatment may exist. It may be that categorical diagnostic constructs are not the best way to describe the condition or gather information of clinical utility (such as outcomes or response to interventions) or research into discovering the causes and underlying processes. The diagnostic construct may thus have some clinical utility but it does not progress to a more scientifically valid construct. Further, it may act like a weed that crowds out the development of more useful blooms of classification that could offer more clinical utility and/or lead to increased scientific understanding.

An established diagnostic construct can accumulate great amounts of attached useful information. If it is replaced by an alternative classification, then there is a potential cost of losing this information. It may be hard to use prior research evidence and clinical experience acquired using the previous diagnostic construct with the new classification. This 'inertial resistance' to adopt a new classification—the entrenched advantages of the established diagnostic construct—has been referred to as 'path dependence' and 'lock-in' (Cooper, 2015). The new classification needs to demonstrate significant advantages to become adopted. An example of a significant advantage could be scientific validity leading to improved utility. Other clear advantages may be markedly improved predictive power in terms of prognosis or treatment outcomes (First et al., 2004), as long as the new proposed classification is not particularly onerous in terms of time and cognitive resources (see Chapter 2).

Absence of a scientifically valid classification is particularly relevant in mental health as our knowledge of the functioning of the mind/brain in acknowledged healthy states is very poor, let alone when people may be regarded as having mental health problems. We have to accept the clinical utility type of diagnostic constructs in the interim whilst awaiting sufficient progress to develop scientifically valid classifications.

A further problem with clinical utility diagnostic constructs is that people may forget—or fail to explain—that they are not scientifically valid. They may regard the diagnostic construct as representing an essentialist construct type whereas in fact it is a nominalist construct type (see Chapter 3). Research grants may only be granted if diagnostic constructs are used as if they are the optimum form of classification, thus reducing the possibilities of gathering information using alternative classifications. This has been referred to as 'reification' that hinders progress (Hyman, 2010).

Differences in structure/process can also occur in spectrum conditions without clear divisions between different diagnostic constructs, or from health, resulting in nominalist rather than essentialist constructs; for example, autoimmune diseases (see Chapter 11).

Determining causality

'Why does this particular person present with this particular problem/condition?' is the question addressed by causality in medicine. Scottish philosopher David Hume doubted we could solve this type of problem by interpreting experience (the problem of induction). Popper tried to resolve this by suggesting that scientists should try to frame theories and explanations in terms that can be shown to be false, that is, falsifiable and testable (see, e.g., Susser, 1998; Weed, 1998). If an experiment shows the 'null hypothesis' (e.g. that a drug is no more effective than placebo) unlikely to be true, then the opposite 'experimental hypothesis' (e.g. that a drug is more effective than placebo) is likely (but still not certain) to be true. Bertrand Russell argued that conclusions about relationships could be drawn independently of experience (Susser, 1991). Some have argued Popper's methods are more suited to sciences like physics and it is still possible to come close to the truth by demonstrating a weight of evidence supporting a conclusion (Chapter 4 in Ghaemi, 2007).

One school of thought is that explanations or causes of events sit at a fundamental level of the natural world. They can be explained first by reference to the laws of physics, which affects the next, chemical, level, which in turn affects the biological, then the psychological, then the sociological. This has been called the 'ontological' level of explanation (Thornton, 2015).

Another type of explanation is that of 'epistemological' levels of explanation (Thornton, 2015). Something may occur at one level without being explained by an interaction or mechanism at a different level. An explanation that occurs at the level of society is not explained by a biological or chemical process. Some researchers have proposed that for certain mental health conditions, the only required level of explanation/causation is the thoughts themselves and their interaction with each other (van den Hout, 2014).

Robert Koch helped isolate and identify the bacteria causing most cases of tuberculosis (mycobacteria tuberculosis). This improved the understanding of tuberculosis, or TB, from primarily 'a social disease' paradigm, according to Virchow, to an 'infectious disease' paradigm (Susser, 1998). Koch is also famous for his 'Postulates' that need to be met before a micro-organism can be identified as the cause of an illness. There is disagreement about which other people contributed to these postulates (Chapter 5 in Bynum, 2008; Susser, 1991) and about the final form of these postulates. Susser's version (Susser, 1991) can be summarized as:

1. The micro-organism must always be present in the disease.
2. The micro-organism must be demonstrated to be a distinctive living organisms from others found in the disease.
3. The micro-organism must be able to the explain the clinical picture and be distributed with the disease's lesions.
4. The micro-organism is proven to cause the disease in experimental animals.

It was often hard to prove this gold standard but even when it *was* met then it was often shown that that these micro-organisms could be present without disease. In TB, it was often necessary for the presence of overcrowding, poverty, and/or malnutrition to be present along with exposure to mycobacterium for the illness to develop. TB is *both* a social disease *and* an infectious disease.

Epidemiologists define causes as being potentially *necessary* and/or *sufficient* (Rothman, 1976; Susser, 1991; Chapter 9 in Schoenberg and Rosamond, 2000). *Necessary* causes are essential for a condition to occur in a person. Without that causative factor the condition cannot develop; for example, a strain of mycobacterium bacillus is *necessary* to be present for someone to develop the disease tuberculosis. Many conditions do not have *necessary* causative factors, such as high blood pressure. It is very rare for a single factor to be a *sufficient* causative factor, that is, the presence of or exposure to the factor *always* causes the condition of interest. (It is not necessary for every case of the condition to have a *sufficient* causative factor.) Many people have exposure to the meningococcus bacteria but not everyone so exposed goes on to develop meningococcal meningitis (Hill, 1965).

For most conditions, a combination of several factors are required to be *sufficient* to cause a condition. These can be thought of as components of an overall causal combination for that individual, and these may vary from individual to individual (Rothman, 1976). This combination of multiple causative factors is therefore *mutually minimally sufficient* and may occur at different time points. Rothman referred to this as the sufficient-component causal model. The visual analogy of a pie is used with each 'component casual factor' being a slice of the pie. Once sufficient factors are present to be therefore *mutually minimally sufficient*, then the condition will develop. (Protective factors may be thought of as being present in the sense that enough causative factors are present to overcome them or their absence is one of the component causal factors).

Two different patients may have some components in common in their particular pie but the component causative factors they do not share may lead to different conditions developing in them. At the simplest level, two individuals may share many components making them vulnerable to infections but were exposed to two different bacteria leading to different type of infections. At a more complex level, certain conditions may share many causative factors in common (e.g. genetic factors or socioeconomic factors) but differ in other factors (sometimes not well understood such as in autoimmune diseases or mental health problems) leading to quite different clinical pictures and thus diagnosed as separate conditions.

Bradford Hill set out influential criteria to help judge if a factor is causal (Hill, 1965).

- Strength (of association)
- Consistency
- Specificity
- Temporality
- Biological gradient
- Plausibility
- Coherence

- Experiment
- Analogy

Hill explained that these factors did not all have to be present to establish causality, but that an expert judgement could be made using these considerations as a framework rather than a checklist. Often in science, statistical tests are performed to examine whether a conclusion can be drawn, but Hill states this may not be necessary in 'weighing up' the evidence using this framework.

Strength of association refers to the relative (not absolute) increased risk of developing a condition when exposed to the proposed causative factors. Absolute risk may not be very informative as they may be small numbers. Relative risk is much more useful often expressed as an odds ratio. Hill gives the example of rates of death due to lung cancer in smokers compared to non-smokers (9–10 times higher for smokers, 20–30 times for heavy smokers), and for rates of death due to coronary thrombosis is about double, or less, for smokers compared to non-smokers.

The lower the strength of association for a proposed causative factor, the more likely that there are confounding factors and/or other factors needed to be present in order for the condition to develop. Even a high strength of association does not prove that a factor is *sufficient* by itself. Not even every heavy smoker develops lung cancer; clearly there are other *vulnerability* factors present, but smoking is still a *potent* cause of lung cancer.

Consistency is whether the evidence of causation for a factor has been 'observed by different persons, in different places, circumstances and times' (Hill, 1965). Hill did not regard this as a particularly important criterion as it may be difficult to gather a wide variety of evidence.

Specificity refers to whether a proposed causative factor is associated with a particular condition, such as a specific site of the condition and specific disease process. Hill also regarded this as an unimportant consideration. If it is present, then it does allow us to draw a conclusion more easily about causation. Many causative factors are not associated with specific conditions or specific disease processes.

Temporality describes the relationship in time between exposure to the proposed causative factor. If there is a close relationship in time to a single exposure to the factor and development of the condition this strengthens the case for a causative relationship. Some conditions seem to be caused by factors long before the condition is detected (sometimes as part of a 'multi-hit' multistage combination of causative factors), however. Other conditions may be caused by long-term exposure to a causative factor; sometimes prolonged exposure in these cases makes the causal link obvious.

Biological gradient is where an increased exposure to the suggested causative factor is associated with an increased risk of developing the condition. (Note that for a protective factor the opposite is true) The presence of a biological gradient is strong evidence for a given factor being a cause of a condition. The gradient does not have to be 'biological', it could be psychological or social; for example, an increased number of negative life events over a short time period has been shown to increase the risk of developing depression in women (Brown and Harris, 1978). We cannot always assume a straightforward linear relationship between the proposed causative factor and risk of developing a condition as this is not always true.

Plausibility. The degree of plausibility that a factor has for causing a condition depends on our state of knowledge. We find it hard to judge how plausible a mechanism is when our state of knowledge of the mechanism underlying the condition is poor. This is doubly so for when we don't even understand the functioning explaining 'healthy' phenomena such as higher mental functions (thoughts, emotions, memories, for example). It is not crucial for establishing causality.

Coherence is where a proposed causative factor should fit with what we know about the condition, such is its course or known biology (as well as psychological and social factors).

Experiment refers to situations where we have information on increasing or reducing the exposure to a proposed causative factor has on the rates of developing the condition of interest. There may be 'natural' experiments when exposure to a suggested causative factor was increased or reduced.

Analogy is the final concept that may be of use in determining causation. If it has been previously shown that a particular type of factor has been causative for a condition, it strengthens the case for a similar factor also being causative. The example of thalidomide causing foetal abnormality makes it more plausible that other drugs taken prenatally may also cause foetal abnormality.

These considerations are meant to taken as a whole when deciding whether a factor is causal in producing a condition. They are regarded as a classic framework model for making judgements about causality in the absence of absolute definitive evidence. The framework also demonstrated the point that determining causality was not just the end in itself, the ultimate goal was to identify a focus for an intervention to improve the health of the population (Hill, 1965; Glass et al., 2013).

Some researchers have tried to reframe these considerations into three broader categories. Direct evidence (incorporating experiment, strength (of association), temporal association); mechanistic evidence (biological gradient and (biological) plausibility); and parallel evidence (coherence, consistency, analogy), with specificity being excluded (Howick et al., 2009).

There are problems with this model of a subjective expert judgement. It can be prone to manipulation of the evidence (Glass et al., 2013). Information contrary to the expert's judgement could be omitted or downplayed. A subtle form is to focus on the shortcomings of evidence that does not fit with the expert's conclusion whilst less attention is paid to problems with the evidence supporting the expert's conclusion. There is a lack of formal basis for making a conclusion, such as a mathematical test (Glass et al., 2013). It does not fit clearly with the Popperian 'falsification' model of establishing conclusions in science (Susser, 1998; Weed, 1998).

Given the problems outlined earlier with this 'classical method', epidemiologists may use different models to examine the question of causality such as the 'counterfactual' model (Hofler, 2005). It compares the likelihood of developing the condition between those exposed and not exposed (the 'counterfactual') to the proposed causative factor. Ideally, you would have data from members of the same population who are identical, apart from whether they were exposed or not to the proposed causative factor.

Mathematical and statistical techniques such as 'bias modelling' may be used with counterfactual modelling to try to correct for *confounding* factors in order to help make judgements on causality that are more reliable than expert judgement using the Bradford Hill criteria (Hofler, 2005).

These epidemiological causative models are used for making decisions about causality in *populations*. This leads to information incorporated into medical knowledge that is then used by doctors when they see *individuals* in clinical practice. Doctors have to be aware of how *transferable* the information is from populations in studies are to the individual in front of them. The information may be drawn from populations that differ markedly from the individual in front of them for example in terms of culture, biology (e.g. diet, genetics) or socioeconomic circumstances.

A framework of three Cs—causes, characteristics, and context—may be helpful for an individual case incorporating both causative and protective factors. These factors may also be interlinked; for example, certain contexts may increase the likelihood of characteristics making people vulnerable or resistant to conditions.

- *Causes* include events or agents that have been shown to increase the chance of a condition arising. Obvious examples are bacteria causing disease or falls causing injuries. They are not necessarily biological; for example, negative life events may increase the risk of developing depression.
- *Characteristics* refer to qualities of the individual that make them vulnerable or less likely to develop conditions. Malnourished people can be vulnerable to a variety of conditions such as nutritional deficiencies or infections (such as TB). People who have low self-esteem or who are prone to worry may be vulnerable to developing a variety of emotional disorders. People can inherit genetic conditions such as sickle cell trait that increases resistance to certain conditions (malaria) but can also make them vulnerable to sickle cell painful crises in certain conditions (e.g. low oxygen levels). Other characteristics can be an absence, such as never having been immunized against particular infections (which would have protected them against infection).
- *Context* is a concept that refers to the relevant factors of a patient's environment such as their culture, their socioeconomic status, or their living environment. People who live in poverty live in unhealthy environments—there may be poor sanitation with high exposure to infectious agents, overcrowding allowing easy transmission of infections between people, or poor diets leading to vulnerability to infection. People who live in poverty are more likely to live stress-filled, demanding lives which can harm their emotional health. Countries with poor public health programmes may have few people immunized against deadly infection. Mental health problems may result from broader societal contextual issues but also from social contexts of their particular 'microclimate'—they may have difficulties in their relationship, may experience bullying or critical or hostile comments from parents or bullying at work. Conversely, environments such as supportive families or wealth may reduce the risk of developing conditions.

Doctors need to be aware of the influence that contexts have on their patients' health. They can offer help in the areas they can influence, such as writing letters which would support the patient's claim to housing or welfare benefits. Public health doctors can try and influence broader social determinants of health, but they are not omnipotent. They have neither the power nor the means to change society, directly, for the better.

Virchow pointed out that whilst it is the duty of doctors to identify the causes of medical problems—often social factors—it is up to politicians to bring about the changes needed to address these causes (Ashton, 2006)

Conclusion

The clinical picture of a patient encompasses the patient's story symptoms, signs, and results of investigations that the doctor is aware of. Apart from an interaction of causative factors as outlined above, other factors significantly affect the clinical picture such as individual cultural factors, experiences, how people view health problems, and personality factors of *both* the doctor and the patient. In addition, the circumstances and contexts in which they interact, as well interpersonal factors operating between doctor and patient, also influence the clinical picture. The degree of commonality between a patient's clinical picture with that of a clinical picture associated with a diagnostic construct allows the doctor to make a diagnosis.

Diagnostic constructs often begin as descriptive, based on certain patterns of the clinical picture. They are used because they can have clinical utility; information can be gathered about prognosis, complications, comorbidity, and responses to treatment (see Chapter 2). The next stage in improving diagnostic constructs is to demonstrate differences of structure and/or processes associated with the diagnosis and not with health or other conditions. These differences can be psychological, social, or biological. The third stage is discovering the cause of the condition and how the differences of structure and/or processes come about. Diagnostic constructs based on the second and the third stages are regarded as scientifically valid. They have several advantages. Investigations can be developed to detect the differences in structures and/or processes to aid in diagnosing the patient accurately. Improved treatments can be developed in order to change the differences in structure and/or processes if this is helpful. If causes are identified, then they can be directly targeted.

Single causative factors are rarely wholly responsible for developing a condition. Some causative factors are necessary for a condition to develop but are rarely sufficient by themselves. Often several causative factors need to be present before a condition to develop and this has been called a sufficient-component cause model (Rothman, 1976). People with the same condition may have different combinations of causative factors. People with different conditions may have some causative factors in common. To help decide if there is sufficient evidence to decide if a factor is causative, people have used the Bradford Hill framework (Hill, 1965), although this doesn't fit with scientific models of testable hypotheses. Causative factors can be organized into a broader framework of causes, characteristics and contexts. Identifying causative factors is important if they can lead to interventions to prevent or reduce the effects of the condition (Hill, 1965).

Chapter 5

Multidisciplinary working, evidence, treatment, and decision-making in medicine

This chapter describes a model of patients presenting to healthcare with various needs. These needs may not all be able to be met using the medical model so doctors may use additional methods or will need to work with others in a multidisciplinary team to meet these needs. There follows a discussion of how evidence is gathered through research as a basis of medical knowledge such as effectiveness of treatments. The different types of treatment objectives and the nature of treatment actions (such as preventative or directly affecting disease) will be outlined. Finally, I will discuss how all these different elements are integrated into a model of medical decision-making that allows doctors to see many patients.

The need for multidisciplinary teams in healthcare

A patient will present to a doctor with needs, something that the patient requires or desires as well as situations (conditions) that can benefit from medical intervention, as shown in Figure 5.1. Some of these needs may require the doctor to use their knowledge and skills related to the medical model. For example, the patient may have a chest infection (that requires the doctor to identify this and begin appropriate treatment) or the patient may be concerned that they have a serious condition and wish the doctor to confirm or exclude this.

Some of the patients' needs—such as their ideas about their problem, their concerns about the implications of their problem, and subsequent expectations of what the doctor can do to help them (Chapter 3 in Pendleton et al., 1984)—may not require knowledge or skills specific to the medical model. For example, the patient may benefit solely from the doctor's interest and concern for their problems.

These other needs may respond more to the doctor's personality traits or communication skills or their professional authority. Sometimes other needs, such as seeking validation for inability to perform usual duties being due to illness or requiring certification from their doctor such as a 'sick note' for work or a supportive letter to change housing for health reasons, rely on doctors' professional authority based partly on their sapiental authority.

The doctor will need to use relational techniques outside of symptom enquiry and physical examination to identify and meet many patient needs (Chapters 1 and 4 in Pendleton et al., 1984). These relational techniques include concern for the patient's

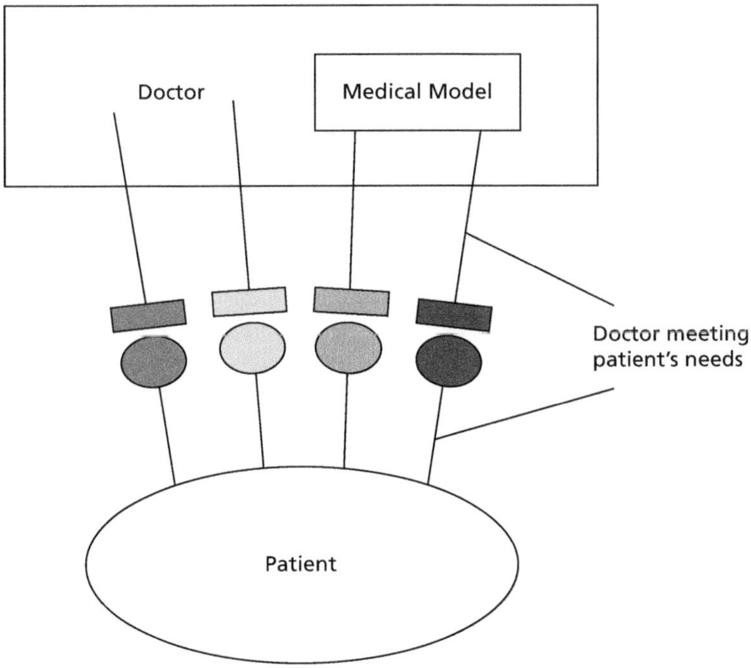

Figure 5.1 Doctor able to meet all patient needs.

point of view, enquiring as to their reasons for seeking medical help, and identifying their ideas, concerns, and expectations. The interaction between doctor and patient—listening to the patient's concerns, validating them as a legitimate matter of medical interest and deserving of help, proving information and support—is itself a therapeutic intervention that can bring some benefit in addition to those from medication or other medical interventions.

The above model is a simplification in that it depicts all the patient's needs being met but this is may not be the case in reality. The doctor may not have identified all the patient's needs. Sometimes the patient has unrealistic expectations, perhaps overestimating the ability of the doctor to change things. Sometimes the doctor will refuse to meet the patient's needs. The doctor may be able to meet the patient's need but due to other restrictions—such as lack of time or not very capable to meet that particular need—they either do not meet the need or refer the patient on to somebody else to do so.

Sometimes a person sees another professional for their problems other than a doctor. These professionals will work to another model (see Figure 5.2) that reflects their own professional training. These other professionals also can use their personal attributes, communication skills, and professional behaviours/authority to benefit the people seeing them.

The professional will need to use their own professional model to meet some of the patient needs. These needs may be difficult for a doctor to meet using a medical model.

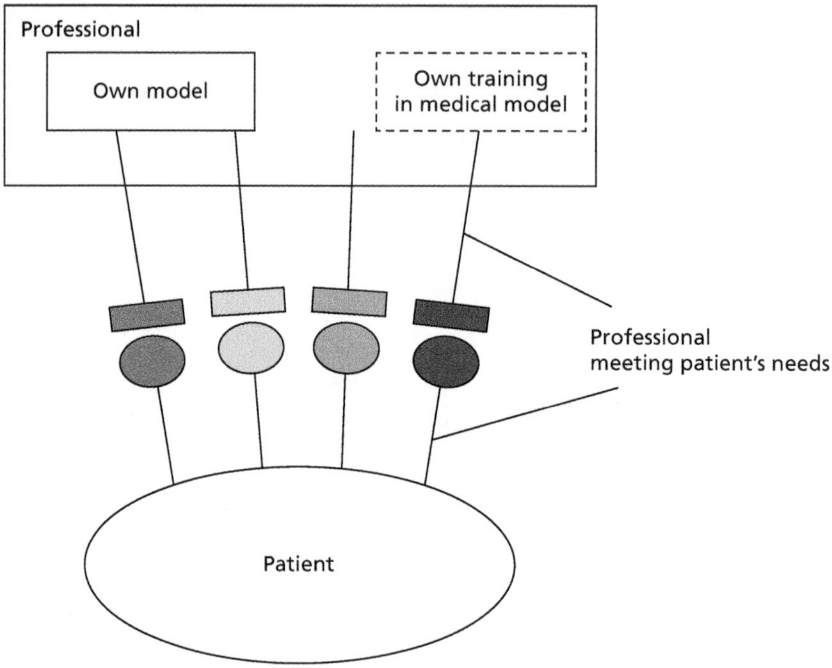

Figure 5.2 Other professional meeting patient needs or doctor not using medical model as their primary model.

For example, if a patient needs to improve mobility of a joint after an operation then a physiotherapist uses their training as a physiotherapist and their treatment model is better placed to help meet this aim. Some needs for help or treatment can be met by using either the medical model or another model. For example, depression could be treated by a doctor with medication or a therapist with psychotherapy.

On many occasions, patient needs' may be met at least as well by other professionals than a doctor, sometimes even better. This may because these other professionals have more time to meet these needs such as the patient being listened to or the professional has access to resources or skills that they have more experience with or training than a doctor. Other professionals may have superior caring and empathy or better communication skills. Their particular professional model and related skills and training may be able to meet a need that the medical model is unable to meet. Sometimes, even if the medical model offers a treatment, other models of care and help may be superior.

There are two slight variations to this to discuss. One is where a professional other than a doctor has had training in the medical model. Some nurses and other professionals have had training in medical prescribing after making a diagnosis. These other qualified prescribers may replace the need for doctors in many situations. Another variation is where a doctor uses another conceptual or therapeutic model other than the medical one described in this book such as where doctors also train as psychotherapists and use psychotherapeutic techniques in their clinical practice.

There are times when a patient sees more than one professional (see Figure 5.3). Multidisciplinary team working occurs when a patient's needs cannot be met by a single individual or professional. An obvious example is hospital care: inpatients get nursing and medical care; pharmacists help with oversight of medications and medication queries; radiographers, occupational therapists, and physiotherapists lend their expertise; receptionists and administrators perform their roles and so forth. Another example is community mental health teams include mental health nurses, social workers, doctors, support workers, and, hopefully, psychologists, all of whom must work together in a coordinated team to help the patient.

This model describes how people with a variety of needs have them met by a variety of different professionals. As in the example shown in Figure 5.2, sometimes similar needs can be met by both the doctor and another professional, sometimes the other professional can meet the need better than the doctor. For reasons of simplicity I have omitted cases where other professionals use the medical model and also when doctors use other models than the classical medical model.

A doctor may have a biopsychosocial understanding of a patient's needs but may only offer primarily biological interventions such as medication or surgery as these are the type of interventions that doctors are best qualified and able in the time provided to deliver. Psychosocial needs will be met by other members of the multidisciplinary team who may be better trained to meet these needs or have superior personal qualities or more time to devote to the case.

Both the models depicted in Figure 5.2 and Figure 5.3 illustrate the concept of 'promiscuous realism' outlined in Chapter 1. That is, there may be multiple ways of viewing the same problem, with the implication being that there may be several different ways of alleviating or helping resolve the same problem. In addition, people's

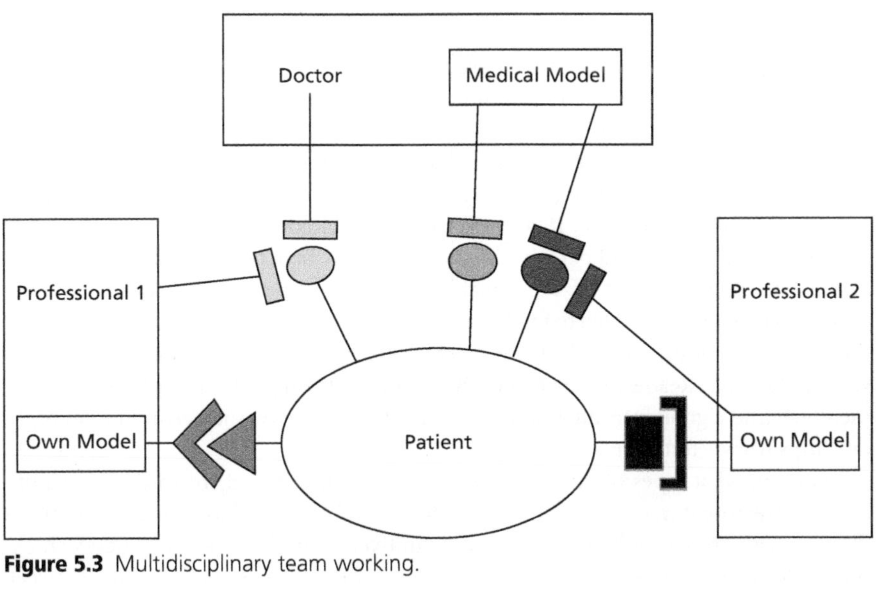

Figure 5.3 Multidisciplinary team working.

needs are often complex and require the help of several different professionals with different approaches or 'models' for these needs to be met.

Even with a multidisciplinary team, not all of a patient's needs may be met. Multidisciplinary teams are expensive and so the amount of resources may be restricted in terms of time given to each patient or availability of interventions by the third party who pays for these teams.

An important omission from all these figures is the support and help patients get from other sources than professionals such as members of their families, partners, and friends. Other people with similar conditions can also be a source of help; their shared experiences can help them empathize and provide information that is useful. Charities, religious groups, and patient support groups can also provide help—empathy, understanding, time to discuss problems, information, campaigning to get needed resources for healthcare, etc.

It is important to note that patients can also experience *harm* at the hands of professionals.

Gathering evidence through research

Doctors' sapiental authority relies on their knowledge of health and illness (see Chapter 1). Historically, doctors relied on a combination of textbooks written by renowned physicians (Chapters 1 and 2 in Bynum, 2008) and their own experience to help them in knowing how to treat patients. The problem with experience is that it can be an unreliable guide to discovering accurate information about conditions (Chapter 6 in Sackett et al., 1991). Medicine moved towards basing knowledge on research rather than reputational authority or personal experience (though experience informs how research is evaluated).

Doctor's evaluations of outcomes, including treatment effectiveness, can be unreliable due to, for example, inaccurate observations or bias caused by expecting a particular result of treatment. A further problem in assessing effectiveness of treatments is the placebo effect. The doctor administered a treatment and the patient reports an improvement. This improvement could be due to a natural fluctuation of severity of the illness, the patient wishing to please the doctor by reporting an improvement, or the beneficial effects of seeing a caring professional leading to an improvement of symptoms (Kienle and Kiene, 1996, 1997), or even a biological effect induced by being offered an inert compound perceived to be potentially beneficial (Encke et al., 2013).

The proper assessment of the effectiveness of treatments AND other types of outcomes (e.g. prognosis) led to medicine harnessing the power first of simple counting the numbers in testing the effectiveness of treatments then the adoption of more advanced statistics. Readers interested in the history of trying to find 'fair tests' for treatment will find a good introduction on the website <http://www.jameslindlibrary.org/> or <https://www.testingtreatments.org>.

Counting what types of outcomes eventuated from different treatments was sufficient if a treatment was greatly effective such as in the early antibiotic trials. Sometimes the numbers are so stark as to indicate definitively causal connections between exposure to factors and subsequent development of conditions such as links between smoking and lung cancer or working as a chimney sweep and developing scrotal cancer (Hill, 1965).

Difference in outcomes due to an intervention, compared to an adequate control treatment (to account for the placebo effect and for the condition's natural course) was hard to demonstrate using simple counting of outcomes in studies of effectiveness of many medical or surgical interventions. This led to an introduction of statistics in the evaluation of research data (Chapter 4 in Bynum, 2008).

Statistical methods were used to establish how probable it was that research results occurred by chance. If a research finding had a 5% or less probability of occurring by chance, then it was 'statistically significant' (described in statistical shorthand as $p < = 0.05$). There are criticisms that the use of the 5% probability threshold still allows too many false positive results (Colquhoun, 2014).

Research deals with probabilities. The aim of the research is to *reduce* uncertainty about the outcome measured, not to provide total certainty (Chapter 3 in Greenhalgh, 2010)). The inevitable flaws in a research study increase the uncertainty with which we regard the conclusions but do not necessarily mean we discard them completely. Interested readers can find good and comprehensible guides to statistics (e.g. Chapter 5 in Greenhalgh, 2010).

Not all studies rely on statistics to test a hypothesis. Some are *descriptive*, that is they describe a state of affairs or describe what happened in a group of participants. Some research studies seek to show an association between two or more factors. The aphorism 'correlation does not mean causation' applies; there may be hidden 'confounding' factors that explain the association. For example, there is an association between later birth order and Down's syndrome. The true (confounding) risk factor for Down's syndrome is maternal age—being born later in the birth order was inevitably associated with older maternal age. Once the effects of maternal age were *controlled* for then later birth order did not increase the risk of Down's syndrome occurring (Hay and Berbano, 1972).

Another important point when evaluating the results of research on, for example, medication or other interventions is that statistically significant results may not be *clinically significant* results (Chapter 7 in Sackett et al., 1991). A large trial evaluating a treatment may find a statistically significant difference between an intervention and a control comparison (e.g. an active drug and placebo), but this effect may be clinically insignificant

There are three main types of interpretational errors when people review the research evidence: uncritical acceptance, unrealistic fastidiousness, and bias. Uncritical acceptance is when we accept a research conclusion too readily. Unrealistic fastidious sits on the opposite end of this spectrum. Any inevitable flaws in the research lead to it being dismissed or ignored. This leads to therapeutic and clinical nihilism as no treatment research or other knowledge based on research can achieve an unrealistically high threshold or is viewed as applying in only very restricted circumstances.

These two types of errors are extreme ends of a dimension. The final type of error is bias. This also lies on a dimension: everybody is biased, to some extent. When the bias is extreme, it leads to problems interpreting a result. Extreme bias is displayed by applying different rules to evidence depending on whether the findings of the research are palatable to the original opinion held. Useful guides to critical evaluation of research are available (e.g. Sackett et al., 1991; Greenhalgh, 2010).

Primary research collects data directly, for example on participants in a trial of drug treatment. Secondary research gathers, synthesizes, and summarizes the results of primary research in a particular area. The varying questions around clinical information are best answered by different types of research studies (Chapter 3 in Greenhalgh, 2010; Chapters 6 and 7 in Sackett et al., 1991).

For evaluating treatment effectiveness, the randomized controlled trial (or RCT)—double-blind, if possible, but at least having the outcome assessments made blind to the intervention group—is the best method to assess effectiveness of an intervention. A good description of why the double-blind RCT is the 'gold standard' can be found in two classic papers (Hill, 1951, 1952). RCTs are the best way to assess differences in outcome between *experimental* and *control* interventions (such as placebo), assuming certain conditions can be met such as adequate control treatments, randomization, and blinded outcome measurements.

It is important that the correct research question is asked–, such as what is the *correct* outcome to be assessed. The question asked and the way the question is assessed—for example, what outcomes are measured and how—can be skewed by interested parties such as pharmaceutical companies or device manufacturers (Chapter 3 in Greenhalgh, 2010; Smilowitz et al., 2016) or researchers who genuinely believe 'their' intervention is useful (and want to prove it to the world) obtain better results than others with less faith or with a (usually unconscious) desire for further research grants. This latter type of bias applies to ALL forms of research, not just RCTs, and to all types of interventions including psychotherapy where 'allegiance' to a type of therapy influences the result (Turner et al., 2014).

Pre-registration of trials and their protocols in trial registries such as can be found at <https://clinicaltrials.gov>. and mandatory publishing of the results has been suggested as a way to address this problem and can be effective in reducing this type of bias and publication bias of only positive results (Smilowitz et al., 2016).

Some people object to the high status given to RCTs because they suit medication trials better than some other type of interventions such as complex psychosocial interventions, for example psychotherapy. This is regarded as an entrenched bias towards biomedical hegemony over other models of care that ignores other types of evidence (Faulkner, 2015). RCTs are not based on the assumption that they are measuring the effect of a medical intervention acting directly on a disease and so are used in other fields than medicine such as education to evaluate different types of educational method (e.g. Jerrim and Vignoles, 2015). Education has been encouraged to adopt the RCT as a research tool to test different methods of educational practice effectiveness (Goldacre, 2013).

An accurate criticism is that most RCTs and medical research is 'top down' in nature (Faulkner, 2015). Measured outcomes are usually decided by researchers (or people who commission the research) without patients' input. This is slowly changing but examples exist where patients had input into the research study design such as what outcomes to assess (Xian et al., 2015)

Qualitative research focuses on the individual-level data that is often lost in studies using quantitative methods. Quantitative methods require standardization of meanings and summarization of data with subsequent loss of individual meaning. The qualitative approach involves asking participants directly about their experiences. Qualitative research is an important type of research that complements more conventional medical research and can also improve quantitative research by improving the questions it studies and the outcomes it measures (Chapter 12 in Greenhalgh, 2010).

Secondary research is where the relevant primary research on a topic (such as the treatment of TB) is sought and described to give an overview of the topic. There are three main types of this type of overview: (expert) review, systematic review, and meta-analysis.

Reviews, sometimes called expert reviews, are where the research evidence is described and summarized. There can be *selection bias* in the research that is included due to the reviewer (sometimes unconsciously) only noticing research that fits their preconceived view. Further *interpretation bias* can occur when the evidence is summarized and described. This becomes more marked the more elevated the expert (Chapter 9 in Greenhalgh, 2010).

A systematic review sets out an explicit information-gathering protocol with clear criteria for including and rejecting research studies for inclusion in the review to try to overcome the information seeking *selection bias* described above, or at least make selection reasons clear.

Meta-analysis (or meta-analytic studies) uses the same techniques of a systematic review to identify research papers. It then extracts numerical data about standardized outcomes for a defined group such as comparing medication against placebo in reducing psychotic symptoms in people who meet criteria for schizophrenia. The result can be affected by what inclusion/exclusion criteria are used to select studies (Taylor and Munafo, 2016).

Next, the data about the same outcome from different studies are combined to give a summary statistic about the outcome in each group, which is usually more reliable and accurate than that from any single research study. This is because the bigger the number of participants involved, the statistically the more reliable the result, so combined results from several studies should produce more reliable results.

Apart from the biases involved in summarizing research, the main problem with secondary research is that it depends on the quantity and quality of the primary research that is accessible. Some primary research is rejected for publication because it is too methodologically flawed. Worryingly, research may be rejected because a similar study has been carried out before (Chapter 3 in Greenhalgh, 2010), even though replicating research is an important part of science.

There is a hierarchy—or pyramid—of evidence based on the methodological strengths of the research (Chapter 1 in Walker et al., 2014), with subsequent 'grades of recommendation' in descending order of methodological strength as shown in Box 5.1. Sometimes the research does not directly answer the clinical question being asked so there needs to be extrapolation from the research that is closest to answering the clinical question. The commonly used GRADE recommendations are often used to

Box 5.1 The evidence hierarchy and grades of recommendation

Levels of Evidence

1a Meta-analysis of RCTs
1b RCT
2a Good quality case-controlled study but no randomization
2b Good quality quasi-experimental study
3 Good quality non-experimental descriptive studies, e.g. case studies
4 Expert opinions including those from expert committees and/or based on the clinical experiences of authoritative sources

Grades of Recommendation

A Level 1 evidence based.
B Level 2 evidence based on or extrapolated from Level 1 evidence
C Level 3 evidence based on or extrapolated from Level 1 or 2 evidence
D Level 4 evidence based on or extrapolated from level 1, 2, or 3 evidence

further 'weight' the quality of the evidence (<http://www.gradeworkinggroup.org/#pub> and Oxman and GRADE Working Group, 2004).

This evidence hierarchy is not to be applied blindly. Well-designed case-control studies carry more weight than poor RCTs and, arguably, meta-analysis/systematic reviews are separate from the hierarchy as they depend on the quality of the studies they analyse (Murad et al., 2016). Some types of questions are best answered by qualitative research.

Clinical decision-making and treatment

After assessing the problems the patient has presented with, resulting in a diagnostic formulation (see Chapters 2, 3, and 4), doctors identify potential objectives of treatment. The term 'treatment' is used broadly to describe interventions from doctors or other professionals designed to benefit the patient.

Unfortunately, the doctor often chooses the treatment objectives themselves without adequate consultation with the patient even in the majority of situations when such consultation is possible (Stovell et al., 2016). The chosen objectives may not match what the patient wants or needs. It is better if the patient chooses the objectives of treatment in partnership with the doctor, who provides advice (Chapter 7 in Sackett et al., 1991; Chapter 2 in Douglas et al., 2009). The patient tends to be more satisfied if this occurs as they have their own objectives of treatment they wish to see fulfilled, they are more likely to follow the suggested plan if they helped choose it, and patient autonomy has been respected. One concern is that doctor's decision-making is influenced by payments from pharmaceutical or other commercial medical companies. Research from the United States suggests that such payments to doctors—for both funding research as well as more direct remuneration—are common (Marshall et al., 2016a). Psychiatry was not amongst the specialties with the highest percentages of doctors receiving these kinds of payments and the total amounts of payments received by practitioners; these were cardiovascular medicine, gastroenterology, and surgical specialties such as orthopaedics.

The treatment plan should be based on the best quality evidence available drawn from research on participants who are similar to the patient (Chapters 6 and 7 in Sackett et al., 1991). It is likely that the doctor is the best source for either remembering this information (having learned it), or searching for the information in the research literature (Chapter 11 in Sackett et al., 1991), or consulting appropriate guidelines.

The patient also brings important information to clinical decision-making, including:

- Their personal experience both of the current problem and past history of problems, and their past experiences of interventions.
- Their particular desires that inform the clinical decisions to be made
- Personal values that make certain interventions undesirable to the patient; for example, Jehovah's Witnesses may reject a blood transfusion.
- Their particular view of what type of help they need or prefer.
- Their personal definition of what constitutes a successful outcome is for them
- The particular limitations of their social circumstances, which might influence their choice of interventions such as ability to pay costs.

Objective(s) of treatment are listed below (adapted from Chapter 7 in Sacket et al., 1998); any changes from the original scheme are italicized). These are objectives and *not* guaranteed outcomes. One intervention might be able to fulfil more than one objective.

Objective of treatment

1. Cure
2. Prevent recurrence/*occurrence*
3. Limit structural or functional deterioration
4. Prevent later complication
5. Relieve current distress/*reduce symptoms*
6. Deliver *appropriate* reassurance
7. Allow to die with comfort and dignity/*avoid overzealous treatment*

Strictly speaking, 'cure' means the elimination of a causative agent or reversal of a disease/illness process. In everyday language, the word 'cure' might mean the resolution of symptoms and/or signs such that the illness is no longer apparent even if the disease/illness process is unknown. Sometimes cure is also used in everyday language to include situations where a treatment is regarded as largely overcoming the problems caused by a condition, even if the condition persists. An example is where insulin is described as a cure for type 1 diabetes, despite the lack of its effect on the underlying disease process. I will use the first, more technical definition, and if I deviate from this I shall endeavour to make this clear.

Preventing recurrence aims to reduce the chances of the condition returning or a new event occurring. Preventing *occurrence* is an appropriate aim where the patient does not have the condition but is vulnerable to developing it.

Limiting structural or functional deterioration refers to both *mitigation* of the effects of the condition (including on functioning and quality of life) and sometimes even *reversal*. Anti-parkinsonian drugs do not reverse the disease process of Parkinson's disease but they do limit the effects of this disease process on symptoms for a period of time.

Preventing later complication describes where a doctor is trying to prevent a likely complication associated with the patient's condition such as preventing heart attacks or strokes in people with high blood pressure.

Relieving current distress/*reducing symptoms* occurs as a treatment objective in situations where the patient is experiencing distressing symptoms and/or signs. Sometimes patient can be experiencing what are clear *symptoms* without necessarily being distressed by them, for example some patients with neurological problems do not recognize they are experiencing problems.

Delivering *appropriate* reassurance is another important role that doctors are expected to perform. The doctor has to avoid being unrealistically over-optimistic; the information she imparts must be realistic.

Allowing a patient to die with comfort and dignity is the final duty owed by the doctor to their patient. They must resist 'heroic measures' where the likely impact is minimal, prognosis is poor, and side-effects unpleasant. *Avoiding overzealous treatment* refers to situations where healthcare professionals are better not giving interventions to patients where the risk of harm is likely to outweigh any benefits to patients.

It may be unavoidable that the doctor chooses treatment objectives with no input from the patient; for example, if the patient is unconscious or too physically incapacitated to engage in discussions and the doctor must choose immediate and necessary objectives (such as starting life-saving treatment to cure or prevent occurrence of a dangerous condition, or even of death). At other times, the patient is said to not have 'capacity' to make a decision about treatment (see Chapter 13). Even in situations of impaired capacity there are ways of incorporating the patient's views into clinical decision-making such as advance directives.

There are multiple types of interventions that doctors and other healthcare professionals can offer to meet objectives of treatment. They can do so through several processes or acting on certain mechanisms listed as follows.

- Reducing exposure to causative factors of a condition or complication
- Increasing resistance to a condition
- Removing the cause of a condition
- Reverse causal mechanism of a condition
- Compensating for effects of condition by direct compensation/replacement
- Compensating for effects of condition by indirect compensation by acting on opposing mechanism

- Compensating for effects of condition by inducing a state that mitigates the effect of condition
- Restoring lost functioning fully or to a degree
- Improving the appearance or improving functioning beyond previous best state
- Unknown (see explanation below)
- Providing information

Reducing exposure describes a variety of interventions including vaccinations reducing exposure to infective agents by decreasing the number of infected cases in a population, making it less likely to encounter infectious people.

Increasing resistance can take several forms. Vaccinations improve the immune system's ability to respond to an infection and defeat it. Good nutrition improves the body's abilities to resist many infections and other illnesses. People with substance misuse problems can be taught relapse prevention techniques to help resist cues triggering substance misuse again.

Removing the cause describes where the cause of the condition has been identified and the intervention aims to eliminate it from the patient. Examples include infections where the intervention's goal is to kill it or the surgical removal of tumours.

Reversing the causal mechanism covers a range of interventions where causal mechanisms for conditions have been identified and interventions target reversing them. Causal mechanism refers to a process identified with producing the clinical picture rather than a cause of the condition developing. Autoimmune diseases are often treated by drugs suppressing the immune system (although the reasons for the autoimmune disease starting is often unknown).

Compensating by direct compensation/replacement includes the use of insulin in type 1 diabetes. Insulin treatment replaces the insulin that the body is unable to produce due to the loss of insulin-producing cells.

Compensating. indirectly through opposing mechanisms is a type of intervention that relies on many body functions being influenced by opposing systems, resulting in a balance; for example, the sympathetic and parasympathetic systems acting in opposition. In Parkinson's disease, anticholinergic drugs can be used to rebalance the body by blocking the effects of cholinergic nerves opposing the action of the depleted dopaminergic nerves in the striatum nigra.

Compensating by inducing a state describes interventions such as anti-epileptic medication. These medications often act by 'stabilizing' the brain's nerve cells thus making them less prone to the over-activity of a seizure. In hypertension—where usually no direct pathological cause is identified—medications are used that lower blood pressure by actions on bodily systems rather than on the (unknown) cause of the high blood pressure. Opioids reduce pain's emotional component, thus making it more bearable. Some have suggested that psychiatric medication may act in this way, inducing some change in psychological functioning that is regarded as therapeutic (see Chapters 7 and 15).

Restoring lost functioning is often how rehabilitative interventions improve outcomes. Physiotherapy to improve mobility after a fracture uses specialized techniques to restore functioning. People with agoraphobia can be helped with a desensitization programme.

Improve the appearance or functioning is how interventions work when there are congenital (from birth) or acquired abnormalities that need medical attention. This can, for example, be congenital heart disease requiring surgery or a poorly healed fracture requiring orthopaedic intervention. People may see a psychotherapist for personal growth reasons (see Chapter 15).

Unknown describes a spectrum of ignorance about the processes of how an intervention works. There may be little or no idea of how an intervention leads to benefits even if there is empirical evidence for its effectiveness. Thiazide diuretics are helpful in high blood pressure but for unclear reasons (see Chapter 15). If the pathway of intervention effects becomes known this can sometimes offer a clue to the processes causing the clinical picture. The intervention may have a direct effect on the condition or an indirect compensating effect. Sometimes, though, we can discover an intervention is effective but we are not able to discover more about the processes causing the condition.

Providing information is the mechanism of action of several interventions. The patient may change their behaviour or point of view after this information is given. Giving advice about the benefits of improving diet and increasing exercise is a commonly used health intervention.

Effectiveness of interventions vary depending on the person and their problems. For people with impairments that medicine is not effective helping, 'social models' of helping may be more effective. These models look at what can be changed about the person's environment and the attitudes of people around them in order to help the person take part in society as much as possible and achieve their aims. Examples include ensuring wheelchair access or changing attitudes to people with learning difficulties to view them as people with agency capable of making choices.

Some people think that medications are chemicals that have specific actions to target diseases. The more complex truth is that medications have effects on bodily systems. These systems are in themselves complex and have complex relationships with other systems in the body. Even if a medication had only a single effect or target of action on the body's systems it is likely not to be confined to a single location in the body where the problem lies. Even if it was, the interconnected nature of the body's systems means there are complex consequences.

The target of action of a medication is often split over several systems and locations. Most medications have several effects and several targets of action. Imagining the body as a pool of water, the effects of medication can be likened to the action of throwing a stone into this pool, the resultant ripples interacting with each other to form complex patterns.

Some medications are artificial chemicals, that is they are not copies of chemicals found in the body. Even medications that are copies of the body's chemicals can still have complex effects, including problematic ones. All medication and chemicals can cause problems if taken in excess. If someone is given too much water, then the fluid overload can cause serious problems such as cardiac failure or swelling of the brain. Even excess oxygen can cause problems such as blindness in neonates or suppression of the hypoxic respiratory stimulus in some people with chronic obstructive pulmonary disease.

There are many variations of bodily systems between different people, thus increasing the complexity of possible variety of effects that can be found when prescribing medications. Penicillin can be a lifesaver for some patients but can cause severe allergic reactions in others.

Medication usually has many effects. Some of them are regarded as therapeutic, some of them are regarded as side effects (or adverse effects). This value judgement is made based on whether the effect is regarded as meeting the objectives of treatment or whether it is regarded as unpleasant or dangerous. Sometimes the doctor and the patient disagree as to whether an effect is therapeutic or an adverse effect.

Sometimes the therapeutic effect is also a side effect or causes a side effect. Drugs to suppress the immune system are used therapeutically in certain situations, for example in autoimmune disease or to prevent rejection of transplants. This immunosuppression has the side effect of making the patient vulnerable to infections.

Medication rarely has effects that work solely on the intended target. Sometimes the target of action is in one area but the drug acts on similar targets in several locations. As an example, many antipsychotic drugs block dopamine receptors all over the brain, including the basal ganglia, causing side effects similar to Parkinson's disease. Another example is antibiotics targeting bacteria in the bladder causing an infection but also killing similar bacteria in the gut that are part of the normal 'gut flora', leading to overgrowth of competing bacteria not harmed by the antibiotic and resulting in diarrhoea or pseudomembranous colitis.

Some drugs have several effects that are regarded as potentially therapeutic depending on the circumstances but may be side effects in different circumstances. Drugs cannot 'switch off' these effects, so all are potentially present. For example, corticosteroids have several effects that can be regarded as useful (Chapter 26 in Harvey et al., 2011): they can reduce inflammation, reduce allergic effects, suppress the immune response, and suppress the production of the person's own corticosteroids (if they have a metabolic defect such as congenital adrenal hyperplasia). Switching off the body's own corticosteroid production is usually regarded as a side-effect, however, and people on high-dose corticosteroids are usually 'weaned off' them gradually to stimulate the body to produce its own again.

Medications also have many effects that are not regarded as therapeutic under most if not all circumstances. Corticosteroids have many side effects (Chapter 26 in Harvey et al., 2011), such as raised blood glucose, increased body fat, hirsutism, peptic ulcers, high blood pressure, or osteoporosis. When deciding with patients what medication to prescribe if the options are roughly equivalent in effectiveness, the choice is often made on the basis the likelihood and undesirability of potential side effects to the individual patient. The doctor must not assume what side effects the patient will dislike.

Sometimes medication targets surrogate outcomes. These surrogate outcomes *may* have an effect of improving the outcomes that are of real clinical interest. We may aim to reduce cholesterol as a surrogate outcome in order to prevent heart disease and strokes. It needs to be proven, for medications acting on surrogate outcomes, that they do have definite benefit on these final outcomes.

The medical model—an important element in healthcare

Healthcare is often paid for by third parties such as health insurance companies or governments. They have an interest in paying for cost-effective high-quality care. They would prefer the care to be based on evidence, as a further guarantee of quality and effective care. Patients have an interest in being seen promptly for care that is effective in meeting their needs without being kept waiting whilst professionals spend all their time with another patient.

An important feature of the medical model is the cycle of medical management. It is summarized in Figure 5.4 as comprising two steps in a cycle, assessment and intervention. A medical assessment is often an intervention in itself; patients may draw reassurance from being assessed.

The first assessment is usually the longest. During this initial assessment, the doctor forms a diagnostic formulation and a management plan, ideally after a discussion with the patient and sometimes after discussion with significant others, other doctors—usually more senior—or other professionals. This will incorporate discussion about the particular risks and how to manage them, what investigations are needed, what interventions should be tried, and other important aspects of care such as whether the patient should be in hospital or not, or whether they should see other professionals or a specialist doctor. This is summarized as the assessment step.

The implementation of this management plan is the intervention step. The doctor's clinical and medical knowledge—informed by research—are used during the assessment and interventions steps.

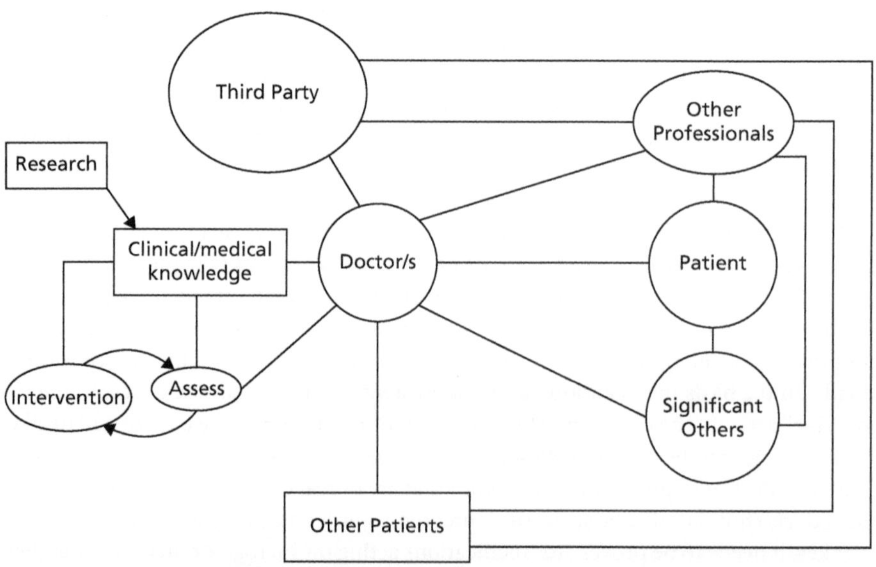

Figure 5.4 The medical model in action.

Sometimes the suggested intervention can take place during this stage, such as advice given or even an operation. On many occasions, the intervention or investigations or other elements of the management plan take place after the doctor's intervention step (such as physiotherapy or psychotherapy). A prescription may be written during the intervention step and medication taken afterwards. This assessment and intervention couplet of steps is a consultation.

After this consultation it is common for the effects of this management plan to be reviewed in a further assessment. This may be done by the same doctor, another doctor (e.g. if the consultation was done by a junior doctor in the middle of the night then reviewed by a senior doctor in the morning), or another professional. Sometimes the patient is discharged with further follow-up arranged, or the patient is told to come back if there is insufficient improvement.

This follow-up assessment by a doctor usually incorporates the previous diagnostic formulation, any relevant investigation results, and collateral information (from other professionals and/or significant others in contact with the patient), and a fresh assessment of the clinical picture presented by the patient which reviews the progress made towards achieving the objectives of treatment. Any fresh information that comes to light is evaluated and acted upon. As a lot of the information has been collected in the initial assessment, subsequent assessments are usually do not take as long. Adjustments to the management plan are made if necessary. Perhaps a complication of the condition has arisen or a side effect needs addressing or the diagnosis changed. This cycle of assessment and intervention is repeated until the patient is discharged.

The duration of this consultation can vary. The assessment usually takes at most an hour for the initial step but can be briefer. In primary care, for instance, GPs typically have ten minutes to complete both assessment and intervention steps. If the intervention takes a long time—such as an operation—then it may exceed the time taken for the assessment. Average times for psychiatric initial assessments are approximately 60 minutes and follow-ups or inpatient reviews 18 minutes (Creed, 1995).

The time of the interval between the cycles of assessment/intervention depends on the clinical situation. It may vary from very brief in urgent emergencies (seconds/minutes), to acute (e.g. 6–24 hours), to longer in outpatients (from weeks to months), to very long (e.g. annual check-ups).

Consultations can be relatively brief or prolonged (such as lengthy operations). If the main therapeutic interventions take place between the consultations (such as taking courses of medication), and in combination with the rapid assessment methods involved in diagnosis (see Chapter 2), then many patients can be seen by the same doctor over time.

This is particularly useful in acute care when there can be unpredictable demand that can result in lots of patients requiring care in short periods of time. Doctors work in teams in acute care with other professionals which means doctors can concentrate on those tasks that are essential for them, and them only, to undertake. The efficiency of the medical model demonstrated by doctors working in a multidisciplinary team means that many patients can be seen, despite large numbers attending for care.

It is also useful in outpatient settings if the review period between consultations is weeks or months (if that is how long the intervention such as a course of medication takes to achieve full benefit). The doctor is thus able to manage and care for large numbers of patients, seeing many patients every week from 15–30 minutes each, then a completely different set of patients the next week, and so on for many weeks until the first set of patients are reviewed. By contrast, a psychotherapist with one-hour sessions will see fewer people per unit time but will then see the same people week after week repeatedly over months.

Health services often prefer doctors in many situations to have large caseloads and focus on providing interventions that require medical input only, with other types of interventions being provided by other members of the multidisciplinary team, because medical time is very expensive. GPs have caseloads of thousands of patients; psychiatry consultants often have caseloads in the hundreds. Consultant psychiatrists may have up to ten times the caseload of other members of the multidisciplinary team (Tyrer et al., 2001).

The other members of the team offer interventions that often require great deals of face-to-face time with their clients. This difference in the amount of time required means doctors can see far greater numbers of people than other members of the multidisciplinary team.

Although this makes sound economic sense it can cause dissatisfaction for both patients and doctors. Due to the high numbers of patients, short appointments are *de rigeur*. During those short appointments, the doctor will need to assess how well the patient has responded to the treatment, review any risk issues, and discuss any changes to the management plan. Detailed discussion of these or other issues is very difficult. Other members of the multidisciplinary team deliver the other aspects of the care plan.

Third-party payers are interested in containing costs. The flexibility to be able to see patients at short notice if required due to concerns about their health and not just assess but also offer interventions in short time periods that is made possible by the medical model is valued by healthcare providers.

In healthcare, the greatest cost is usually staff—their wages, cost of training, providing infrastructure such as buildings, and associated costs (maintenance, power, 'hotel costs'). The cost of medication is usually small in comparison. There are exceptions to this; some cancer drugs are very expensive and there is a wide variety in costs of artificial hip replacements.

Mental health is no exception, and staff and facility costs are the most expensive items of expenditure. An economic analysis of costs of schizophrenia in England showed staff costs were the largest item in the budget; the costs of psychiatrist time alone cost more than medication (Mangalore and Knapp, 2007). In South Korea, medication costs were 3.17% of the total direct healthcare costs compared to outpatient care costs contributing 18.56% and inpatient care 78.27% of direct healthcare costs (Chang et al., 2008). In the United States, 22% of direct healthcare costs of schizophrenia were due to medication, 35% to long-term care, 12% inpatient care, and 31% outpatient care (Wu et al., 2005). In the CUTLASS trial comparing older cheap antipsychotics with new expensive antipsychotics (Davies et al., 2007), total medication costs were a fraction of direct healthcare costs over a year; older medications cost £576 out of £18,858 total direct healthcare costs, and the newer medications cost

£929 out of £20,118; again, inpatient care was by far the biggest item of expenditure at £17,170 for older medications group and £16,953 for the newer medications group.

Doctors provide care at all hours as part of their professional culture. Working at nights and weekends can be taxing—the medical model (as described in Chapter 2) helps minimize this effect on assessment and decision-making. Doctors recognize a previously described problem then recall the appropriate information and steps to take. It would be hard for a psychotherapist to get out bed at 2 a.m., do a psychological formulation and initial therapeutic session, and then go to work all day and see their regular therapy patients.

Junior doctors provide direct out-of-hour care—alongside other colleagues such as nurses—with senior doctors providing advice or coming in if necessary. The pay for on-call is often at reduced rates, although seniors may be paid more if they have to attend. UK consultants usually have a 3% supplement to their wages for doing on-call work, say one day in ten (including Bank holidays and weekends), in addition to their regular work. If they have to come in to see patients, this may be compensated for by either time off in lieu (e.g. one afternoon off per fortnight) or about 5% supplement to their normal pay. This relatively cheap way of arranging senior cover at all hours is another reason why doctors are regarded as vital members of staff for mental health services.

In mental health services there is the virtue of 'horizontal integration', including administrative compatibility, with the rest of the health service where the medical model is prevalent (see Chapter 2). Physical health problems may present with mental health symptoms; the general medical training of doctors helps with detecting physical conditions presenting in this way. The effectiveness of the medical model for an individual patient depends on the doctor having effective interventions for their condition.

Conclusion

Doctors often work in multidisciplinary teams because patients frequently have complex needs that doctors may not have either the time or the expertise to help effectively. Research methods to minimize bias in collecting information of clinical interest have been developed. Use of randomized controlled trials—especially where the researcher is *blinded* as to which intervention group the participant belongs to—is the best method of assessing the effectiveness of interventions. It is important that researchers ask the correct questions and measure the right outcomes.

Research gives degrees of confidence, not certainty. No research is perfect. Interpreting research avoiding being either too cynical or too trusting and certainly avoiding bias as much as possible is crucial. There is a hierarchy of quality of research evidence that leads to strength of grades of recommendations based on this research.

Doctors should decide with their patients what the objectives of treatment are. Once the objectives are agreed, the next step is to discuss what interventions are best to achieve these objectives

Medications interact with the complex interconnected systems of the human body. They very rarely have only limited effects in one area of the body. They usually have multiple effects distributed throughout the body. These effects are regarded as a therapeutic effect or a side effect dependent on whether they help achieve the objectives of treatment.

The medical model can be very cost-effective in terms of time and being able to see many patients and offering interventions e.g. medication, this allows more patients to be able to be offered care. Doctors offer care at all hours. These factors, along with horizontal integration with the rest of health, explain why the medical model is an important part of mental health care so long as the doctor can offer effective interventions for a patient's condition.

Chapter 6

Criticism of psychiatric diagnosis

I have outlined the concepts underpinning the medical model in general medicine and mental health as well as its strength. These depend on diagnostic constructs having useful attached information and effective interventions (if available). It is now time to look at criticisms of the medical model in mental health.

Philosophical criticisms—such as whether the mental health problems are really 'health' problems—I leave aside as I am not best qualified to discuss them, and I urge the reader to consult Cooper's work, which offers a good introduction to this (Cooper, 2007). Power relationships and social discourses offer another kind of criticism of medical models; these issues occur in all medical specialties, indeed all interactions with professionals. However, I am not particularly qualified to offer an evaluation of these arguments and so do not provide a critique here.

I am qualified to discuss those criticisms presented within scientific or clinical frameworks on how to appraise scientific and clinical terms and research. I will try and present information fairly and in a balanced way.

The medical model often involves making a diagnosis and prescribing medication as an intervention. Criticism of the medical model in mental health in terms of a clinical or scientific discourse will focus on these two areas of diagnosis and medication. This chapter will focus on diagnosis. Chapter 7 focuses on psychiatric treatments.

Rather than presenting an exhaustive review of the literature on the topic, I want to look at Kinderman's 2013 article, which to my mind summarizes best the concerns leading critics have of the medical health model as applied to psychiatric diagnostic constructs.

Criticisms of psychiatric diagnosis

'Drop the language of disorder' (Kinderman et al., 2013) was written by three clinical psychology professors, Kinderman, Read, and Bentall, and an academic psychiatrist in the 'critical psychiatry' tradition, Moncrieff. All authors published a number of articles and books criticizing psychiatric diagnosis, treatment, and the 'biomedical model'. This paper is, therefore, perfect for summarizing criticisms of psychiatric diagnoses because it collates prominent critics' views. These criticisms may be based on an inaccurate view of medicine by people without medical training but one of the authors, Moncrieff, is a medical doctor so if her recall of medicine is reasonable and not skewed by ideological bias, this information deficit ought to be minimized.

The criticisms could be wholly correct or wholly incorrect or they may be correct to a degree but the problems they identify in the psychiatric diagnostic system may also be present in the diagnostic system used in general medicine. Clinical psychologists and psychotherapists may also be correct in that the psychiatric diagnostic model may not be useful to them in the way they work with their clients (people who see psychotherapists are more likely to describe themselves as clients rather than patients; McGuire-Snieckus et al., 2003), but that does not mean that psychiatric diagnostic constructs are not useful to psychiatrists in consultation with their patients.

Kinderman and colleagues (2013) outlined several problems identified with psychiatric diagnostic constructs (the more technical terms will be explained later in this chapter):

- Poor reliability, but the authors accept that psychiatric diagnoses can be reliable although they assert that this is only under carefully controlled conditions, not found in routine clinical practice.
- poor validity (i.e. the constructs do not correspond to an objectively validated entity)
- poor utility
- poor epistemology (in particular, that the psychiatric problem must be caused by a bodily disease)
- poor humanity
- thresholds may be set too low, thus inflating the numbers of people regarded as needing help, with a subsequent potential bonanza for drug companies but at the cost of exploiting vulnerable people
- medicalization of everyday and normal reactions to stressful life circumstances with 'no easy "cut-off" between "normal" experience and "disorder"' (Kinderman, 2013)
- people with the same diagnosis may be very different, even to the extent of not having the same symptoms
- lack of acknowledgement of social factors as a context for causing the problem, including traumatic events and social adversities
- that the diagnosis in itself is not useful for planning treatment without including other clinically relevant information in a formulation
- other alternatives to the psychiatric diagnostic construct can be used for administration and research purposes as well as for communication between clinicians
- specified problems are a better construct for research into causes and planning treatment of mental health problems.

The last two points I will address briefly. I will focus on the usefulness of diagnosis in clinical practice. This is an extensive 'rap sheet' for psychiatric diagnostic constructs. How do we decide whether the verdict of the accusations of Kinderman (2013) on psychiatric diagnosis is guilty, not guilty, or not proven? The preferred method is to gather evidence and then adjudicate on the basis of this evidence rather than on the aesthetic value of the rhetoric used to make this argument.

Similar criticisms of 'functional psychiatric diagnosis' are made in a position statement by the official body of British clinical psychologists, the Division of Clinical Psychology (Division of Clinical Psychology, 2013). The phrase 'functional psychiatric diagnosis' refers to mental health problems without an identified biological cause, such as an underactive thyroid gland causing depression. To avoid repetition, the criticisms of this position statement will be mentioned where they differ or expand upon the long list above. They make explicit an objection to the 'disease-based model' and the assumption that biology has the primary role in causing 'functional' mental health problems.

The position statement states that diagnosis should not be 'presented as objective statement of fact' as it relies on many subjective factors but this ignores the fact that in all medicine, diagnosis should always be provisional, open to revision, is often used to describe nominalist concepts, and is influenced by subjective factors (see Chapters 1, 2, 3, and 4). The authors may be criticizing the tendency of some psychiatrists to minimize the inherent uncertainty of all diagnosis. They may also be referring to the lack of laboratory tests or other objective proofs to confirm many psychiatric diagnoses (see discussions about 'validity' later in this chapter). The position statement assumes that a diagnosis must follow the Sydenham model of underlying disease causing symptoms and that it ignores the possibility that diagnostic constructs sometimes just describe either a collection of symptoms that go together (a syndrome) or a zone of the spectrum of states possibly continuous with good health that is not necessarily caused (or predominantly caused) by a classic disease, or a zone of the spectrum of conditions, or just denoting a problem that is thought to benefit from medical or other health professionals' interventions (see Chapter 3).

The rest of this chapter will discuss reliability, validity, and utility, and will generate questions to ask about psychiatric diagnosis.

Reliability of psychiatric diagnosis

Achieving reliability in making a psychiatric diagnosis is a crucial issue affecting both clinical practice and research (Spitzer et al., 1978) which led initially to drafting the Research Diagnostic Criteria (Spitzer et al., 1978), then to the publication of the DSMIII diagnostic manual (APA, 1980) and later editions issued by the American Psychiatric Association.

Reliability in this sense means 'reproducibility of distinctions made between some aspects of persons' (Shrout et al., 1987), in this case is referring to the process of assessing a patient and then arriving at the diagnosis (also see Chapter 4). The same article makes the point that it is not just about replication but discrimination, in the sense of placing order and categorizing these distinctions. A clinician can make the same diagnosis all the time but this is likely to lead to problems in clinical practice if, for example, all cases of pneumonia, asthma, and pulmonary embolism are all diagnosed as asthma. Reliability is also context-specific; an example is given that a test of intellect designed to identify people with learning difficulties from people without learning difficulties may be less useful in separating out top college students (who may all score very high marks on this test).

A diagnosis is said to be reliable if it is 'stable'; it does not change all the time without good reason, such as change in the clinical picture of the patient. More commonly it is also said to be reliable if two 'raters' agree on the same diagnosis (inter-rater reliability).

Commonly this is measured by two clinicians assessing the patient separately or even both at the same time with one clinician interviewing and another observing (or less satisfactorily, reading case summaries known as 'vignettes') and measuring how often they agree on the same diagnosis.

A diagnosis may also be said to be reliable if there is some reference test (that is said to offer definitive proof of the diagnosis being present) and a comparison of the clinician's diagnosis with the result of the test is made. An example is surgeons diagnosing acute appendicitis and whether the appendix removed after an appendectomy shows signs of inflammation under microscopic examination by the pathologist. It should be noted that this still involves some subjectivity—obviously so in the case of the surgeon making the diagnosis but also in the case of the pathologist interpreting the cellular and tissue features under the microscope.

Sources of unreliability in making a diagnosis (Shrout et al., 1987) can be divided into separate categories:

- Information variance, when there are differences in information gathered about the patient between different doctors. For example, the doctors may ask different questions, may forget to ask about important information or to perform a specific element of the examination, misinterpret a clinical sign, the relationship between a patient and a doctor may mean the patient feels able to discuss an important and sensitive topic with one doctor but not the other.
- Occasion variance. This is where the information varies on occasion. This may be because of biological factors. For example, if the pulse is checked when the patient is sleeping it remains high in hyperthyroidism but reverts to normal if the patient is anxious instead—assuming, of course, that you don't startle the patient awake by checking their pulse! Other examples are measuring hormones in the blood, which may vary depending on time of day, or if a patient is asked a question equally skilfully by two doctors and gives different responses to each.
- Criterion variance. If doctors use different criteria to make a diagnosis or place different emphasis on the same criteria (weighing them up differently) then they draw different diagnostic conclusions. They may have completely different theories or models of what causes mental disorders and so prioritize different information to arrive at a diagnosis. Confusingly, they may use similar names as their colleagues for completely different concepts. (One way of remedying this is to use standardized diagnostic criteria.)
- Performance variance (not the term used by Shrout and colleagues). If the doctor is lacking in carefulness, is inconsistent or incompetent then their diagnosis may differ from another doctor—perhaps this doctor was tired from all-night working?
- Instrument or measurement variance (not included by Shrout and colleagues). This refers to the fact that all instruments or measurements, including lab test results, have a possibility of error, often within a known range. If the test results differ even though what they are measuring remained constant, then this can lead to different conclusions being drawn by different doctors as to the diagnosis.

Without reliable agreement regarding whether a diagnosis (or any construct) is absent or present then its usefulness in research is limited and makes any decisions or inferences made on the basis of that research uncertain. Without being able to agree that the diagnosis of participants in one study is equivalent to the diagnosis made of the participants in another, we cannot compare the results of different studies either. We will also find it difficult to match the patient with the diagnosis in the clinic to participants reliably with the diagnosis in the research.

The questions we should ask about psychiatric diagnostic systems to assess their reliability in terms of agreement between a clinician's diagnosis and a reasonable reference standard as well as ability to discriminate between different clinical problems are:

- What is the reliability of the diagnosis when compared to a relevant reference criterion?
- What is the reliability of discriminating between different diagnoses?

Validity of psychiatric diagnosis

Validity is a complex concept that some people argue is 'all or nothing' (Kendell and Jablenksy, 2003); a diagnosis is either valid or it is not valid. Validity can also be thought of as representing something 'real' or 'true'. How should we judge the validity of a psychiatric diagnosis?

In the article by Kinderman and colleagues (2013) validity issues with psychiatric diagnostic constructs are:

- include no unique correspondence with biomarkers
- not objectively verified entities
- are not essentialist entities (e.g. indistinct boundaries between different diagnostic constructs, symptoms can be present in more than diagnostic construct, high co-occurrence rates)
- have poor prediction of course and treatment effectiveness (these are arguably utility issues)

Kraepelin, one of the German-speaking giants who helped create the concepts used in modern psychiatry (others include Eugen Bleuler, Kurt Schneider, and Karl Jaspers, not to mention Sigmund Freud and Carl Jung as pioneers of psychotherapy) felt that a psychiatric diagnostic system should identify disease entities with identical symptom pictures, identical pathology, and an identical aetiology, and incorporate observations of the course, outcome, and treatment of the condition (Kraepelin and Diefendorf, 1904/1907).

Robins and Guze (1970) outlined five interacting phases to develop and demonstrate valid diagnosis in psychiatry.

1. Clinical description of a distinctive clinical picture or syndrome including demographic or course features.
2. Laboratory studies such as biological markers detected in tests that confirm the presence of a psychiatric disorder or psychological tests that are reliable and accurate.

3. Delimitation from other disorders. This includes using exclusion criteria for the diagnostic criteria based on clinical picture or test results to separate out similar, but different, illnesses. This serves to make the group described by the diagnosis as homogenous as possible (i.e. cases with the same diagnosis are similar to each other).
4. Follow-up study. Follow-up of cases with the same diagnosis completed to show that they had similar outcomes (prognosis). If outcomes vary greatly for the same diagnosis, it would suggest that the group described by the diagnosis was not homogenous and includes different illnesses or conditions. The authors acknowledge that there can be variable prognoses even in cases of the same illness, but markedly differing outcomes suggest we should think again. Another important outcome would be diagnostic stability, that is that the diagnosis remained the same throughout time.
5. Family study. If family members were assessed for mental health problems and increased prevalence (i.e. a higher number of cases than expected) of the same disorder in close relatives were found, this would indicate a valid entity. On the contrary, if no increased prevalence of the same disorder was found in close relatives, this would suggest that the diagnostic construct was not a valid entity.

These phases were further expanded by Kendler (1980). Antecedent validators (before onset of the problem) include familial aggregation (i.e. the same disorder is found in close family members more than would be expected than by chance); premorbid personality (the personality of people with the diagnosis have similar features before they became unwell), and precipitating factors (people with the same diagnosis have similar causes or preceding events before the diagnosis). Concurrent validators (during the problem) includes psychological tests and laboratory tests (although Kendler stated few were available in psychiatry). Finally, predictive validators (of the outcome of the problem) included diagnostic consistency over time, rates of relapse and recovery, and response to treatment.

Both these suggestions are methods of proving that the separate clinical diagnostic constructs are indeed linked to discrete disease entities in the classic Sydenham model of disease leading to unique clinical syndromes (see Chapter 3). In the absence of methods that accurately measure underlying functioning of a complex organ, as the mind/brain, these 'validators' are taken to be a proxy indicator for this. For example, if it can be clearly shown that a unique clinical syndrome runs in families, this indicates a genetically inherited disease entity (or social causes repeating in families). Steps are suggested to refine and improve the diagnostic criteria into more valid entities, a process referred to as epistemic iteration. Note that these proxies of validity also have clinical utility (usefulness).

The article that stated that validity is either present or not (Kendell and Jablensky, 2003) gave two main criteria for validity. A psychiatric diagnostic construct has validity if its defining characteristic is a syndrome (a collection of clinical features that seem to go together or cohere) that is separated from 'neighbouring' syndromes and also from normality by a 'zone of rarity'. Another example of validity is when the diagnostic constructs uses a more 'fundamental' definition based on pathology (examples given are genetic, physiological, cellular pathology, or molecular differences) with a zone of rarity between that diagnostic construct and other conditions with similar syndromes. This zone of rarity means a clear difference between the diagnostic construct and normality as well as other diagnostic constructs—'carving nature at the joints'.

Validity in this case is not based on the cause (or aetiology) of the diagnosis as this may be unknown. The establishment of aetiology can also be complex so that syndromes can be discovered before aetiology and this can lead to further research on aetiology based on cases identified by the syndrome. Finally, without clear-cut syndromes it may be impossible to find the underlying biological causes of the disorder. The authors then concede that many psychiatric diagnostic constructs lack validity.

Several ways of determining validity of a diagnostic construct have been suggested (Rodrigues and Banzato, 2015), (proofs of validity of diagnostic criterion will be omitted):

- A test independent of the diagnostic criteria is used to confirm the diagnosis, for example use of laboratory tests.
- If the construct is a fair or representative depiction of the important features of a condition (for mental health this would include behavioural or psychological features).
- If the construct describes a syndrome of clinical features including common prognosis.
- If the construct carries useful information about the clinical picture, clinical management, and treatment of a condition not based solely on the construct's definition.
- If the construct describes a coherent group; for example, for mental health conditions, psychometric testing of people meeting diagnostic criteria gives one-dimensional results.
- There is a common unique cause (preferably biological) for all people meeting diagnostic criteria.
- If there as an associated objectively verifiable and harmful dysfunction.
- If the construct describes a pattern or structure of symptoms found in the natural population.

It should be noted that these are mainly medical psychiatric concepts of validity. Psychologists have also been interested in the concept of validity, initially in whether the use of questionnaires and their interpretation can be said to be measuring something that exists outside the questionnaire itself and whether their tests really are measure what they are intended to measured Some of these aspects of validity are face validity (the construct seems a good description of the condition or phenomena), predictive validity (the accuracy of information attached to the construct on outcomes, complications, and responses to treatment), and external/construct validity (the degree of correspondence with external factors such as biomarkers) (First et al., 2004).

It can be seen from this review of the concept of validity that it seems to comprise several different but overlapping concepts. In language, we may know what we mean but we struggle to define it in a water-tight, comprehensive manner.

There may be drawbacks with a nosology (system of classification) that places validity or scientific accuracy at a premium but at the expense of usefulness (Kendler, 1990). It may exclude concepts from the historical tradition and clinical experience of psychiatry that may still be useful and other concepts that are difficult to measure scientifically. It may prioritize highly complicated diagnostic criteria with higher reliability and/or validity but may be too cumbersome for everyday clinical use. Aiming to be comprehensive, it may introduce diagnostic categories that have little validity. Finally, it may not be helpful for the administrative purposes of a diagnostic system.

Kendler further makes the point (1990) that subjective judgment, even if based on demonstrated expertise on the subjects, is still required over several issues and not everyone will agree with these 'non-empirical' or value-based decisions. Areas of contention could include defining the proper construct (or defining criteria) of a diagnosis; how to weight the importance of different validators; how to separate conditions into separate categories (e.g. subtypes of same condition, different types of an overarching category of conditions, or completely different conditions altogether); and how to balance reliability and validity. Another bone of contention could be the balance of validity versus utility as well as the usefulness of a diagnostic system to different methods of clinical practice.

It is debatable whether many psychiatric diagnostic constructs are truly separate from each other—indicating that they are often 'spectrums of illnesses/conditions' (see Chapter 3)—often referred to using terms like 'high degree of comorbidity'. This may not be true comorbidity, and co-occurrence may be a better term (Widiger and Samuels, 2005). A common definition used in medicine of comorbidity identified it as the presence or potential presence of an additional condition whilst a patient already has an identified 'index' condition (Feinstein, 1970).

The implication may be (falsely) taken that the two conditions involve two separate causes or differences of structure or process. Again, given the lack of knowledge of these, in psychiatric diagnostic constructs this would be an unsafe assumption. Even in general medicine, separately identified conditions may be different aspects of the same underlying causes or differences in structure/process (see Chapter 3).

As discussed in Chapter 10, in order to avoid people assuming that separate causes/differences of structure or process are involved in producing the different diagnostic constructs, the term 'co-occurrence' has been suggested as a better alternative in mental health (Widiger and Samuel, 2005). 'Consanguinity' can also be used to indicate closely related constructs that should be thought of as part of a single condition (Tyrer, 2017). 'Co-occurrence' is preferred in this book as it makes no assumptions about the nature of relationship between different conditions.

The recognition of a condition may lead to further investigations increasing the chances of recognizing further conditions (Feinstein, 1970). Co-occurrence may also affect the prognosis or outcome of the index condition as well as affecting the treatment choices (the preferred treatment of the index condition may be contraindicated in the presence of the second condition), and treatment outcomes may be altered by co-occurrence (Feinstein, 1970), although the actual effects of co-occurrence may be under-researched (Muth and Glasziou, 2015).

The causes of co-occurrence may be diagnostic (i.e. where symptoms may be found in both diagnostic constructs and are non-specific to those diagnostic constructs), pathogenic (i.e. one condition can be recognized to cause another condition as a complication or other aetiological relationship, either locally or in another area through disseminated effects or spread of disease), or prognostic (where one condition increases the chances of developing another condition) (Feinstein, 1970; Kaplan and Feinstein, 1974; Dell Osso and Pinni, 2012).

The reason for prognostic comorbidity is not necessarily aetiological (i.e. diagnosis *x* directly causing diagnosis *y*). It may be that two conditions share similar or overlapping causes or differences of structure or process such that developing one condition indicates a situation where the second condition is also likely to develop. In these situations, the term co-occurrence may underplay the relationship between the two diagnostic constructs—that they share similar underlying causes or differences of structure or process (though they may not be identical in both conditions, leading to differences in the clinical picture; see Chapter 4). This situation may also explain the 'spectrum of illnesses/conditions' (see Chapter 3) where several conditions are more likely to be diagnosed together.

Diagnostic co-occurrence may be artefactual (where a broader entity has been split into numerous, smaller diagnostic categories, and so people who present with the broader entity may fit several of the diagnostic categories) or even spurious (where a broadly defined entity contains more narrowly defined categories and the patient is given a diagnosis of both the broader entity AND the more narrowly defined category) (First, 2005a).

Several of the concepts associated with validity overlap with those that are felt to be features of utility as described later in this chapter (First et al., 2004). If we concentrate on features that do not overlap with utility, we can identity several questions to ask of psychiatric diagnostic constructs:

- Is the condition described by a diagnosis clearly separated from other conditions in terms of clinical features?
- Is the condition clearly separated from normality? (the absence of boundaries separating 'normal' human experience and mental health conditions)
- Is the condition clearly identified with a causal mechanism (aetiology)?
- Is the condition clearly associated with a proven and detectable difference in structure or process? This difference acts as a proof of the diagnosis and can be identified with some sort of test such as biochemical or radiology tests?
- Is there little co-occurrence of conditions (i.e. conditions are separate clinical entities)?

Utility of psychiatric diagnosis

We have seen that some of the components of validity addressed also have clinical utility (usefulness). A diagnostic construct can be said to have utility for clinical practice if there is useful information attached to it (e.g. about prognosis and responses to treatments), and for research if it allows hypotheses to be tested about associated factors such as causes or mechanisms (Kendell and Jablensky, 2003). Psychiatric diagnostic constructs were noted to be heterogeneous in terms of causes, mechanisms, and outcomes, resulting in uncertainty of the associated information (Meehl, 1973, p. 92).

Examples of utility given include information on likelihood of relapse of the condition, of the success rates of different potential treatments (all these could be regarded as predictive validity, demographic information such as usual ages of onset, and in what gender or social groupings the disorder is more commonly found. The diagnostic construct's prototypical clinical picture will give information about what types of symptoms the patient will present with and how they may change.

Two main criteria for utility of a specific diagnostic construct are suggested (Kendell and Jablensky, 2003). First, whether the diagnostic construct has allowed good quality information to be generated from research based on adequate criteria for this diagnostic construct. Second, whether the diagnostic construct gives useful information on aetiology (cause), prognosis (range of outcomes), and treatment that separates it from other diagnostic constructs (particularly closely related or similar diagnostic constructs). The authors also state that this information is more context-sensitive than validity, which is supposed to operate more objectively. This means a diagnosis may be useful to a psychiatrist who works in a particular way but not so useful to a clinical psychologist who works in a different way. For instance, schizophrenia may be a useful diagnostic construct to clinical psychiatrists but less useful to genetic researchers, for whom a broader psychosis diagnostic construct maybe more useful in research.

Noting the lack of definitions of clinical utility except in Kendall and Jablensky's article, Michael First and colleagues (First et al., 2004) produced the following suggestions for clinical utility for uses of diagnostic constructs: forming concepts of diagnostic constructs such as what they represent; allowing communication of relevant information between professionals, patients, carers, and for administrative purposes; a common definition of diagnostic constructs for clinical use; providing information on treatment responses and likely outcomes/complications guiding clinical management. Use of diagnostic constructs for purposes such as charging third-party payers was not included in clinical utility.

Rodrigues and Banzato (2015) describe a 'pragmatic conception of validation' which is similar to utility. They state that it does not matter how or why a diagnostic construct is useful, just that it is. This usefulness is a legitimate justification for the diagnostic construct even if it does not represent a valid separate disease entity on the basis that medicine is practical.

Tennant and Thompson state that for diagnosis, utility is more important than validity (Tennant and Thompson, 1980). The utility they refer to is the ability to predict (presumably as outlined earlier in the book) clinical features, outcomes, and responses to treatment. They describe disease as not true or false but possessing utility, and that classifications of disease should be viewed as being predictive rather than in terms of causality.

Of course, validity can help to improve the utility of the diagnostic construct, for example if tests are developed to confirm the diagnostic construct and distinguish it from other diagnostic constructs, or by identifying common mechanisms/causes allowing better prospects of developing treatments. However, doctors have been using invalid diagnostic constructs and models for centuries (the humoural model, for instance) but still found them useful. The purpose of diagnosis is usefulness, not truth. Truth aids usefulness but diagnosis may still have utility without validity.

The DCP position statement on 'functional psychiatric diagnoses' (Division of Clinical Psychology, 2013) defines utility as providing information on guiding treatment, clinical management guidelines, and effective planning of services and research.

In contrast to their statement that many psychiatric diagnoses lack validity, Kendall and Jablensky state that psychiatric diagnostic constructs often have utility to psychiatrists when seeing patients (Kendell and Jablensky, 2003). This conclusion about psychiatric diagnosis having utility is in opposition to the claim that psychiatric diagnostic constructs lack utility (Kinderman et al., 2013). The DCP position statement (Division of Clinical Psychology, 2013) also states that psychiatric diagnostic constructs lack utility. How do we understand this opposite view?

Many clinical psychologists find that a psychiatric diagnostic construct is not helpful to *them* when they see their clients with the methods *they* use. Remember it was stated that the utility of a diagnosis is context-specific, so in the context of the way some clinical psychologists work, a psychiatric diagnosis could be of little use. The American DSM psychiatric diagnostic system explicitly states that it is also for use by psychologists, psychotherapists, and mental health social workers. However, diagnostic systems are primarily designed by psychiatrists for use by psychiatrists, with less regard for how other professionals work. This psychiatric classification has a powerful effect on what research is done, how mental healthcare is organized, and how services are delivered.

There are benefits to cross-talk between professionals to ensure that they are referring to the same types of conditions, but having to translate from another profession's classification into another is an additional cognitive burden to hard-working professionals, an imposed 'bilingualism'. Professionals can feel that their 'professional space' has been intruded upon by another profession. It is unsurprising, therefore, that resentment builds up towards a psychiatric diagnostic system that often lacks validity and has little utility for professionals not using the medical model. The DCP position statement (Division of Clinical Psychology, 2013) only makes statements from the point of view of clinical psychologists and does not explicitly state that they mostly apply to clinical psychologists.

Another objection that some clinical psychologists have may lie in the historical development of their profession. As a profession that grew out of a science (psychology) applied to benefit their clients, clinical psychologists may be attracted, quite naturally, to the notion that scientific validity is paramount. They may tend towards a paradigm that it is essential to the primacy of scientifically valid concepts in order for any method or model to achieve proper usefulness such as the Periodic Table in chemistry.

Clinical psychologists also have greater experience than psychiatrists in measuring psychological attributes in both 'healthy' and 'clinical' populations and finding the results often sit on a spectrum rather than there being clear-cut differences between the two groups. Thus, their prior experience tends to have them view psychological concepts as dimensions, in contrast to doctors whose initial experience in general medicine with classifying begins with categories including clear-cut syndromes or diseases (Keeley, 2015).

Some psychiatrists may use the word 'disease'—when other psychiatrists say 'illness'—to highlight their medical credentials to colleagues in other specialties. Medicine, on the other hand, is a practical art that uses science with the end goal of benefitting patients. To that end, it has a long history of being of benefit long before it had scientifically accurate concepts to support the benefits it brought. Doctors may therefore be more willing to accept practical measures so long as they are useful in some way, even if not scientifically valid. Science is embraced by medicine as the best way to ensure patient benefit, not as an end in itself.

Notwithstanding these questions on disputes about the utility of psychiatric diagnostic constructs, what questions should we ask to test utility? To state that a psychiatric diagnostic construct has poor utility for prognosis (or outcome) if it is associated with a range of outcomes we are implying that we expect a diagnostic construct to be associated with a certain single outcome. We would also like to see if information beyond the diagnostic construct ('meta-diagnostic' information) is needed to help predict outcomes, as that would suggest that diagnostic constructs may have some but limited utility. Is the diagnostic construct in itself sufficient for managing the patient in terms of predicting outcomes and making treatment decisions? In other words, do we have to use additional clinically relevant information beyond the diagnostic construct in our clinical practice? Looking at the various definitions of utility as addressed earlier, the following questions seem reasonable:

- Does the condition have uniform prognosis (does the condition have a predictable unitary outcome)?
- Does the condition have different outcomes from other conditions?
- Does the condition predict differences in treatments given and their effectiveness?
- Is the use of the diagnosis justified due to some utilitarian reason, such as relieving distress or reducing risk?
- Is there a need for clinical information beyond the diagnosis in clinical decision-making?

Other criticisms about psychiatric diagnosis

To discuss epistemology of disorders, we have to understand what epistemology means. Epistemology is the study of what we know and how we acquire that knowledge. Both Kinderman and colleague's article, 'Drop the language of disorder', (Kinderman et al., 2013) and the DCP position statement (Division of Clinical Psychology, 2013) clarify that in the context of mental health, by epistemology of disorders they mean the assumption underlying knowledge of mental health that biology is the primary cause of mental health problems.

They believe that understanding treating and researching mental health problems as if there is an underlying disease cause, as in the Sydenham disease model, is a fundamental mistake. If we conceive of mental disorders in completely the wrong way, then our treatments, research, and how we manage these problems will be based on incorrect knowledge in the past (because research and experience was based on false premises), untenable practice in the present (because it is based on incorrect knowledge), and pointless research in the future (because it is heading in the wrong direction, due to being based on false assumptions).

This criticism of diagnosis is based on viewing diagnostic constructs only denoting only a classic Sydenham style syndrome clearly separate from health and separate from other syndromes/diseases caused by an underlying disease process. As seen in Chapter 3, this is only one of the different types of condition described by a diagnostic construct. Sometimes a diagnostic construct is used to describe a problem for which a health professional is thought to be helpful and may not involve a disease process at all. Some diagnostic constructs—for example, conversion disorder—are based on assumptions about psychological mechanisms. A diagnostic construct may describe a clinical picture caused by a network of interconnected symptoms rather than an underlying cause (Borsboom and Cramer, 2013; Borsboom, 2017).

The humanity of the psychiatric diagnostic construct is the next issue raised, and the vaguest. If something is intended to benefit and does so (which the questions above should allow us to answer), then can it be this inhumane? The greatest cost to people given a psychiatric diagnosis, unrelated to questions of side effects of treatment given for that diagnosis, may be the stigma associated with the diagnosis, as well as potential restrictions of liberty (such as being given treatment without consent). The following two questions seem relevant.

- Is the diagnosis associated with stigma?
- Is the diagnosis associated with a restriction of liberty?

Concerns about the diagnostic threshold being set too low for mental health disorders will be addressed by the question of continuity with normality already listed. Discussions of concerns about the medicalization of everyday life will be touched on in the questions of using a diagnosis for a disorder based on utilitarian reasons.

Other concerns centre on the variable clinical pictures that can be built from different people given the same psychiatric diagnosis, particularly where the diagnostic criteria are 'polythetic'. This is a category with broad criteria, where none of the criteria are necessary nor sufficient. This means that two people with the same diagnosis (if it is defined with polythetic criteria) can have different symptoms. For example, a diagnosis may be given if *either* criteria A or B is met or if *both* criteria A and B are met. Thus, some people will have criteria A met, some people will have criteria B met, and some will have both A and B criteria met. In this case, some people with the same diagnosis do not have all criteria in common. Sometimes in diagnostic criteria, some features *are* essential but others are optional. It is possible to have situations where two people with the same diagnostic label have completely different symptoms.

Diagnostic constructs with variable clinical pictures, particularly if they use polythetic criteria, rely on a 'family resemblance' (Rosch and Mervin, 1975) between different 'cases' of the same diagnosis. Remember that in the classic Sydenham disease model a disease process should produce a distinctive syndrome. This leads to a natural and understandable question: 'how can people with different symptoms have the same diagnosis?' This means the following questions should be asked:

- Is the condition associated with variable clinical pictures?
- Is the condition diagnosed with polythetic criteria?

We come now to the accusation of downplaying of social factors such as adversity and traumatic events in favour of biological explanations. This relates also to the issue of medicalization raised earlier. Are we merely applying a medical band aid to what are understandable normal to social stressors? This suggests the primacy of social factors as a cause of conditions, albeit with psychobiological factors also involved.

The issue also relates to an extent to boundaries or turf wars between professions. I mentioned earlier about how some psychologists may feel that doctors have *invaded* their professional space. If psychiatric conditions are uniquely strongly related to social factors as compared to other medical conditions, then perhaps this is an illegitimate invasion. If social adversity or trauma cause many types of medical conditions, then the presence of the medical profession in mental health is perfectly legitimate and we should welcome collaboration between the professionals.

- Is the condition caused by social difficulties and/or traumatic events?

Testing the criticisms of psychiatric diagnosis

Now that we have framed the concerns of the critics of psychiatric diagnostic constructs into a series of questions, how do we answer them? First, we will use examples of psychiatric diagnostic constructs. This means that concerns may be found to be justified for some particular psychiatric diagnostic constructs but not the whole overarching system.

What would be the best way of judging the merits of psychiatry? We could attempt to devise some numerical method, using our judgment to arrive at what seems a reasonable threshold. However, any numerical method usually involves making assumptions, and these assumptions may make the test unrealistically hard or too easy to pass. Many kinds of numerical assessments rest on a value judgment made by an 'expert' that is then regarded as an objective standard. Statistics is a complicated business; an overlooked assumption easily leads to a false conclusion.

Many numerical methods may also use examples from the 'hard sciences' such as chemistry, biology, and physics which are good at separating elements, species, or subatomic units. These methods may not be appropriate in the applied sciences of medicine and psychology. Medicine is a practical art that harnesses the power of science for its ultimate purpose of helping patients. A better comparison of methods would, in my view, be to compare psychiatry with general medicine in the issues raised by psychiatry's critics.

We are using general medicine as an external criterion. Why? Few people would deny the value of general medicine as a whole as a therapeutic model (whilst still allowing people to question certain specific treatments and practices) and few would question general medicine's continued existence as a medical specialty. It represents a large chunk of medical activity. Diagnostic constructs are used for the same purposes in general medicine as they are in psychiatry—to provide attached information used in clinical decision-making (see Chapters 2 and 5). Given general medicine's credibility and centrality to medical practice as a whole, it stands as a good yardstick by which to judge psychiatry.

This book will thus concentrate on looking at how psychiatry compares with general medicine in the issues raised by the critics. Can we identify 'zones of rarity' between psychiatry and general medicine? (This is similar to demonstrating a diagnosis is valid, as suggested by Kendell and Jablensky, 2003). Can we separate psychiatry from general medicine as completely different entities? Or is there partial or even complete overlap between psychiatry and general medicine in the nature of their diagnostic constructs?

To use a geographical parallel, if medicine as a whole can be regarded as the European continent and general medicine is the heart of this continent (Germany or Austria), where would psychiatry lie (see Figure 6.1)? If there is little to separate psychiatry from general medicine, then psychiatry will be at the heart of Europe too (perhaps Slovakia or Switzerland). If there were no overlap then psychiatry would be akin to Britain's relationship to the continent, once part of medicine but now separated from the main medical specialties by a sea of difference (Britain was united with the continent until the English Channel flooded. Perhaps psychiatry has been separated from the rest of medicine by scientific progress in other branches of medicine?). If there is a partial overlap, then psychiatry still be a part of the continent but located at the periphery, like Norway or Italy.

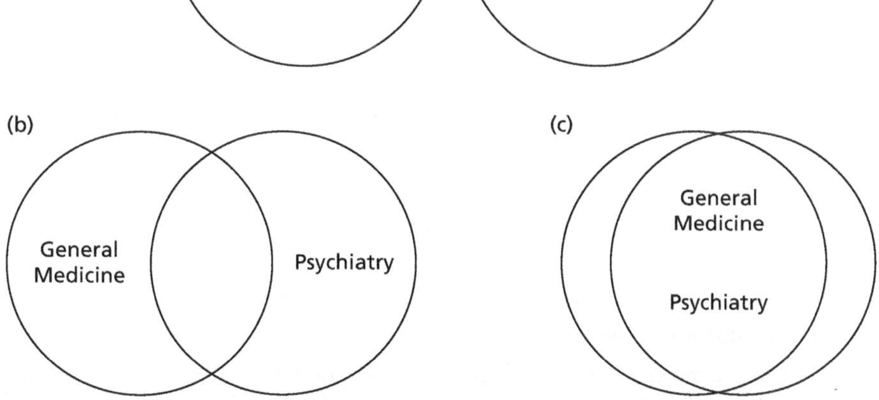

Figure 6.1 Three scenarios of medical model compared in general medicine and psychiatry: no overlap/some overlap/near total overlap.

Conclusion

Ironically, we will be classifying psychiatry and its sub classifications. We will see if it should remain within the 'family' of medical specialties or whether we should diagnose psychiatry as a 'non-medical entity'. We will mention briefly other forms of classification that could be used as an alternative in mental health. The questions we will ask in the comparison are repeated below (see Box 6.1) in an order that will be easy to answer.

Box 6.1 Questions to compare the medical model in mental health and general medicine

- What is the reliability of the diagnosis when compared to a relevant reference criterion?
- What is the reliability of discriminating between different diagnoses?
- Is the condition clearly separated from normality?
- Is the condition associated with variable clinical pictures?
- Is the condition diagnosed with polythetic criteria?
- Is the condition described by a diagnosis clearly separated from other conditions in terms of clinical features?
- Is there little co-occurrence of conditions; that is, are conditions separate clinical entities?
- Is the condition clearly identified with a causal mechanism (aetiology)?
- Is the condition clearly associated with a proven and detectable difference in structure or process? This difference acts as a proof of the diagnosis and can be identified with some sort of test, such as biochemical or radiology tests?
- Is the condition caused by social difficulties and/or traumatic events?
- Is the diagnosis associated with stigma?
- Is the diagnosis associated with a restriction of liberty?
- Does the condition have uniform prognosis (does the condition have a predictable unitary outcome)?
- Does the condition have different outcomes from other conditions?
- Does the condition predict differences in treatments given and their effectiveness?
- Is the use of the diagnosis justified due to some utilitarian reason such as relieving distress or risk?
- Is there a need for clinical information beyond the diagnosis in clinical decision-making?

Chapter 7

Criticism of psychiatric treatment

It is important to discuss criticism of psychiatric treatment as this is an crucial part of the medical model in mental health. As in Chapter 6, I will focus on one source of criticism in the form of a book and articles written by Joanna Moncrieff. She is a psychiatrist and thus understands the intricacies of general medicine and medication. The criticisms are used to generate a set of questions that can be used to compare psychiatry with general medicine, as in Chapter 6. Treatment in general medicine is used as a comparison for the same reasons as for diagnosis in the previous chapter.

Criticisms from *The Myth of the Chemical Cure*

One place to start is Moncrieff's *The Myth of the Chemical Cure*, whose subtitle, 'A critique of psychiatric treatment', indicates that it is well-suited for the purposes of this chapter (Moncrieff, 2009a). A broad critique is further described in an article jointly written by Moncrieff (Yeomans et al, 2015). To help identify useful questions to evaluate psychiatric medication, Moncrieff has written several articles criticizing several 'classes' (or types) of psychiatric medication: antidepressants (Moncrieff and Kirsch, 2005); antipsychotics (Moncrieff, 2009b, 2015a); and lithium in the treatment of bipolar disorder (Moncrieff, 1995, 1997).

Unfortunately, *The Myth of the Chemical Cure* relies on an information deficit on the part of the reader or a prior willingness to view psychiatric medication as particularly ineffective/harmful. Rather than list every problematic statement in the book, only a few will be described.

Moncrieff mentions the role of medication in psychiatry and emphasizes its central role, but this is, in part, due to the use of medication as an intervention which allows doctors to see more patients than using psychotherapy (see Chapter 5). Data from outpatient activity of doctors collected in the United States (NAMC, 2012) indicate that psychiatrists mention medication in outpatient records at similar rates to other specialties such as internal medicine physicians, cardiovascular doctors, and GPs, at about 80% of outpatient appointments.

Current use of drugs is compared to use of medication before the 1950s. With the advent of antidepressants and antipsychotics it is stated that drugs were prescribed because they made psychiatry 'scientific' and promoted theories of specificity of treatment for specific illnesses, and that their use supported the claim that psychiatrists could 'cure' people. Psychotherapists have used the term 'talking cure' from the very late nineteenth century but a patient initially coined the term (Launer, 2005). 'Curing' mental health problems is, therefore, a concept that belongs to both psychotherapy and treatment by medication.

The new medications were observed to be markedly more effective than previous ones for mental health conditions. This observation was later confirmed by research, initially crude research by contemporary standards but eventually by randomized controlled trials (RCTs), unlike other treatments that psychiatrists believed were effective based on their clinical experience such as insulin coma therapy. Thus, the evidence of effectiveness is more certain in the modern era than in previous eras due to the relatively recent introduction of better research methods (Tansella, 2002). We may not know the mechanism of action (see Chapter 15) for many treatments but we have greater justified confidence in current treatments than had those in previous eras. Indeed, it was the use of modern research methods—the RCT—that demonstrated insulin coma treatment was ineffective in schizophrenia (Ackner et al., 1957).

Moncrieff can still present useful questions to ask, without being used as a source of answers. The points made in her book about the mechanism of action of psychiatric medication not usually reversing a disease process and that it is often unknown how any benefit is produced are both useful. If we understand the mechanism of action of a medication, then several potential benefits arise. We may learn something about the condition. This can occur even if the medication does not act directly on the causative mechanism of the condition. We may also be able to develop more medications that act in the same but superior way, either more effectively or with fewer side-effects. As a result, we arrive at our first question:

- Does the treatment used have a disease-reversing mechanism of action that produces the clinical benefit?

On the other hand, we may sometimes have medication that works but we do not know how. If a medication works we should continue using it but we should keep trying to discover why medication is effective (Shah and Mountain, 2007). The purpose of gaining knowledge of mechanisms of action is to benefit the patient further. An unknown mechanism of action of a given medication may be frustrating, but the benefit derived should not be devalued.

Moncrieff discusses how drug actions are evaluated by examining research methodology, and she highlights the fact that even RCTs cannot eliminate 'extraneous' factors that can influence the results. Early papers on RCTs (e.g. Hill, 1951, 1952) discussed how RCTs reduce the effects of bias but did not claim to eliminate these effects completely.

The claim by Moncrieff that drug RCTs rely on the assumption of disease-centred mechanism of action by the medication is misleading (Chapter 2 in Moncrieff, 2009a).

First, RCTs—as discussed in Chapter 5—are used in education to evaluate the effectiveness of different teaching methods (e.g. Jerrim and Vignoles, 2015) and promoted as an evaluation technique for education research in Goldacre (2013). They have also been used to evaluate website designs and interventions for people receiving benefits (see Part 1 in Haynes et al., 2012). The comparisons used in this type of research are different types of interventions rather than placebos, but clearly there is no disease involved. The use of a placebo in the RCT is to control for the non-specific effects of being given treatment and the natural course of the condition (see Chapter 5). RCTs are used to compare the effect of different interventions on outcomes for different situations, not necessarily only diseases, so no there is no assumption of acting on 'specific diseases'.

Second, the RCT is used to evaluate the effectiveness of different interventions on outcomes by minimizing the effect of various biases on this evaluation (see Chapter 5). It is *not* dependent on how the intervention achieves this outcome. Thiazide diuretics are an example of medication that has been proven effective in RCTs for hypertension, despite not acting in a 'disease-centred way' (ALLHAT, 2002; Musini et al., 2014).

Third, even if an assumption is incorrect (e.g. we may be misled in thinking we know how a medication works in a 'disease-centred way' whereas in fact the mechanism of action is unknown), if an RCT demonstrates that a medication improves an outcome for a condition then this result not devalued by it being based on a false assumption as to how the result was achieved. An improved outcome for a patient is an improved outcome, no matter what.

Fourth, doctors see many conditions that are not 'diseases' (see Chapter 3), and there are placebo-controlled RCTs carried out for interventions in these conditions. These RCTs are the basis of NICE Guidelines for the treatment of high blood pressure, for example (NICE, 2011).

Moncrieff lists a series of reasons why any apparent difference in outcomes between a medication and placebo in an RCT may not solely be due to the action of the medication. These are not in themselves controversial; subjectivity of measurements, participants, or researchers measuring outcomes realizing they are on the active drug because participants experience side-effects are all normal occurrences. Thus, these trials become *unblinded* and this can influence the outcomes. This can happen to some extent in research on all types of medication. Moncrieff's own meta-analysis (Moncrieff et al., 1998) showed antidepressants were still significantly more effective than 'active placebo' (i.e. the placebo was an active drug that had side effects similar to the antidepressant to maintain *blinding*). Subjectivity and psychological factors also influence outcomes in general medicine.

The 'drug-centred model' and 'disease-centred model' of treatment

Yeomans, Moncrieff, and Huws (Yeomans et al., 2015)) discuss the 'drug-centred model' and 'disease-centred model' constructs in less misleading language than used in *The Myth of the Chemical Cure* (Moncrief, 2009a). Nevertheless, the arguments made in this paper were refuted in an accompanying article (Taylor, 2015). Yeomans and colleagues' work does make a good starting point for us to examine critiques of psychiatric treatment.

They contrast the drug-centred model with the disease-centred model, but only the first five points made are relevant for the purposes of this chapter.

1. Both models require good knowledge of psychopharmacology
2. In the drug-centred model, medications are thought to have multiple effects through various pathways, whilst the disease-centred model separates therapeutic effects from side effects.

3. The drug-centred model presumes that medication is harmful and should not be used if it can be avoided, whereas the disease-centred model assumes that because a disease-causing abnormality is being reversed then medication must be helpful.
4. In the drug-centred model, some of the effects of medication (e.g. on behaviour) may be beneficial, whereas in the disease-centred model, undesirable effects of medication (e.g. sedation) are regarded as not central to the medication's action.
5. The drug-centred model uses a pragmatic style based on how the medication affects the individual, but in the disease-centred model, the hypothesized abnormality of functioning/mechanism justifies prescribing medication.

Point 1 is clearly not a point of difference. As regards Point 2, in Chapter 5 it was stated that drugs have complex effects on complex systems but we regard these effects as beneficial or harmful depending on the situation (sometimes the same effect can be regarded as beneficial or harmful depending on the location or clinical situation). Thus, both points of view can be held at the same time and are not relevant to whatever prescribing model the doctor uses.

Point 3 is the first point of proper contrast. In the drug-centred model, medication is *always* harmful but in the disease-centred model, medication is *always* beneficial. The more accurate view is that all medications are *potentially* harmful; one may be allergic to drugs or may experience a side-effect, the drugs may interact badly with other medication, or a person could be prescribed too high a dose. Even if we restrict this statement to psychiatric medications it would be hard to prove harm was caused to everyone who took them. What some people may interpret as harm—such as slowing of thoughts—may be experienced as beneficial, for instance to someone experiencing racing thoughts.

Similarly, medication is not *always* beneficial. In general medicine, many people do not experience benefit from medication even where a clear disease is present. It is better to state that medication is *potentially* beneficial. We are more confident of *potential* benefit if there is good quality research that demonstrates that the medication was more effective than placebo for the patient's condition. Not everyone will benefit from a given drug, even if research shows that it is effective for a condition.

Point 3 is a good example of an overly *rigid* viewpoint stating that medication is either *always* harmful or *always* beneficial. Universal absolute rules like this are rare in medicine; people, their conditions, and their interactions with interventions are simply too variable for *universal absolute rules*. The best we can often hope for is probability statements such as what frequency and types of harms and types of benefits a patient can expect from medication

If we regard medical interventions as a whole, then some forms of interventions are associated with *always* causing harm. Interventions that involve cutting tissue, such as surgery, do cause harm, however these types of harms are believed to be outweighed by the benefits (e.g. removing an inflamed appendix).

Point 3 is useful as it suggests a good question. Moving away from the *absolute* of medication being *always* harmful we can examine the question of it being potentially *relatively more* harmful than treatments in general medicine. This type of harm needs to be evaluated in terms of the frequency of risk of causing harm as well as the nature and severity of these harms.

- How harmful are the treatments used?

Point 4 is the crux of how the drug-centred model views how psychiatric medication can be useful at times. Drugs are viewed as psychoactive compounds (they are active on the *psyche* in the same way cardioactive drugs affect the heart) and these psychoactive effects may have some benefits. Emotional indifference caused by antipsychotics may help with people with psychosis, emotional blunting caused by SSRI antidepressants may help people with depression. It should also be noted that psychoactive effects may vary according to the person's current mental state; for example morphine, an opioid used primarily as a painkiller, is more likely to have unpleasant psychoactive effects if people are pain-free (Chapter 14 in Harvey et al., 2011). These psychoactive models are inadequate to describe all the clinical benefits from psychiatric medication, such as reducing hallucinations (Taylor, 2015).

The disease-centred model regards the drug's *primary intended action* as reversing a hypothesized abnormality of function in order to reduce symptoms, and any other mental effects (such as sedation) are *unintended actions* and do not have a therapeutic function, and so they are regarded as side effects. There is little evidence that psychiatric medications act this way (see Chapter 15).

Point 5 seems to be referring to two different time frames. The description of the drug-centred model depicts a situation where the patient has had *prior* experience of psychiatric medications and can give input into which medication suits them best. The disease-centred model seems to describe a doctor choosing a medication for a new patient based on which medication would reverse a hypothesized abnormality causing the diagnosed condition. When prescribing, doctors are expected to take a history which includes past responses to medication, so doctors using a disease-centred model would be expected to take into account the patient's previous responses to medication.

Point 5 also omits another method of choosing medication to prescribe, a model that takes into account research evidence that a medication has been shown to be beneficial in a condition, even if it does not act by removing a cause or reversing a disease process (see Chapter 15). This research evidence is combined with the patient's past experiences, clinical situation, and shared objectives of treatment to decide which medication to use (see Chapter 5).

The distinction between the drug-centred model and the disease-centred model seems to rely on misleading statements (drugs being regarded as *always* harmful or *always* beneficial, or making statements of differences in attitudes that can in fact be held by doctors using both models of drug actions).

These are the only two models of prescribing that are presented by Yeomans and colleagues as being used by psychiatrists, with the disease-centred model stated as the commonest (Yeomans et al., 2015) without sufficient evidence that this is true. The two models presented in the article are possibly extremes of psychiatrists' beliefs around psychiatric medication stated as being 'rigidly' applied in all circumstances.

The best way to discover what the prevailing prescribing models of psychiatrists are is to ask them. I asked a group of 88 consultant psychiatrists to fill in an online questionnaire and over 60% replied. They were questioned about their general attitude to medication in psychiatry and specific types of medication in specific situations (antidepressants in adult depression, antidepressants in adult anxiety, antipsychotics in non-manic psychosis, lithium in bipolar disorder, benzodiazepines for short-term treatment of anxiety, stimulants for ADHD, and thiamine for prevention of Wernicke–Korsakoff in alcohol withdrawal). The options for the prescribing models given were of four types: 'drug-centred', 'disease-centred', 'outcome-centred' (medication was shown to have benefits in outcomes in research, but the mechanism was unclear), and 'medication not indicated' (that medication type not useful for that situation). The results were analysed by myself and two of my trainees (Dr Adam Moreton and Dr Mawada Adam).

By far the commonest model in terms of general attitude to prescribing in psychiatry is outcome-centred; medication can be beneficial and can also cause harm, *not* a certainty of benefit or harm but not necessarily by acting to reverse a disease process (Chapter 3 in Cookson et al., 2002). Only two psychiatrists (3.63%) had a general disease-centred model, and the rest (96.37%) had a general outcome-centred model. For almost all clinical situations, the outcome-centred model was the commonest chosen—from 70.59% (the use of benzos in short-term treatment of anxiety) to 96.15% (the use of lithium in bipolar disorder), with results around 85% for outcome-centred model for antidepressants and antipsychotics. Even if all the missing respondents had chosen the disease-centred model for these situations, then the outcome-centred model would still be the commonest choice.

The exception was the use of thiamine to prevent Wernicke–Korsakoff syndrome in alcohol withdrawal because thiamine deficiency is the cause of this condition (Chapter 5 in Walker et al., 2014). In this instance, 70% of psychiatrists reported using a disease-centred model. There were also situations when individual psychiatrists thought that the specified medication should not be used.

The obvious conclusion that can be drawn is that that Moncrieff and co-authors are wrong: the disease-centred model is not the commonest model used by psychiatrists (Moncrieff, 2009a; Yeomans et al., 2015), at least for this sample of psychiatrists. The other conclusion is that psychiatrists are flexible in their rationale for using medication, depending on the medication and the patient's condition . Psychiatrists tend to have an outcome-centred model, except if there is clear evidence in favour of a disease-centred action.

Criticism of specific medication classes—antidepressants

Moncrieff has criticized the effectiveness of antidepressants (Moncrieff and Kirsch, 2005). The paper quotes Kirsch's finding that the *mean* (average) difference between participants in RCTs comparing antidepressants with placebo was 1.7 points on the Hamilton Rating Scale for Depression (HAMD). This is a very small difference and of limited clinical significance in itself. The difference between antidepressants and placebo was statistically significant.

What does this difference mean in terms of effectiveness of antidepressants? The problem with this paper is that it asserts that this average small difference is *uniform* across *all* people taking the medication compared to placebo. In other words, *everyone* taking the antidepressant experiences a very small advantage in taking it, compared to taking a placebo. The authors use a graph demonstrating this uniform difference across the whole range of HAMD scores. A *hypothetical* graph without supporting evidence is not *proof*, however. In her book, Moncrieff stated that reaction to medication varies a great deal between people (Moncrieff, 2009a).

The mean difference figure given is an average over a whole group; it does not tell us what is happening at an individual level. For many medications, not just psychiatric ones, the level of response varies greatly between individuals. An average of a small difference in a group may reflect some individuals having a large response, some a small response, some no response, or the condition worsening.

Depression is a *heterogeneous* diagnostic construct with many different causes and different processes amongst people with the same diagnosis (Goldberg, 2011). This means we can expect that antidepressants will have a different response and effectiveness amongst individuals with the same diagnosis (Stein, 2015). Even if we take people sharing a homogeneous medical diagnosis, such as urinary tract infection caused by the same bacteria given the same antibiotic, we can see variable response. The different people's causative bacterial strains may have differing levels of sensitivity to the antibiotic. Some people may therefore respond better to the same antibiotic than others with the same diagnosis. This variability of response will be greater for *heterogeneous* diagnostic constructs like depression (Stein, 2015).

Furthermore, the brain comprises very complex inter-related systems whose interactions vary according to the individual. We can expect that introducing a chemical that affects the brain such as an antidepressant will also have complex effects that vary between individuals, including variable effectiveness in reducing HAMD scores.

Clinical experience also confirms that people prescribed antidepressant have variable effects in response to the medication; some of these effects are regarded as therapeutic, others are regarded as side-effects (sometimes both). Some patients seem to respond very well to the medication, others less well, others feel worse.

It is therefore unlikely that antidepressants have a uniform effect on all people. However, this raises an important point: does the *average* effect of antidepressants for a group of people with depression prescribed them indicate it is a *sufficiently effective* treatment to be useful? This produces the following question:

- How effective are the treatments used?

We shall again compare the effectiveness of medications used in medicine. In addition, we will compare the effectiveness with psychotherapy as an alternative to psychiatric medications.

Criticism of specific medication classes—antipsychotics

Moncrieff accepts that antipsychotics are effective at reducing psychotic symptoms in some patients (Moncrieff, 2015a). She also points out that there is evidence for alternative treatments for acute psychosis (Moncrieff, 2009b). She highlights adverse effects of antipsychotics before discussing what she considers serious flaws in research studies demonstrating antipsychotics effectiveness in reducing relapse.

Moncrieff contends that any apparent advantage of antipsychotics for reducing relapse in people with psychosis is due to a methodological error. People with psychosis are stabilized on antipsychotics. Some continue on antipsychotics whilst others have their antipsychotics stopped (sometimes replaced with placebo). This withdrawal from antipsychotics causes states that are either mistaken for psychosis or *are* psychotic states due to withdrawal ('dopamine supersensitivity psychosis'; Chouinard and Jones, 1980), or these withdrawal states in themselves are a stressor that causes a relapse of psychosis.

The advantage for antipsychotics in reducing the risk of relapse was very large in a meta-analysis of comparing antipsychotics to placebo in preventing relapse (Leucht et al., 2012a); 64% relapsed on placebo compared to 27% on antipsychotics over 12 months, albeit including some studies that were not double-blind RCTs—this is over twice the reduction in rate of relapses consistent with a likely clinically significant benefit (Chapter 7 in Sackett et al., 1991)). This means that withdrawal-induced psychosis would have to be responsible for a large proportion of relapses in the placebo group to make the benefit clinically *insignificant*. When Moncrieff reviewed the evidence for psychosis caused by antipsychotics, there was a small effect on numbers of withdrawals from antipsychotics causing psychosis, except in the case of clozapine (Moncrieff, 2006), but insufficient to explain the large difference in relapse rates between antipsychotics and placebo. A recent review of dopamine supersensitivity induced by antipsychotics identified several studies with high rates of antipsychotic-induced dopamine supersensitivity withdrawal psychosis in participants (except those prescribed clozapine), using varying criteria to identify the phenomena (Chouinard et al., 2017). The rates seemed higher than those I encounter in my clinical practice but I mostly see patients early in the course of their illness so my experience may not be representative. It may be that in patients on antipsychotics for years these drugs may eventually cause relapse by dopamine supersensitivity, but that is still a delay in relapse compared to not taking any antipsychotics at all.

Early relapses after stopping medication do not always imply a withdrawal cause, it may simply reflect the fact that the antipsychotic was reducing the symptoms but that whatever is causing the psychosis is still active. When the antipsychotic is reduced or stopped then the psychotic symptoms become apparent again. Another alternative is that the antipsychotic has a protective effect against psychosis relapse and without it the patient relapses.

Relapse rates do not seem to differ much between studies where antipsychotics are stopped abruptly and studies where antipsychotics are withdrawn gradually; tapered antipsychotic withdrawal resulted in a 22% relapse rate, abrupt antipsychotic withdrawal resulted in a relapse rate of 28% compared to placebo 64% (Leucht et al., 2012a). The taper period was over three weeks and thus short, but this is still strong evidence that the only a small proportion of difference in relapse rates between antipsychotics and placebo is caused by withdrawal-induced psychosis.

To illustrate, I will discuss a study which was open-label (both participants and researchers knew whether they were taking antipsychotics or not) and where participants chose either to discontinue medication or continue it after a period of 'clinical remission' for 12 months and 'functional recovery' for 6 months (Son et al., 2016). This study is chosen to demonstrate the time course of relapse after discontinuation of medication. Forty-six participants opted to discontinue antipsychotics—withdrawn gradually—and twenty-two participants opted to continue antipsychotics. Relapse was defined as an increase in psychotic symptoms according to certain items in the PANNS questionnaire measuring psychotic symptoms. These items were clearly psychotic symptoms, not just non-psychosis withdrawal symptoms. Relapse was also defined as suicide or hospital admission. The two groups were different in terms of duration of being on medication and starting dose (both higher in the discontinuation group suggesting they may have had a more severe condition on average).

Taking into account unblinded assessments, that treatment status was not randomized, and that there were some differences at baseline between the two groups, there was still convincing differences in relapse rates after three-year follow-up; 67.4% in the discontinuation group and 31.8% in the maintenance group. In fact, there were no relapses in the maintenance group in the first 12 months. Interestingly, the median time to relapse was 122 days and the mean time to relapse was 209 days in the antipsychotic discontinuation group. The median time is the point at which half the relapses in the discontinuation group have occurred, so half the relapses occur *after* four months in the discontinuation group. The mean is higher than the median, which indicates that a proportion of the relapses (at least half) took place long after the four-month period. The implication is that half the relapses took place four months after gradual antipsychotic discontinuation so are not due to antipsychotic withdrawal, as suggested by Moncrieff.

Given the small absolute difference between relapse rates in tapered versus abrupt withdrawal (Leucht et al., 2012a), and at least half the relapses occur outside a time period consistent with withdrawal-induced psychosis, a scenario where 50% difference between antipsychotic and placebo relapses are due to withdrawals is unlikely, and still would have a 20% absolute reduction and about a 40% relative reduction, which is still a clinically significant benefit (Chapter 7 in Sackett et al., 1991). The research evidence supports the view that antipsychotics do reduce relapses in people who meet schizophrenia criteria (Leucht and Davis, 2017).

My clinical experience is that withdrawal states do occur, particularly with short-acting drugs like quetiapine. They can usually be distinguished from acute psychosis except in the case of clozapine, where a clear withdrawal psychosis can be seen with florid psychotic symptoms and features of confused states (but I have seen a similar state in quetiapine withdrawal psychosis). In both my clinical experience and in the research evidence, the withdrawal states from antipsychotics are not a sufficient reason to account substantially for increased rates of relapse of psychosis on stopping antipsychotics.

Moncrieff makes the valuable point that psychiatric research tends to focus only on relapse as an outcome measured in long-term studies, whereas other types of outcomes such as social functioning may be more important to patients (Moncrieff,

2015a). This lack of research means it is hard to judge the impact of antipsychotics on these other outcomes.

Criticism of specific medication classes—lithium in bipolar disorder

Moncrieff has expressed grave doubts about the effectiveness of lithium in the treatment of bipolar disorder, both in the acute phase and in the prevention of relapse of bipolar disorder (Moncrieff, 1995, 1997). She points out that what may appear to be a protective effect of lithium on relapse may actually be patients withdrawn suddenly off lithium and onto placebo having episodes of 'withdrawal mania'; up to 50% risk in three months after stopping lithium suddenly (Suppes et al., 1991). These additional withdrawal episodes of mania in the placebo group increase the chances of participants remaining on lithium having fewer episodes of mania, by contrast. These criticisms will be answered by using papers contemporary with Moncrieff's criticisms.

Moncrieff reviewed evidence from earlier trials that showed lithium was effective in milder cases of acute mania but that it was less effective than antipsychotics for more severe cases of mania with marked behavioural disturbance (Moncrieff, 1997). She dismissed a double-blind RCT comparing the effectiveness of lithium, divalproex, or placebo in the treatment of acute mania (Bowden et al., 1994) on several grounds (Moncrieff, 1997). First, the trial had sufficient statistical power to demonstrate effectiveness of lithium but only did so at one of four time-points. Second, the use of additional (or supplementary) medications during the trial complicates interpretation of the results. Third, that the rate of premature terminations from the trial was similar between lithium and placebo, suggesting they were similarly effective.

This interpretation of the trial was shown to be unnecessarily negative (Cookson, 1997; Jefferson, 1998). The first point about lack of statistically significant results ignored the fact that roughly twice as many participants were given divalproex (68) or placebo (73) as were given lithium (35). This was a deliberate feature of the study, which was intended primarily to demonstrate effectiveness of divalproex in acute mania. Lithium was able to demonstrate a statistically significant improvement compared to placebo at the ten-day assessment point but not at other time-points, but the average difference between the change in mean mania rating scale scores between lithium and placebo was similar to the average difference between divalproex and placebo at these other time-points. In other words, lithium had similar effectiveness in reducing mania as divalproex, but the trial was *underpowered* to show lithium having a statistically significant result at all time-points.

The use of supplementary medications was limited to two sedatives during the first ten days of the study and was reduced over the time period, and supplementary medication was not used for the eight hours before assessment of participants, so the effect of supplementary medication was unlikely to alter the result significantly (Cookson, 1997; Jefferson, 1998).

Moncrieff oversimplified when describing premature terminations—56% for lithium participants and 61% for placebo—excluding participants who recovered early (Moncrieff, 1997). A more detailed breakdown of these figures shows that 33% of the participants receiving lithium left the trial early due to lack of effectiveness, compared to 51% of the participants receiving placebo for the same reason. Eleven per cent of the participants given lithium had to leave the trial early due to side effects compared to 3% of the placebo group. This suggests not equivalence of treatment but that lithium was more effective than placebo but that it was also more likely to give side effects. Lithium dosage was high, with a maximum allowed serum lithium level of 1.5 mMol/L when the usual maximum in the United Kingdom is 1.2 mMol/L. This may have increased lithium's effectiveness but it also increased side-effects.

A final point that Moncrieff ignored was that 48% of the participants given lithium had a previous history of not responding to it (Bowden et al., 1994; Jefferson, 1998). This was borne out by the results of the trial. Participants given lithium with a previous history of not responding to it did a little worse than those given placebo, whilst those with previous history of response had the greatest response to lithium of any treatment group. Despite this, lithium showed an advantage over placebo in the whole group of participants at multiple time-points (but significantly only at ten days), thus reasonable confidence can be held that lithium is effective in the treatment of acute mania.

Moncrieff makes legitimate points about the methodological limitations of the earlier studies on the effectiveness of lithium in preventing further episodes of bipolar disorder ('prophylaxis') (Goodwin, 1995; Cookson, 1997; Jefferson, 1998). Lithium requires monitoring of its serum level because high serum levels are associated with toxic, and even dangerous, side-effects (such as kidney and brain damage). This means that a doctor needs to be aware of the serum levels of a participant in the research study and to adjust the dose if necessary, which can 'unblind' assessments by that doctor. The problem of lithium withdrawal causing mania (Suppes et al., 1991) also complicates interpretation of studies where participants who were on lithium have it replaced with placebo.

An example of this type of discontinuation study (Baastrup et al., 1970) was a double-blind study. Participants with either bipolar disorder or recurrent depression who had been on lithium for at least a year were randomized to continue lithium or placebo. Relapse was defined as either hospital admission or increased support at home due to worsening of mental health. As the participants had been on lithium for a long time, there was no need to alter dosage to reach therapeutic levels or to avoid dangerous levels of serum lithium. For those who did not relapse, the trial lasted on average nearly five months. None of the participants who continued on lithium relapsed, but 12 out of 22 participants with bipolar disorder on placebo relapsed, and 9 out of 17 participants with recurrent depression relapsed. Although the results seem clear-cut, it is possible that the relapses in the bipolar group were due to lithium withdrawal-induced mania (Suppes et al., 1991).

The authors stated that the relapses occurred spaced out throughout the follow-up months and were not due to withdrawal-induced mania (Baastrup et al., 1970), but only gave an unpublished paper as a reference to prove this. In a later paper (Schou, 1997), it was stated that all the relapses were preceded by a psychological event such as marital problems or difficulties at work; Schou suggests the possibility that the placebo was unable to protect the participant from relapsing under psychosocial stress but that lithium could have done so. It could be these psychological events were actually caused by a withdrawal-induced mania which could then have led to these difficulties.

A possible indicator that the relapses were not all due to withdrawal-induced mania is the similar rate of relapse in the recurrent depression participants given placebo, as lithium is less likely to cause withdrawal-induced depression (Suppes et al., 1991).

A large prospective study compared lithium or imipramine (antidepressant) with placebo for two years in participants with either recurrent depression or recurrent bipolar disorder (Prien et al., 1973). The participants were started on lithium for a short period but withdrawal-induced mania was not a feature of their condition (Prien et al., 1973; Goodwin, 1995). Only participants given imipramine had increased manic episodes. Those given lithium or placebo tended to have depressive episodes.

The treating doctors knew which treatment the participants were given and were allowed to increase the dose of lithium if suspecting relapse. Single blind increases the risk of bias in a study. Moncrieff reports that the 28% of participants who had lithium increased due to early signs of relapse should be excluded (she contends that including them makes the results less scientifically valid). Furthermore, all participants who dropped out early (who tended to be on placebo) should also be excluded. This way of analysing the results very strongly favours the placebo and is more likely to make lithium seem ineffective. This leaves a comparison of 29% in the lithium group having a good outcome versus 19% in the placebo group. This difference was no longer statistically significant.

The justification for excluding participants who had their lithium dose increased when there were signs of early relapse would suggest that lithium does have a benefit in treating acute mania. Increasing the lithium if early relapse is detected is normal clinical practice; this may have reduced the scientific validity of the study but increased its clinical validity as it reflects usual clinical practice (Goodwin, 1995). Excluding this group is likely to underestimate how useful lithium is in reducing relapse of bipolar disorder.

Failure to achieve statistical significance is more likely a reflection of the study becoming *underpowered* after the exclusions to show a statistically significant result for the size of the effect of lithium compared to placebo. This results in the analysis being biased towards placebo (Goodwin, 1995). The study by Prien and colleagues gives us a moderate amount of confidence in lithium preventing relapse in bipolar disorder but this effect may be modest in degree (Prien et al., 1973).

Moncrieff (1995) criticizes a double-blind RCT of lithium versus placebo to prevent relapse that did not feature lithium discontinuation (Coppen et al., 1971) for only reporting on participants who managed to complete at least 16 weeks of the trial. There is also criticism that the main outcome measure was proportion of time spent in relapse, not number of relapses or time to relapse, and for being affected by numbers who dropped out which may make this measure unreliable. The research study included both patients with recurrent depression as well as recurrent bipolar disorder, with many of the outcomes broken down into recurrent depression (unipolar) and bipolar groups.

Regarding the criticism of the higher drop-out rates amongst placebos, it has been argued that this favoured the placebo group as they were in the study for a shorter period and thus had less opportunity to relapse (Goodwin, 1995). The use of data from participants who completed 16 weeks is not terminal to the usefulness of the study. It means we apply the findings of the study to patients in clinical practice who can complete 16 weeks of lithium treatment.

This trial also assessed several types of outcomes: a global assessment of outcome from a doctor blind to treatment group, and a global assessment of outcome from a psychiatric social worker again blind to treatment group and the use of additional treatments. These additional treatments included electroconvulsive therapy, antidepressants, and anti-manic medications. All these separate outcome measures showed that lithium was more effective in both the whole group and bipolar participants, with statistically significant differences.

The study by Coppen and colleagues had a number of strengths (Coppen et al., 1971). One doctor managed the dosage of lithium levels to help preserve blinding of the separate assessing doctor. Steps were taken to try to maintain blinding of the patients on placebo. There were checks to see if the assessing doctor was successfully blinded to treatment group. Multiple types of outcomes were measured to confirm that improvement was reflected from several perspectives. Consequently, contrary to Moncrieff's dismissal, reasonable confidence can be held as to the value of lithium in preventing relapse of bipolar disorder so long as a patient can continue it for at least 16 weeks.

A non-experimental follow-up study over many years compared 41 patients with recurrent bipolar disorder prescribed lithium and 40 patients with recurrent bipolar disorder who either did not take lithium for long or were not prescribed it all. It concluded that the lithium's benefits on relapse prevention in this clinical sample were 'modest' and less than expected from experimental studies (Markar and Mander, 1989).

Relapse was defined as admission to hospital with mania or depression. Participants were only included in the lithium group if they were concordant for at least six months and had a mean serum lithium level of 0.4 Mmol/l (this is the lower end of the therapeutic range). This is not a large sample size and it failed to identify statistically significant differences in mean number of admissions per year or mean number of weeks spent as an inpatient per year.

The authors also included a life table (Figure 1 in Markar and Mander, 1989) depicting the probability of remaining relapse-free. There is a clear advantage favouring lithium of remaining relapse-free from about 20 months that reaches its maximum at 72 months, then narrows but persists until the end of follow-up at 160 months. Visual reading of the graph shows that at 72 months about 30% of the lithium group are relapse-free but only about 10% of the controls are relapse-free. Therefore, the odds of remaining well on lithium seems 2.5–3 times better at 72 months on lithium than the controls. None of the control group are relapse-free after about 150 months, but approximately 10% of the lithium group have managed to remain relapse-free until follow-up at 160 months.

The statistical tests were not significant but this is a reflection of the small sample size and lithium not having a large size of effect. The study was *underpowered* to demonstrate a statistically significant result for this size of effect. The results fit with the observation that lithium needs to be taken for at least two years before a benefit can be shown in preventing relapse in bipolar disorder (Goodwin, 1994).

It has been suggested that the differences in results between experimental trials of lithium and observations of results in clinical practice can be explained by differing levels of concordance—taking the medication reliably and consistently—with better concordance with lithium in experimental trials as compared to the studies observing clinical practice (Guscott and Taylor, 1994). There is a difference between conceptual *efficacy*—a potential size of effect as demonstrated in research such as double-blind RCTs—and *effectiveness* in ordinary clinical practice. *Efficacy* is usually greater than *effectiveness* as the participants in clinical trials are often less complex and more concordant with treatment than patients in ordinary clinical practice and the treatments may be delivered to a higher standard.

A recurrent theme in the lithium research is that the studies are underpowered for lithium's degree of effectiveness because RCTs are expensive to carry out and the need for the RCT to carry on for many months to show any benefit for lithium increases the expense still further. Lithium is not a patented drug and it is relatively cheap, which means there is no incentive for drug companies to fund this type of research (Bernadt and Stein, 1997).

Meta-analysis can solve this problem by pooling results from these underpowered trials (see Chapter 5). One meta-analysis of lithium's effectiveness at preventing relapse (Davis et al., 1993) was available at the time of Moncrieff's two articles from 1995 and 1997 but it is unclear as to why Moncrieff did not mention it. This meta-analysis showed a pooled advantage in relapse rates for lithium versus placebo of 55% from ten placebo-controlled studies that was highly statistically significant (Jefferson, 1998). Clearly, the methodological issues of these studies mean that that difference between lithium and placebo has been overestimated, but it seems likely that that there is some benefit for lithium in preventing relapse in bipolar disorder.

The later review by Moncrieff (1997) also analysed the evidence for lithium's effectiveness in depression as an 'augmentation' treatment when added to depression. Moncrieff concludes the evidence is limited for the effectiveness of lithium in this regard. The authors of one of the papers that Moncrieff quoted to demonstrate lithium was ineffective in this role criticized Moncrieff's interpretation of the paper (Bernadt and Stein, 1997). They point out that amongst multiple misinterpretations, she only quoted part of their results, and that their results showed lithium was effective as an augmentation to antidepressants for depression. In fairness, the authors agreed with Moncrieff about uncertainties about the use of lithium in clinical practice.

There does seem evidence that lithium is effective in treating acute mania and also offering a modest benefit in preventing relapse in bipolar disorder in those who can continue to take it for two years or more.

Conclusions

Moncrieff's criticisms of psychiatric medication are undermined by several flaws—such as not fitting with the evidence—of which several examples have been given throughout this chapter. For example, Moncrieff's model of disease-centred versus drug-centred prescribing describes extremes of attitudes to prescribing, whereas in reality, most psychiatrists adopt a more flexible approach based on effectiveness demonstrated in research which does not make assumptions about reversing hypothesized mechanisms.

Moncrieff does, however, make several valid points. Most psychiatric medications are not 'cures', in the sense of eliminating a cause or reversing a disease process. They have complex effects which are described as therapeutic or adverse depending on the value judgements of the clinician or patient. Psychoactive effects, as described by Moncrieff, may explain therapeutic benefits in *some* patients but not in *all* patients experiencing therapeutic benefit. There should be more research on the long-term consequences of psychiatric medication as well as the subjective experiences of taking psychiatric medication and the mechanisms of how they may benefit patients.

Moncrieff's criticisms of antidepressants are based on the assumption that a small average benefit over placebo in a group of patients given antidepressants represents a *uniform* small benefit for everyone prescribed antidepressants compared to placebo. Anyone with clinical experience of using antidepressants will notice a highly variable response to antidepressants; some patients respond very well but others barely respond or not at all. The average small benefit over placebo in a group represents some patients in a group having a large benefit but others very little response, creating an average of small benefit.

Moncrieff accepts antipsychotics are effective in acute psychosis but implies that apparent benefits in preventing relapses of psychosis are due to withdrawal states caused by ceasing antipsychotics. Unfortunately for this theory, the time pattern of relapses as well as the rates of observed withdrawal states and lack of major differences between gradual and sudden discontinuation of antipsychotics all prove that withdrawals are insufficient to explain all the large difference in relapse rates between placebo and antipsychotics.

She provided detailed criticism that there was lack of evidence for lithium in the acute treatment of mania or the prevention of relapses of bipolar disorder. There is evidence for withdrawal of lithium leading to a high risk of mania. In fact, there is reasonable grounds from a double-blind RCT to be confident that lithium is effective in acute mania. Examining the evidence from RCTs and naturalistic studies, there is evidence that lithium does have a modest benefit in preventing relapses in bipolar disorder so long as the patient takes it for over two years.

Despite this rejection of many of Moncrieff's assertions, useful questions have been identified to compare psychiatric medications and interventions with those used in the rest of medicine (see Box 7.1).

Box 7.1 Questions to compare psychiatric treatments with treatments in general medicine

- How effective are the treatments used?
- How harmful are the treatments used?
- Does the treatment used have a disease-reversing mechanism of action that produces the clinical benefit?

Chapter 8

Reliability of diagnosis

Box 8.1 Questions used to compare diagnostic constructs of psychiatry with general medicine

- What is the reliability of the diagnosis when compared to a relevant reference criterion?
- What is the reliability of discriminating between different diagnoses?

These two questions (see Box 8.1) appear similar: if we assess patient's clinical picture as matching diagnosis *X*, we are implicitly saying it is *not* diagnosis *Y* which may produce a similar clinical picture. The difference applies when there are 'gold-standard' reference criteria such as a reasonably objective test proven to be definitive in establishing the presence of a diagnosis. The second type of question applies where there is no such gold standard and reliability is measured as agreement between clinicians about the diagnosis in the same patient.

Agreement between a doctor's diagnosis and a reference standard, such as a lab test result, in a sample of participants can be described using statistics (Chapter 4 in Sackett et al., 1991; Takwoingi et al., 2015) such as:

- Sensitivity (number of patients diagnosed with condition / total number meeting criteria for condition according to reference standard)
- Specificity (number not diagnosed with condition / total number not meeting criteria for condition according to reference standard)
- Positive predictive value (PPV) (number diagnosed with the condition that actually meet criteria for the condition according to the reference standard / total number diagnosed with the condition)
- Negative predictive value (NPV) (number not diagnosed with the condition that do not actually meet criteria for the condition according to the reference standard / total number not diagnosed with the condition)

Looking at the second type of situation, which is more common in mental health due to the lack of gold-standard references, the simplest measure of reliability is the percentage of agreement between clinicians as to the diagnosis. Unfortunately, there are several flaws with this (see Spitzer et al., 1967): it takes no account of the effects of agreement by chance and it gives no indication of the degree of disagreement over diagnostic categories (e.g. the difference between asthma and chronic obstructive airways disease is less than the difference between asthma and myocardial infarction).

The kappa concordance statistic was proposed as the best measurement of 'shared discrimination' between two doctors as to the diagnosis (see Chapter 6; Spitzer et al., 1967; Shrout et al., 1987). The simplest version is calculated by

{(probability of observed agreement – probability of expected agreement by chance)/
(1 – probability of expected agreement by chance)}

with probabilities expressed as fractions of 1.

It can be 'weighted' to reflect degrees of diagnostic disagreement—called weighted kappa (Spitzer et al., 1967). Agreement between multiple observers can be calculated (Shrout et al., 1987) using a modified version of kappa (Fleiss, 1971). The usefulness of the kappa statistic is affected by the base rate occurrence of the diagnosis: if it is infrequent then the kappa may become more unreliable, but this problem occurs with all alternatives to kappa (Shrout et al., 1987).

Kappa exists within a range of −1 (total disagreement between observers) to 0 (only chance agreement between observers) to +1 (total agreement between observers). Clearly, a value of 0 or less for a diagnosis indicates that its reliability is useless, but what do values > 0 mean? A commonly used interpretation of kappa values, based on judgement rather than objective measures, is given below (Viera and Garrett, 2005).

- < 0 less than chance agreement
- 0.01–0.20 slight agreement, *better than chance*
- 0.21– 0.40 fair agreement
- 0.41–0.60 moderate agreement
- 0.61–0.80 substantial agreement
- 0.81–0.99 almost perfect agreement

To understand what these kappa figures mean in real life, a couple of examples will be discussed. If a diagnosis was present in about 50% of cases seen by two doctors, and if the kappa value was 0.5, then the two doctors had agreed on the diagnosis about 75% of the time. If a diagnosis was present in 5% of cases seen by two doctors and the kappa value was 0.2, then two doctors had agreed on the diagnosis 24% of the time (Kraemer et al., 2012). There are alternative interpretations of kappa values (including weighted values) and intra-class correlation values (ICC), which is another measure of agreement often used in assessing reliability of psychological assessments including psychiatric symptoms (Cicchetti, 1994).

- < 0.40 poor agreement
- 0.40–0.59 fair agreement
- 0.60–0.74 good agreement
- 0.75–1.00 excellent agreement

The first set of interpretations will be employed here as they seem the most commonly used, but the latter will be used for discussing ICC values as Cicchetti's paper explicitly stated that they can be used to interpret ICC values (Cicchetti, 1994).

Factors that affect reliability of a diagnosis have been discussed in Chapters 4, 5, and 6 such as criterion or information variance and cultural and interpersonal factors. This chapter will present data on the reliability of diagnostic constructs in common psychiatric diagnostic systems before discussing the reliability of diagnosis in general medicine. It ends with a brief outline of reliability of alternative classifications.

Reliability of psychiatric diagnosis

The first step in increasing reliability of a psychiatric diagnosis is to have a common understanding of each diagnostic construct (Chapter 1 in Cooper and Sartorius, 2013) to reduce criterion variance. This led to developments including a glossary describing each construct in a prototypical case description (see Chapter 3) from ICD-8 onwards (Chapter 1 in Cooper and Sartorius, 2013). Reliability data for the most recent version of ICD (ICD-10) psychiatric diagnostic constructs based on this type of prototypical clinical case description are available (Regier et al., 1994).

Differences in diagnostic constructs of schizophrenia and other diagnoses led to differences in which diagnosis was chosen by UK and US psychiatrists when viewing videotapes of the same patients (Kendell et al., 1971). The reliability of psychiatric diagnosis in several early studies was collected and a mean calculated for the kappa of several diagnostic categories of 0.24–0.77 (Spitzer and Fleiss, 1974). These used a variety of methods and criteria thus mean kappa value is not the most valid measure but it gives the most practical method of summarizing this data.

In the United States, the St Louis Group promoted operational criteria, a set of rules with checklists that define each diagnosis (see Chapter 3) to reduce criterion variance. This led to the development of the Research Diagnostic Criteria (RDC) (Spitzer et al., 1978) which was the initial step towards DSMIII (APA, 1980) published by the American Psychiatric Association, whose explicit aim was to provide reliable psychiatric diagnosis for research, clinical, and administrative (including reimbursement) purposes. This was followed with further editions (DSM-IIR, DSM-IV, and DSM-5). Reliability data are available for most editions (Spitzer et al., 1978; Williams et al., 1992; Regier et al., 2013). I was unable to obtain any data for DSM-IV as these were found in 'DSM-IV Sourcebook Volume 4' which I could not obtain.

Different methods have been used for assessing participants, with two raters (usually psychiatrists or psychologists) then allocating a diagnosis. Both raters being present at the same interview of the participant (by one of the raters) or all raters being given the same information—either in the form of a written vignette, a videotaped interview, or a summary of the clinical details presented at a case conference—reduces information and occasion variance. Test and re-test methods involve the same participant being interviewed by two raters at separate times—this is a more realistic scenario and it does not reduce information or occasion variance.

Standardizing the questions that a rater asks the participant (a 'standardized interview') may reduce the information or performance variance. This can be markedly different from a typical clinical interview and may hinder collecting vital clinical information. A 'semi-structured standardized interview' may help with this problem by allowing the rater some flexibility in the questions asked (Chapter 9 in Cooper and

Sartorius, 2013). Some studies have the raters using their own method of assessing the participant, sometimes with guidance as to the best methods to adopt.

Rather than giving a mean kappa value for the entire diagnostic system (Spitzer et al., 1978; Kirk and Hutchins, 1994), it is more informative to present data on kappa for separate diagnostic categories under each type of diagnostic system. Most psychiatric diagnostic criteria shown in Table 8.1 are based on the clinical picture without laboratory (including imaging) test confirmation, although in clinical practice tests may be used to exclude some conditions (e.g. drug intoxication as cause of psychotic symptoms) or to confirm other conditions (e.g. Alzheimer's disease)

Several points that must be borne in mind. Not every psychiatric diagnostic construct in psychiatry is listed in this table. It is easier for clinicians to agree on a broader diagnostic category such as schizophrenia than a narrower category such as 'paranoid schizophrenia'. Most psychiatric diagnoses are in the moderate to substantial agreement range, which is reasonably impressive. There are exceptions to this; DSM-5 major depressive disorder and generalized anxiety disorder are in the slight to fair agreement range. Not listed in the table are examples such as DSM-5 mixed anxiety disorder, in DSM-5 with kappa value −0.004 (worse than chance) and in ICD-10 schizoid personality disorder with kappa value 0.2. A study with psychologists using standardized clinical interviews and DSM-5 found higher kappa values than the DSM5 field trials; for example, kappa value 0.72 for major depression (Tolin et al., 2016). Finally, differences in kappa values for the same diagnosis between different diagnostic systems may be due to methodological differences in the studies measuring reliability.

These figures for reliability are from research studies and may overestimate reliability in routine clinical practice. On the other hand, the reliability data shown below from general medicine will also include those from research which are similarly likely to be more reliable than routine clinical practice thus making it an equivalent comparison. One study (Miller et al., 2001) compared the psychiatric diagnosis of 56 participants based on routine clinical assessment ('traditional diagnostic assessment') plus other information compared to two standardized psychiatric interviews (the SCID-CV and CADI). Agreement and kappa values were compared with 'consensus' diagnosis (made using a structured method involving all psychiatrists using all the information). Using consensus diagnosis as the reference standard, traditional diagnostic assessment had 53.8% agreement and kappa = 0.4325 (fair agreement); the SCID-CV had 85.7% agreement and kappa = 0.8189 (excellent agreement); the CADI had 85.7% agreement and kappa = 0.8147 (excellent agreement). The main disagreement between traditional diagnostic assessment and consensus agreement was the high proportion of schizoaffective disorder diagnosis made by consensus (over one-third of the sample), which suggests either criterion variance or missing information from traditional diagnostic assessment or an unusual sample. In addition, schizoaffective disorder is a much less reliable diagnosis than schizophrenia or bipolar disorder (Santeman et al., 2016), thus its high prevalence in this sample reduced reliability in the whole sample. Taking this into account, the kappa in the fair agreement range seems acceptable.

Table 8.1 Reliability of psychiatric diagnosis in different classification systems.

	System	**DSMIII**	**DSMIII**	**DSMIIR**	**ICD-10**	**DSM-5**
	Reference	Spitzer et al, 1979	Spitzer et al, 1979	Williams et al, 1992	Regier et al., 1994	Regier et al., 2013
	Method	JNT	TR	SI/TR In patients	JNT or CC	TR
Diagnostic Broad category	Diagnostic Narrow category					
Childhood/Adolescence Disorders		0.66	0.81		0.71–0.85	
	Conduct disorder				0.6–0.78	0.46 (very imprecise estimate)
	ADHD					0.61
Learning Difficulty		0.66	0.85		0.77–0.79	
Organic brain syndrome		0.74	0.83		0.66–0.76	
	Chronic brain syndrome, e.g. dementia	1.0	0.74			0.78
Alcohol Problems				0.75	0.71–0.82	0.40
Drug problems		0.9	0.7	0.84		
Schizophrenia		0.82	0.82	0.65	0.79–0.81	0.46
	Paranoid SCZ				0.74–0.76	
Delusional disorder		1.0	1.0	0.69	0.52–0.68	
Schizoaffective		0.56	0.53	0.63	0.51–0.57	0.50
Mood disorder		0.70	0.65		0.66–0.79	

	Major depression			0.64	0.48–0.69single episode; 0.53–0.72 recurrent	0.28
Manic-depression/Bipolar type I				0.84	0.69–0.83	0.73
	Manic episode				0.69–0.77	
Personality disorder		0.61	0.54		0.51–0.52	
	Sociopathic/Psychopathy/Antisocial				0.43–0.65	0.20
	Borderline/Impulsive-EU				0.38–0.43	0.54
Neurosis/anxiety		0.74	0.43		0.68–0.73	
	Panic disorder			0.58		
	Agoraphobia			0.57		
	OCD			0.59	0.77–0.79	
	Generalized anxiety disorder			0.56	0.30–0.49	0.20
	PTSD				0.52–0.76	0.67
Eating disorders		–0.01	0.85			
	Anorexia nervosa			0.72		
	Bulimia nervosa			0.86		
Somatization/Somatoform	Briquet's/Somatoform/ Somatization Disorder	0.53	0.66		0.45 –0.68	

JNT = participant interviewed in presence of two raters, usually by one of the raters

Mixed = variety of different methods used

CC= participant interviewed by one rater, then clinical information presented to group of raters in case conference

SI = Standardized interview used by rater

TR= Test/Retest Participant interviewed on one occasion by a rater then on another occasion by a different rater

LT = lifetime diagnosis (when appropriate to designate as such)

Problems with identifying the correct diagnosis in general medicine

Chapter 4 discussed reasons for lack of reliability in diagnosis and how this affects psychiatric diagnosis in particular. In general medicine, conditions can also be difficult to diagnose correctly; that is, the diagnosis is unreliable. A few examples will now be given to illustrate this point. On some occasions, laboratory tests may be able to improve diagnostic reliability but they may not be ordered if the doctor is wrongly convinced that they have made the correct diagnosis or they may be misinterpreted due to an inaccurate diagnostic hypothesis. Some general medical conditions, such as epilepsy (Chapter 26 in Walker et al., 2014), are identified on the basis of the clinical picture, although tests may help to confirm the diagnosis. Other general medical conditions—often called functional or medically unexplained—are identified solely on clinical picture in the absence of confirmatory laboratory tests (see Chapter 12).

Pulmonary venous thromboembolism (PE) can have a similar clinical picture to other conditions (Chapter 19 in Walker et al., 2014). The differential diagnosis (see Chapter 2) for an acute massive PE includes myocardial infarction, pericardial tamponade, or aortic dissection. For an acute small/medium PE, the doctor must bear in mind the potential for the diagnosis to be a pneumonia, pneumothorax, or a musculoskeletal chest condition. An apparent chronic PE may instead be explained by other causes of pulmonary hypertension.

Excess glucocorticoids (Chapter 20 in Walker et al., 2014), often known as Cushing syndrome, has a very varied presentation (e.g. high blood sugar, centripetal obesity, high blood pressure), and can be confused with other common conditions with some similar features that also affect secretion of cortisol (e.g. obesity and depression). Gastro-oesophageal reflux disease (GORD) is a common condition that is classically associated with heartburn (Chapter 22 in Walker et al., 2014), but up to 50% of patients present with other symptoms such as chest pain or chronic cough.

Pyogenic liver abscess (Chapter 23 in Walker et al., 2014) often presents in an atypical fashion and the diagnosis is often only made at post-mortem. Necrotic colorectal metastases can be wrongly diagnosed as a liver abscess. Acute cholecystitis (acute inflammation of the gallbladder) can be confused for diseases located in the chest, oesophagitis, myocardial infarction, dissecting aneurysm, or biliary colic (Chapter 23 in Walker et al., 2014). Anaemia can be hard to diagnose (Chapter 24 in Walker et al., 2014), especially in the elderly, as the clinical features such as symptoms may be hard to detect and slow in onset.

Computed tomography (CT) scans of the head can detect up to 85% of subarachnoid haemorrhages (SAH) but can miss the rest as these scans struggle to detect small amounts of blood in the subarachnoid space (Chapter 26 in Walker et al., 2014). Lichen planus (Chapter 28 in Walker et al., 2014) is a condition of the skin and mucosa that can be hard to recognize as it may present in an atypical form. Lesions are commonly found in the mouth; they may not have been noticed by the patient or the doctor unless specifically sought.

Erythropoietic protoporphyria (Chapter 28 in Walker et al., 2014) is a rare porphyria that is often diagnosed late, despite being very symptomatic on exposure to sunlight, as the physical signs are often subtle. Associated anaemia can be confused for iron-deficiency anaemia. The accurate diagnosis of cardiac conditions is made more difficult because the range of possible cardiac symptoms is limited and so different disease processes often present with similar symptoms (Chapter 18 in Walker et al., 2014). The clinical pictures of dilated cardiomyopathy and specific heart muscle diseases (e.g. connective tissue disorders or sarcoidosis) are very similar. Other conditions that are hard to distinguish include amyloidosis, eosinophilic heart disease, and obliterative or restrictive cardiomyopathy. Hypertrophic cardiomyopathy has a similar clinical picture to heart disease associated with Friedrich's ataxia.

Chest pain can be caused by multiple conditions, many of them not cardiac in origin (Chapter 18 in Walker et al., 2014). Common causes of chest pain include emotional (e.g. anxiety), cardiac (e.g. angina or myocardial infarction), aortic (e.g. aneurysm), oesophageal (e.g. oesophagitis), respiratory (e.g. pulmonary embolism or pneumothorax), musculoskeletal (e.g. rib fracture or intercostal muscle injury), or neurological (e.g. herpes zoster).

The diagnosis of myocardial infarction (MI) can be made more complicated by the effects of gender and ethnicity on the presenting clinical picture, leading to the MI either receiving delayed treatment or being missed, with grave implications for outcomes (Barakat et al., 2003; Elsaesser and Hamm, 2004). Ethnic minorities such as Bangladeshis are less likely to present with classic central crushing chest pain even when the effects of diabetes are taken into account (Barakat et al., 2003). Women are also more likely to present with atypical clinical pictures (Elsaesser and Hamm, 2004). Using more sensitive lab tests (troponin-A) helps improve the diagnosis of MI in women (Shah et al., 2015).

Both syphilis and TB can be described as 'great imitators' in that their clinical pictures can resemble other conditions. In Chapter 4 there was a discussion of varied presentations of TB where the diagnosis was long delayed and even laboratory tests for TB were initially unhelpful in making the diagnosis (Sievers, 1961). Abdominal tuberculosis (Chapter 22 in Walker et al., 2014) can be confused for Crohn's disease, with similar clinical picture and radiological features. There may not be any signs of TB on the chest X-ray or pulmonary symptoms.

The diagnosis of von Willebrand's disease (Chapter 25 in Walker et al., 2014) can be more difficult in those with blood group O as they have lower circulating factors of von Willebrand factor than those with the condition who do not have blood group O. This needs to be taken into account when interpreting lab test results. Copper deficiency is a diagnosis that is easily missed (Chetri et al., 2014). The clinical picture is often hard to separate from subacute combined degeneration of the cord due to vitamin B12 deficiency and can also co-occur with this latter condition. This means that if vitamin B12 deficiency is confirmed in a patient then the doctor may not check for copper deficiency which may also be present. Copper deficiency can also be mistaken for myelodysplastic syndrome due to similar haematology test results.

An acute inflammatory arthritis called acute pseudogout resembles both gout and septic arthritis in its clinical picture (Chapter 25 in Walker et al., 2014). It is important to check for infection of the joint (e.g. Gram stain and culture of joint fluid) as a patient can have *both* septic arthritis and acute pseudogout, and the treatments and outcomes are very different.

Acute disseminated encephalitis (Chapter 26 in Walker et al., 2014) has a very variable clinical picture and can be confused with a first attack of multiple sclerosis. A variant of Huntingdon's disease —the Westphal variant—may present with parkinsonian symptoms instead of the more usual chorea, making diagnosis difficult and unreliable (Chapter 26 in Walker et al., 2014). Transient ischaemic attacks (TIA) is a diagnosis that may be unreliable if a history is not properly taken. Conditions with brief temporary symptoms, such as syncope or amnesia, may wrongly be diagnosed as TIA (Chapter 26 in Walker et al., 2014).

These general medical conditions illustrate the fact that even when a known mechanism/cause exists or there is a helpful diagnostic laboratory test for a general medical diagnostic construct, reliable diagnostic practice is not always possible due to similarities in clinical picture between different diagnostic constructs.

Reliability of general medical diagnosis

There is less focus on the reliability of medical diagnosis in the form of agreement between different doctors or other professionals. More often, the interest is in the error rate, using objective validating gold standards such as laboratory test results to determine how often a doctor gets the diagnosis wrong. Often people overestimate the reliability and objectivity of medical diagnosis compared to psychiatric diagnosis (Pies, 2007, the source of several papers cited below). Koran's review of the reliability of the clinical method included a variety of different methods of measuring agreement used by the included studies such as percentage of agreement between observers and the kappa statistic (Koran, 1975a, 1975b).

Research focusing on agreement between clinicians is more useful if it uses the kappa statistic to allow a better comparison with the research on reliability of psychiatric diagnosis summarized earlier. Sometimes this research is based on agreement of a diagnosis based on viewing the same test result—for example, X-ray or pathology slide—to reduce information variance (e.g. Weidow et al., 2006). Other studies may measure diagnostic agreement based on either clinical signs, such as conjunctival paleness to diagnose anaemia (Wallace et al., 2000), or diagnostic agreement based on interpreting two tests, such as ECG and troponin blood test results to diagnose myocardial infarction (Lim et al., 2006).

A more realistic type of study is where the participant is interviewed and examined by the doctor and a diagnosis made, but a diagnosis decided before laboratory results are known may underestimate the reliability of medical diagnosis in clinical practice. A study of this kind had both doctors present at the same interview and examination (Marin et al., 2010), which tends to give better reliability than doctors interviewing and assessing the participant separately.

One study used discharge summaries and interviewed medical students, senior doctors in management positions (medical managers), and coding specialists (professionals employed to allocate diagnostic codes using medical notes and discharge summaries for administrative/reimbursement purposes) (Stausberg et al., 2008). Using discharge summaries reduces information variance, but without actual contact with the patient, thus potentially reducing the amount of useful information to the clinician. This study used discharge summaries from patients who tended to have renal problems as the primary diagnosis. Kappa values are given for the medical managers. The terminal digit ICD-10 code is highly specific. The three-digit code corresponds more closely to the narrow diagnostic categories for psychiatry and the group codes match broader diagnostic categories for psychiatry. Incidentally, the coders were better for terminal digit codes (but still moderate reliability) than the medical managers (kappa = 0.42) and similar to medical managers for three-digit code and group code (kappa = 0.63 and 0.71, respectively).

There are some studies on the reliability of agreement over presence of signs on examination (e.g. Close et al., 2001). These are included to demonstrate that even what we regard as more objective clinical examinations in general medicine compared to psychiatry can still vary in their reliability. Psychiatry is not unique in that multiple factors can affect agreement between clinicians as to the presence of clinically important information (see Chapter 4), or that reliability is not perfect (see Tables 8.2, 8.3, and 8.4).

Appendicitis has a high degree of diagnostic unreliability with about 20% of surgically removed appendixes not showing pathological signs of inflammation in a large audit based on the United Kingdom. Use of CT scans can reduce this rate to 4.5–8.7% (D'Souza, 2015). In one study (Golden et al., 2016; see Table 8.4 for details), given that the female prevalence was 60%, the combined PPV was approximately 60% of a doctor's diagnosis of likely appendicitis being confirmed as appendicitis. (PPV was even lower in participants under 18 years old and was closer to 50%).

A study measuring kappa values for respiratory signs (Spiteri et al., 1988) looked at the agreement of physician diagnosis after examination compared with established diagnosis based on history, examination, and tests results. The accuracy in making the diagnosis varied with the condition but also with the skill and competence of the clinician. All the physicians had passed the MRCP, the postgraduate examination for general medicine and related specialties in the United Kingdom.

Koran's review (Koran, 1975a, 1975b) included studies featuring both kappa and percentage agreement (e.g. diagnosis of angina based on the history). One large study looked at three studies measuring diagnostic error (Singh et al., 2014) and extrapolated an error rate of 5% of US outpatient consultations. Like all extrapolations, this estimate may not be very accurate. Identifying errors relies on the presence of a gold standard validating external criterion. Another large review examined the usefulness of a variety of methods of estimating diagnostic error (Graber, 2013); autopsy studies are likely to give overestimates of rates of diagnostic error.

An examination of the data on reliability of diagnosis in medical specialties (including surgery) presented earlier shows a degree of overlap with reliability of psychiatric diagnosis. Reliability as measured by the kappa statistic tends to show moderate to substantial reliability—similar to psychiatric diagnosis—but some measurements are in the poor to fair range. Reliability as measured by judging comparison with a gold standard validating criteria is variable, dependent on the condition, but does seem high for many medical diagnostic constructs.

Table 8.2 Kappa values for diagnosis in medicine.

	Reference	**Weidow et al., 2006**	**Marin et al., 2010**	**Detre et al., 1975**	**Vobecky et al., 1989**	**Andrion et al., 1985**	**Stausberg et al., 2008**
	Method	Inspection of knee x-rays to stage osteoarthritis (OA) by two orthopaedic surgeons and two radiologists	Two doctors At same interview and examination	22 physicians viewing 13 angiogram 'cines', i.e. moving films	Three expert pathologists reviewed slides (no history) previously agreed criteria For diagnosis	Five pathologists reviewed slides (no history) 29/88 went for consensus review and results of these used as part of final analysis	34 medical managers reviewed five discharge summaries each (vignettes) coded for ICD10 codes kappa values for primary diagnosis
Broad category	Narrower category						
	Ahlback OA staging classification	0.11–0.12 Inter-observer					
Paediatric Skin/soft Tissue	Diagnosis of abscess		0.39				
	Need for drainage		0.43				
Vessel disease on angiogram films				'level of observer agreement for most angiographic items found to be approximately midway (dotted line) between chance expectation and 100% agreement' Interpreted as approx. 0.5 (Kraemer et al., 2012)			

Inter-pathologist agreement colorectal adenocarcinoma	Adenocarcinoma diagnosis	0.78		
	Gradation of differentiation	0.75		
Inter-pathologist agreement malignant mesothelioma	Overall		0.46	
	Necropsy and surgery		0.57	
	Endoscopy biopsy		0.54	
	Needle biopsy		0.21	
	Unspecified Biopsy		0.30	
ICD10 code	Terminal code (exact diagnostic subcategory)			0.27
	Three-digit code (diagnostic category)			0.56
	Group (broad diagnostic category)			0.64
	Chapter (system, e.g. digestive system)			0.71

Table 8.3 Kappa values for signs and diagnosis in medicine.

	Reference	Wallace et al., 2000	Gao et al., 2008	Close et al 2001	Koran 1975a & 1975b	Spiteri et al., 1988	Lim et al., 2008
	Method	Surgeons and ophthalmologists: consultant and registrars both specialties	One surgeon and one radiologist reviewed seven mammogram films per 101 participants	Agreement in bimanual pelvic examination findings between two doctors in the ED	Review of studies on reliability of clinical method (Table reference given)	24 physicians with MRCP of varying experience examined 24 patients	ECGs and troponin results assessed by two raters from patients admitted to ICU (results for troponin used as more representative for of clinical practice)
Broad category	Narrower category						
Diagnosis anaemia on conjunctival examination		0.36, 0.55, 0.39, 0.60 (no benefit for specialization or experience)					
Mammographic density indexes	Wolfe scale		0.87				
	Boyd scale		0.86				
Posterior tibial pulse/ dorsalis pedis pulse					A Table 8.1 0.605/0.513		
ECG normal or abnormal					B Table 8.4 0.725		
Joints considered 'diseased'					B Table 8.5 0.348		

Joints considered 'normal' or doubtful			B Table 8.5 0.471		
Signs of ulcerative colitis	Frequent 'reliable' signs		B Table 8.5 0.733–0.826		
	Frequent 'unreliable' or infrequent signs		B Table 8.5 0.500–0.568		
Pyelonephritis present or not			B Table 8.5 0.425		
Pyelonephritis present or not (undecided films included)			B Table 8.5 0.277		
Heart valve lesion present			B Table 8.6 0.601 (equivalent to 92% agreement)		
Chest signs (18 in total)	Six most reliable signs			0.43–0.52	
	Six intermediate reliability signs			0.32–0.41	
	Six least reliable signs			0.0–0.28	
Primary outcome	Myocardial infarction/ ischaemia				0.41
Secondary outcomes (six outcomes)	Three most reliable				0.44–0.84
	Three least reliable				-0.00–0.24
	Pelvic exam adnexal tenderness, adnexal mass, uterine size	0.07–0.26 (calculated in Kraemer et al., 2012)			

Table 8.4 Diagnostic errors/agreement in medical specialties not measured with kappa.

	Reference	**Hampton et al., 1975**	**Singh et al., 2014**	**Graber, 2013**	**Koran, 1975b**	**Spiteri, et al., 1988**	**Golden et al., 2016**
	Method	Physician agreement with referring GP's diagnosis after history/ examination tests	Three observational studies of outpatient care in the United States Diagnostic error is failure to recognize despite strongly indicative lab tests or take appropriate action	Review of variety of research techniques estimating diagnostic error	Review of studies on reliability of clinical method (Table reference given)	24 physicians with MRCP of varying experience examined 24 patients and making diagnosis. Compared with diagnosis made by own team based on history, examination, and lab tests	287 participants > 11 years old referred for CT scan to diagnose appendicitis Appendicitis confirmed by surgical findings/CT scan/ pathology report or clinical follow up – Prevalence =30% Accuracy of physician estimate of risk of appendicitis >60% Based on Clinical Picture 60% participants were female
Broad category	Narrower category						
Physician agreement with GP		46.25% agreement					
Primary care where correct diagnosis should be made earlier or abnormal test results followed up			6.3% errors				

	Lack of follow-up for abnormal tests indicative of colorectal cancer	0.009% errors	
	Lack of follow-up for abnormal tests indicative of lung cancer	21.64% errors	
Autopsy reports-clinically significant discrepancies in diagnosis			10–20% autopsies significant discrepancies
Standardized patients with common conditions			Internists misdiagnosed 13%
	Case reviews		12–51% of patients with subarachnoid haemorrhage are misdiagnosed in the emergency department

(*continued*)

Table 8.4 Continued

	Reference	Hampton et al., 1975	Singh et al., 2014	Graber, 2013	Koran, 1975b	Spiteri, et al., 1988	Golden et al., 2016
	Diagnosis of angina from history				Table 8.6 75% agreement		
	Agreement on cardiac valve lesion				Table 8.6 16–31% complete agreement 53–69% partial agreement		
Five to eight diagnoses for each patient, physician agreement on all Diagnoses					77% agreement For all diagnosis		
Accuracy of doctors' diagnosis compared to reference standard						72% correct diagnosis (from 0% for bronchiectasis and 36.3% for pneumonia to 100% for asthma and pneumonectomy)	Sensitivity Males 65%/Females 74% Specificity Males 74%/Females 68% PPV Males 69%/ Females 43% NPV Males 70%/Females 89%

PPV = Positive Predictive Value, NPV = predictive value

Reliability of alternative mental health classifications

This section will look at the reliability of three proposed alternatives to the psychiatric diagnostic systems (formulation, symptom-based, and dimensional). It should also be noted that these different types of classification are not mutually incompatible (see *promiscuous realism* in Chapter 1). Clinicians will often use more than one model during their clinical practice to help inform clinical decision-making. For example, DSM-5 has an explicit combination of a broad schizophrenia diagnostic category with five psychotic symptom dimensions and three additional dimensions (APA, 2013).

Psychological formulation is different in nature from diagnosis, symptom-based, and dimensional classification. The Division of Clinical Psychology has published a useful summary to explain psychological formulation (DCP, 2011) based on an earlier DCP publication (DCP, 2010). A psychological formulation is the summary of what relevant biopsychosocial factors have been learned during assessment placed in a framework using knowledge of psychological theories and research to help the clinician meet the client's needs.

The formulation also involves intuition, flexibility, and critical evaluation of one's experience, and is jointly constructed through a shared understanding between therapist and client of the latter's predicament (Chapter 6 in DCP, 2011). It differs from a psychiatric diagnostic formulation, which includes a preferred diagnosis and possible alternative diagnoses and a summary of the clinically relevant biopsychosocial factors (Chapter 9 in DCP, 2011).

A systematic review of the research on reliability of psychological formulations broke down the results into different theoretical models of psychotherapy (Flinn et al., 2015; see Table 8.5). Reliability was measured in terms of agreement between participants of the formulation of cases presented in various formats.

Two conclusions can be drawn from this systematic review. First, psychodynamic formulations provide the best evidence for reliability (Integrative psychotherapy formulations' reliability may have been inflated by the use of pooled judgments). Second, apart from psychodynamic formulation, the reliability of psychological formulation is inferior to that of psychiatric diagnosis (mostly in the slight to moderate/substantial range rather than the moderate to substantial range of psychiatric diagnosis).

The inferior reliability of psychological formulation compared to psychiatric diagnosis suggests that it is unable to replace psychiatric diagnosis in all situations (see Chapter 2 for a description of these roles of diagnosis). It may still have clinical utility as a *technique* when working using a psychological model, for example when providing psychotherapy. Even when listing the purposes of psychological formulation (Chapter 7 in DCP, 2011), the DCP guidelines do not include classification for purposes of research, administration, or statistics but suggest this may be an area of further development (Appendix 1 in DCP, 2011).

Symptom-based classification (an alternative term to symptoms is 'complaints' or 'experiences') classifies patients/clients based on the presence of individual symptoms. There are several advantages:

Table 8.5 Reliability of psychological formulation.

Flinn et al., 2015	**Psychotherapy Model**				
Reliability	**Cognitive**	**Behavioural**	**Psychodynamic**	**Integrative**	**Overall**
Virtually none to Moderate	One study				
Virtually none to Substantial					One study
Slight to Fair		One study			
Slight to Moderate	Two studies				
Slight to Substantial			One study		Six studies (two studies used pooled judgements which inflated reliability)
Slight/Fair to Substantial				Two studies (both used pooled scores which may have inflated reliability)	
Fair to Moderate			One study		Two studies
Moderate					Two studies (One study used pooled judgements which inflated reliability)
Moderate to Substantial			Five studies (Two studies used pooled scores which may have inflated reliability)	Three studies	Four studies
Substantial	One study				One study

- The classification is based on what is present in the patient (some patients with the same diagnosis may have different symptoms), so people classified on the basis of a symptom may be more homogenous than those based on a diagnosis. Mental health symptoms themselves can be quite heterogeneous, especially the more unusual experiences or beliefs associated with psychosis—the content of one person's paranoid delusion may differ markedly from another person's paranoid delusion.
- Some argue that symptoms should be (Bentall, 2006) and have been the primary focus of psychiatry/mental health as 'the basic unit of analysis' rather than conditions (Berrios, 2013).
- It may be easier to research the processes leading to a symptom, especially in complex systems like the mind/brain, rather than using heterogeneous diagnostic constructs (Bentall, 2014). On the other hand, it is customary to differentiate patients with similar symptoms if different causes are present (e.g. if someone experiences visual hallucinations as a result of taking LSD then their outcomes and treatment are likely to differ from somebody who has visual hallucinations in the absence of an obvious cause). This type of categorical decision-making then allocation to a group is a process I refer to as 'diagnosis by proxy'.

Rather than focus on disadvantages of a symptom-based classification that relates to utility, I will briefly examine the information available for reliability of symptoms.

One study controlled for information and criterion variance by asking three assessors to examine case notes, case abstracts, and case vignettes of 54 participants and used predefined descriptive criteria of symptoms to determine if a list of symptoms was present (McGuffin et al., 1991). This checklist included 57 symptoms and 17 other items (such as duration of illness); the symptoms covered psychotic symptoms and mood symptoms, including elated mood. The kappa values between different assessors for almost all the symptom items was in the moderate to substantial agreement range (but three symptoms such as 'loss of pleasure' had kappa values in the fair agreement range). Incidentally, agreement on the diagnosis had kappa values of 0.57–0.87 (mostly in the substantial range).

A review of the characteristic symptoms of schizophrenia (Andreassen and Flaum, 1991) found that many symptoms of schizophrenia had moderate to substantial or good to excellent inter-rater reliability (if the suggestions for ICC values are used), although some symptoms had only poor to fair reliability in occasional studies (such as 'flat affect' or 'bizarre delusions').

A systematic review of studies that used the Hamilton Rating Scale for Depression 17-item version (Bagby et al., 2004) examined the psychometric properties of this rating scale. A rating scale should reduce criterion variance for evaluating symptoms. The inter-rater reliability for depressive symptoms measured using this scale was found to be poor for many items and only adequate for some of the rest. Using standardized interviews improved the inter-rater reliability to excellent agreement, however trained psychiatrists differed 20–90% of the time on the same items. These problems in reliability may be due to the flaws in the Hamilton Rating Scale rather than great unreliability in assessing depressive symptoms per se (Bagby et al., 2004).

The large DOSMED study examined the outcomes of psychotic illness across 12 centres in 10 countries across several continents (Jablensky et al., 1992). This study used the Present State Examination-9 which is a semi-structured standardized interview schedule comprising 138 items covering a broad range of symptoms, for example, psychotic, depressive, and anxiety symptoms. A glossary defining symptoms and training reduced criterion variance. Reliability figures for agreement on ratings for symptoms between raters within each research centre and between research centres were ascertained (Chapter 1 in Jablensky et al., 1992).

Within ten research centres, joint assessments of participants by two raters (alternating in the role of interviewer and passive rater, reducing information variance) at initial assessment and follow-up assessment allowed assessment of reliability using the ICC statistic and Pairwise Agreement Rate. One symptom ('conversion') showed particularly poor reliability, but for 137/138 symptoms, the Pairwise Agreement Rate was 0.80 or more (or agreement as to presence of symptom between two raters was 80%). At the initial assessment, 67.4% of symptoms had ICC values in the good to excellent range (0.60+). Thirty-four case summaries were used to test reliability between research centres: 40 raters in 10 centres took part. The mean Pairwise Agreement Rate was 0.73 and the mean ICC across symptoms was 0.82 indicating excellent agreement.

Reliability of agreement for most psychiatric symptoms is in the moderate to substantial range; as in general medicine the reliability of agreement is less for certain symptoms. The reliability for most psychiatric symptoms is at least as good as that for diagnosis. Borsboom and colleagues calculated there are 439 symptoms listed in DSM-IV (Borsboom et al., 2011). As most patients have more than one (and indeed have many) symptoms, the usefulness of symptoms for statistical or administrative purposes is limited. The usefulness of symptoms based approach in clinical practice will be briefly discussed in Chapter 14.

The final type of classification that we shall examine is a dimensional classification. This is based upon the research evidence that certain symptoms tend to associate together in 'dimensions' in both the general population (e.g. Wright and colleagues suggested three dimensions: internalizing, externalizing, and psychotic experiences (Wright et al., 2013)) and in patients attending mental health services (e.g. Kotov and colleagues described five dimensions: internalizing, externalizing, thought disorder (equivalent to a broader psychosis grouping), somatoform, and antagonism (Kotov et al., 2011)). The names of these dimensions are *chosen* by the researchers based on what types of symptoms are associated with the dimension. These dimensions are sometimes referred to as factors after the statistical method—factor analysis—used to identify them. Dimensional classifications still involve categorical decision-making in a similar way to symptom-based classifications.

Within these larger dimensions can exist hierarchies and a number of smaller dimensions within dimensions or broad groups. Some have suggested that the psychosis dimension can be split into five smaller dimensions (van der Gaag et al., 2006b) or a more complicated hierarchical structure of a general psychosis dimension with five sub-dimensions (Reininghaus et al., 2013). Similarly, there is a suggested 11-dimension model for anxiety and depressive symptoms incorporating personality temperament (Brown and Barlow, 2009).

Symptoms may associate together but this does not necessarily mean that a categorical diagnosis is the best classification for research and clinical practice. Dimension-based classification is said to have certain advantages for the following problems with a categorical psychiatric diagnostic system (Widiger and Samuel, 2005):

- Many/most patients qualify for more than one diagnostic category; that is, high co-occurrence which may be due to similar underlying processes
- Boundary disputes between 'neighbouring' diagnostic categories such as bipolar I, bipolar II, and cyclothymia where the exact demarcating criteria are hard to determine reliably, if indeed they exist at all (see Chapter 3)
- Frequent use of 'Not otherwise specified' (or NOS) subcategory of a broader diagnostic category. Many diagnostic criteria describe a prototype of a concept (see Chapter 3). Many patients in clinical practice do not match easily to the prototypes described in the mainstream diagnostic categories so the NOS subcategory is used instead.

These criticisms are partly based on an assumption that a categorical diagnosis should always represent essentialist separate syndromes or diseases (see Chapter 3) rather than be used for nominalist description of an area of a spectrum of health/conditions. Some have argued that because categorical or dimensional classifications can be converted into each other they are essentially equivalent (Kraemer et al., 2004). In other words, they can both be used as classification methods and which is used depends on needs of the users of the classification.

Some studies have examined reliability of dimensional models in mental health. It is possible to measure dimensions using detailed questionnaires or complex assessments combined with formulae to produce dimension ratings or scores (see van der Gaag et al., 2006b for an example using the PANNS psychosis rating scale). This is a more complex type of assessment than is useful for brief appointments used in the medical model or when people are seen in emergency situations. There are studies examining the reliability of simple dimensional ratings made after assessments that are typical of the duration possible during the brief time of a medical appointments (see Chapter 5).

The CGI-SCH rating scale (Clinical Global Impression Schizophrenia scale) classifies psychosis in four dimensions and provides an overall global severity score (Haro et al., 2003). In three centres in Spain, Greece, and the United Kingdom, 114 patients were jointly assessed in outpatient-type durations on two separate occasions with one psychiatrist interviewing the patient whilst the other observed. This reduced information variance, and a manual describing how to use the rating scale reduced criterion variance. Intra-class correlations of inter-rater reliability for the four dimensions and global dimension (0.64–0.82) was substantial, except for the depressive subscale which was close at 0.64.

An older brief rating scale—commonly referred to as the 'KGV' scale—that can be used to assess different dimensions of psychosis was developed in Manchester (Krawiecka et al., 1977). An accompanying manual reduces criterion variance and tapes of ten patients being interviewed (reducing information variance) were rated by two psychiatrists who interviewed the patients and three psychiatrists who had trained themselves using the manual. Four symptom/dimension items were rated on basis of replies to questions, and four items—either symptoms or side effects—were based on observation. Kendall's efficient of correlation was used as a measure of agreement and varied between 0.58–0.87 for all items between the five psychiatrists (it was higher usually for items based on replies to questions than those based on observations). This seems a more than adequate degree of reliability.

The previous two studies examined brief dimensional measures of psychosis. The Health of the Nations Outcomes Scale (Wing et al., 1998) was designed as a practical, brief outcome scale for use in routine clinical practice (e.g. medical appointments). It measures several areas relevant to mental health that can be regarded as dimensions of symptoms, such as hallucinations and delusions (combined), cognitive symptoms, or depression. It also incorporates other important areas of assessment for mental health such as risk (aggression, self-harm), and social areas of concern such as relationships and residential environment. Less common mental health symptoms are rated under 'other symptoms', with separate subheadings. Physical health is also given a global rating. HONOS is used across the globe; when I worked in Australia it was widely used as a routine outcome measure.

An Australian study compared intra-class correlations from a variety of studies in Australia and the United Kingdom using various methodologies (Brooks, 2000). The UK trials were part of the development of the HONOS instrument and had far higher ICC scores than those run in Australian.

Overall, the ICC ratings for the different symptoms' dimensions scores varied from 0.40 to 0.81, that is, from less than satisfactory to excellent. The ICC was particularly low in the Australian trials. For the social items as a whole, the ICC was lower and ranged from 0.12 to 0.82. Differences in reliability is to be expected in psychometric assessments when comparing use in research centres or centres that develop the assessment to other centres where it may be used in routine clinical practice.

Dimensional assessments have been recommended as an alternative to the use of categorical diagnostic systems for classification in mental health. The number of dimensions to be measured varies depending on the nature of the presenting clinical problem. This great number may make it difficult to use dimensions for the administrative or other non-clinical roles of diagnosis (First, 2005b; see also Chapter 2). Brief assessment systems for dimensions that can be used in medical appointments are available. Their reliability appears equivalent to psychiatric diagnostic constructs.

Conclusion

The reliability of most psychiatric diagnostic constructs is in the moderate to substantial range in research studies but is likely to be lower in clinical practice. Some diagnoses in general medicine are not very reliable and in research studies reliability of diagnosis in medicine is similar to that of psychiatric diagnostic constructs. There is a degree of overlap between diagnosis in general medicine and psychiatry that but not near total overlap (see Table 8.6) due to the greater use of more objective tests in general medicine.

There are alternative classification systems for mental health problems. Psychological formulation—except psychodynamic formulation—is less reliable than psychiatric diagnosis. Symptom-based classification has at least equal reliability to psychiatric diagnosis. Dimension-based classification has equivalent reliability to psychiatric diagnosis. These alternative classifications may not as useful for administrative, statistical, or other functions of diagnosis. In clinical practice, a combination of these different classifications is often used to guide clinical decision-making.

Table 8.6 Reliability of psychiatric diagnostic constructs compared to general medicine.

	No Overlap	Some Overlap	Near Total Overlap
What is the reliability of the diagnosis when compared to a relevant reference criterion?		X	
What is the reliability of discriminating between different diagnoses?		X	

Chapter 9

Spectrums of health

Box 9.1 Questions to compare diagnostic constructs of psychiatry with general medicine

- Is the condition clearly separated from normality?

Are conditions that are given a diagnostic label capable of being separated from normality (see Box 9.1)? If a state is clearly separated from normality, does this automatically mean it is a condition of medical interest or an illness?

To answer this, we must have a definition of normality so that we can separate conditions from it clearly and dependably. Some conditions are identified by extremes of a range of values existing in a population—such as blood pressure—where every member of the population has a value and normality is defined as a statistically typical value. Other states are regarded as normal because they are regarded as typical or acceptable or a non-harmful individual variation of experience/process or structure. The term normality can also be used to refer to the usual state of affairs in most individuals in a population. Can a clear 'zone of rarity' (Kendall and Jablensky, 2003) be established between people meeting criteria for a diagnosis and the rest of the population? Is the demonstration of this 'zone of rarity' reliable and is it as objective as possible? A definition of normality does not imply people with states labelled normal are in some way superior to, or imply greater status or possess greater humanity than people in different states than those labelled normal or healthy. It also does not mean people in states different than those labelled normal or health are 'abnormal'.

This chapter begins with a discussion of whether psychiatric diagnostic constructs are clearly able to be separated from normality and then considers general medicinal diagnostic constructs that are difficult to separate from normality. Finally, there will be a brief look at alternative classification models in relation to their ability to separate mental health problems clearly from normality.

Psychiatric diagnostic constructs and separation from normality

This section will examine the broad groupings of emotional disorders (anxiety and depression), psychotic disorders (such as schizophrenia), and personality disorders and discuss whether they can be clearly separated from 'normality' or health.

In general medicine, conditions that are on spectrums of health are often defined based on directly measured variables such as blood pressure or plasma glucose. In mental health, conditions are often not measured directly (we do not have machines that measure how depressed someone is) but are assessed indirectly instead, such as asking about symptoms or completing questionnaires. The construct that is being measured indirectly—such as depression or schizophrenia—is said to be *latent* (Lubke and Miller, 2015). Apart from the use of this indirect measurement, there is usually the added complication that people from different cultural backgrounds will experience and describe distress or mental phenomena in different ways (see Chapter 4; Marsella, 1978; Kleinman, 1987, 2004; Berrios, 2013). Blood pressure is blood pressure, whether the person is from Derby or Dhaka. However, the latent construct labelled depression may be experienced or described differently (or not at all) in Newcastle compared to Nairobi.

There are several different statistical methods used to identify the best way to classify psychopathological entities (Haslam, 2003; Haslam et al., 2012; Lubke and Miller, 2015; Miettunen et al., 2016)- such as personality traits, psychosis, or depression- as discrete categories or as dimensional spectrums (see Chapter 3). Taxometric procedures, model-based clustering, and latent variable mixture modelling are different statistical methods, and which one that should be used depends on the nature of the data that are available (Lubke and Miller, 2015).

Depression is a heterogeneous diagnostic construct (Goldberg, 2011; Shorter, 2014) with many different types of distress subsumed under a single category and it frequently co-occurs with anxiety (Goldberg, 2011). Some believe melancholia should be separated out from depression (Cole et al., 2008); other terms such as endogenous depression may also be used to label this condition. It is said that this ancient diagnosis (the word 'melancholia' stems from the Greek for 'black bile', an excess of which was said to be the cause) more clearly distinguishes a qualitatively different experience of low mood and distress from that of normal sadness which at the severe end may meet the criteria for a depressive episode (Fink and Taylor, 2007; Carroll, 2012). Further differences that differentiate melancholia from other depressions include a higher chance of experiencing further episodes of low mood after the first episode without preceding severe life events (Brown et al., 1994). Other differences from other depressions include the use of biomarkers as part of the diagnostic criteria, such as REM sleep abnormalities or high cortisol production (Fink and Taylor, 2007; Parker et al., 2010), although the dexamethasone suppression test—the commonest measure of high cortisol production—has a mixed evidence base as a biomarker, including differentiating between different psychiatric diagnostic constructs (Arana et al., 1985).

Statistical techniques such as taxometry have been used to examine the question of whether depression best fits a discrete categorical model (like syndromes) or a dimensional model (like spectrums of health and other conditions, as described in Chapter 3). These largely agree that depression fits better with a dimensional model, but that there may be categories equivalent to endogenous depression or melancholia (Haslam, 2003). A more recent review of the taxometric evidence using the comparison curve fit index (CCFI) measure has confirmed this dimensional model of depression has more studies supporting it than the categorical model (Haslam et al., 2012).

Mario Maj suggested that the current diagnostic constructs of depression such as DSM-IV include dimensional elements (e.g. varying severity—mild/moderate/severe) as long as a threshold of number of symptoms and associated impairment is crossed, but this threshold may not be defined at the correct level and that severity of symptoms rather than number may be a better method of deciding if depression should be diagnosed (Maj, 2012).

For generalized anxiety disorder in both adults and adolescents, varying the diagnostic thresholds, such as duration of symptoms, greatly alters the condition's prevalence, indicating that this condition exists on a dimensional spectrum in the population rather than as a discrete category (Burstein et al., 2014).

Three nationwide surveys of psychiatric morbidity (symptoms and diagnosis) have taken place in the United Kingdom, for which data are available (Jenkins et al., 1997, Singleton et al., 2001; McManus et al., 2009) included 7,400 to 10,100 participants each, interviewed by lay interviewers (i.e. not mental health professionals) using standardized interviews (the Revised Clinical Interview Schedule (CIS-R)) to identify the presence of common mental disorder (CMD). These participants were chosen as representative of the national population. Additional assessments were carried out, including those looking for relatively rare conditions such as schizophrenia. Depending on the assessment results, a smaller number of participants were chosen for the second phase of interviews by psychiatrists or psychologists using more detailed standardized assessments to identify rarer psychiatric conditions.

The CIS-R assesses symptoms lasting at least a week, such as depressive or anxiety symptoms as well as sleep, fatigue, and irritability, collectively referred to as 'neurotic' symptoms. The threshold for CMD was a CIS-R score of 12 or more and an algorithm was used to decide which CMD was present depending on which pattern of symptoms was present. From 14.4 to 16.4% of adults aged 16 to 64 across the three surveys (McManus et al., 2009) met this criterion for CMD.

Diagnostic constructs such as depression or generalized anxiety may be different aspects of a broad spectrum of conditions (see Chapters 3, 4, and 11), therefore it will be helpful to examine total number of neurotic symptoms within the population. The range of CIS-R scores can be broken into four bands and from the three surveys for adults aged 16 to 64 (McManus et al., 2009) the percentage of participants in each band were as follows

- 66.1–67.1% had CIS-R scores 0–5
- 17.0–18.8% had CIS-R scores 6–11
- 7.2–8.4% had CIS-R scores 12–17
- 6.9–8.5% had CIS-R scores 18+

This distribution of scores is consistent with a spectrum of neurotic symptoms distributed throughout the population, albeit with lower numbers of symptoms being the most common. There is no clear 'zone of rarity' of CIS-R scores between those meeting the criterion for CMD and those not. This is consistent with the evidence of taxometric studies that neurotic symptoms follow a dimensional spectrum within the population instead of a categorical model (Haslam, 2003; Haslam et al., 2012).

Schizophrenia is another heterogeneous diagnostic construct comprising many different conditions (Eugen Bluler referred to the 'schizophrenias' to emphasize this (Hoenig, 1983)). The question of whether the different psychotic diagnostic constructs are separate entities is discussed in Chapter 11. The Schizophrenia Library in Australia regularly reviews the evidence about people meeting the criteria for schizophrenia (Matheson et al., 2014). It noted high-quality evidence for several differences, comparing participants meeting criteria for schizophrenia and 'healthy control' participants (apart from the presence of psychotic symptoms).

- Large effect sizes (see Chapter 15 for an explanation of this term) for increased presynaptic dopamine function (but not presynaptic dopamine transporter density) in participants diagnosed with schizophrenia.
- Large effect sizes for a variety of cognitive impairments in participants diagnosed with schizophrenia such as information processing, theory of mind, and working memory.
- Medium effect sizes for differences in sizes of brain structures and white-matter abnormalities.

There was also high-quality evidence for differences found in relatives of participants meeting criteria for schizophrenia and for participants who may be in the early stages of developing a psychosis condition.

- Medium effect sizes of similar cognitive impairments in first-degree relatives of participants meeting criteria for schizophrenia.
- Small effect sizes for cognitive impairments in people at risk of developing psychosis/in the prodromal stages.

Many other differences are recorded, often with lower quality evidence, for participants meeting criteria for schizophrenia compared to healthy control participants, such as higher numbers of minor physical anomalies (Matheson et al., 2014). These are differences *averaged* over a group and there can be an *overlap* between individuals in two different groups even with large effect sizes. For example, even though there is a large effect size difference of cognitive impairment between participants meeting schizophrenia criteria and healthy controls, some people meeting schizophrenia criteria achieve first-class university degrees whilst other people regarded as healthy may struggle to get passing grades at school.

Despite evidence of many differences, none are sufficiently clear-cut to be used as the basis of tests which reliably identify schizophrenia and that can be used to supplement or replace clinical interviews and assessments. Even using the latest brain-scanning techniques analysed using sophisticated classification schemes gives insufficient inaccuracy to diagnose individuals with schizophrenia (Kambeitz et al., 2015).

Famously, Rosenhan concluded that even with clinical assessments and interviews it is clear that we cannot distinguish the sane from the insane in psychiatric hospitals (Rosenham, 1973). In this famous experiment, eight people presented to different hospitals complaining of hearing a voice saying 'thud', 'empty', or 'hollow'. They were admitted to hospital and proceeded to act normally and were kept in hospital for days, sometimes weeks, and were almost always diagnosed with schizophrenia.

Assuming the experimental subjects were truthful in their reports of their behaviour, this experiment measures whether clinicians can distinguish between people falsely reporting psychotic symptoms and those truly experiencing psychosis. It then tests whether clinicians can overcome an initial faulty conclusion. It does demonstrate the value of reliable tests to aid diagnosis and the fact that their absence causes problems. On the other hand, as Clare points out, it is a very different healthcare environment where somebody with one symptom and little evidence of risk or impaired functioning gets admitted to hospital easily and stays for long periods when UK clinicians struggle to get people admitted with high levels of distress, obvious impairment of functioning, and/or risk (Chapter 3 in Clare, 2011).

If psychotic symptoms identified at clinical assessment are used as the basis for meeting criteria for a diagnosis of schizophrenia (or other psychosis diagnostic construct), then what is the evidence for their distribution across the population? Various arguments exist as to whether the distribution of psychotic symptoms in the population fits categorical or dimensional models better. The debate is complicated by disagreements about the degree of *continuity* between milder psychotic like experiences and those experiences regarded as full-blown psychotic symptoms; that is, are they really on the same spectrum (Sommer, 2010)? There is also the complication that some commentators wish to emphasize continuity between psychotic symptoms and everyday experience for *moral* reasons to reduce stigma by demonstrating psychosis is not different from 'normality' (David, 2010).

Some studies have suggested a dimensional structure for 'paranoia' or persecutory beliefs in the population (Freeman et al., 2005; Bebbington et al., 2013). However, these studies often include everyday suspicious thoughts (e.g. 'do you find it hard to be "open" even with people you are close to?') as well as descriptions of experiences that are more likely to be clinically paranoid ('have you ever felt that your thoughts were directly interfered with or controlled by some outside force or person?'). They found that those who reported symptoms of clinical paranoia also tended to report far more suspicious thoughts, so an apparent continuum may be a continuum of everyday suspicious thoughts with an overlapping additional population of clinically paranoid individuals who also have many everyday suspicious thoughts as well. It has been suggested that an apparent continuity of psychotic symptoms between 'normality' and severe psychosis may in fact be an overlap of two separate populations, one with psychotic or psychotic-like experiences with low need for care and another population with psychotic experiences/symptoms associated with motivational and cognitive impairments associated in turn with a higher need for care (Kaymaz and van Os, 2010).

A study using data on psychotic symptoms collected from the National Comorbidity Survey (NCS) in the US (broadly similar to the UK National Psychiatric Morbidity Surveys mentioned earlier except using the Composite International Diagnostic Interview (CIDI)) concluded after using latent variable mixture modelling that psychotic symptoms in the population followed a dimensional model (Miettunen et al., 2016). Concerns remain about the quality of data obtained as the CIDI interviews were carried out by trained interviewers who were not clinicians; their judgement as to whether the interviewed person was describing a psychotic symptom or not may differ from that of clinicians. This reduces the confidence one can hold in the result of the study.

A review of the evidence for the underlying structure of psychosis discussed several points (Linscott and Van Os, 2010). The prevalence and incidence of individual psychotic symptoms was far higher in the population than the incidence and prevalence of schizophrenia; some symptoms were 3 to 28 times more prevalent. There was a great degree of variation of the incidence and prevalence of psychotic symptoms related to social and demographic factors such as unemployment, immigration, and exposure to trauma. This fits with the dimensional model of psychosis throughout the population, but against this the analysis of variation in incidence and prevalence of psychotic symptoms showed that about 50% of this variation was due to different methods of assessing and classifying experiences as psychotic symptoms.

Linscott and Van Os then summarized the results of statistical analysis of psychometric studies of a boundary between schizophrenia and health based on questionnaires measuring 'schizotypy' and concluded that there was good evidence for such a boundary. This boundary, however, created a larger group of people than just those who met the criteria for schizophrenia, that is these schizophrenia diagnostic criteria may identify a severe end of a psychosis spectrum that was itself separated from health. 'Schizotypy' is a concept based on a model proposed by Meehl (1962) and summarized by the study authors (Linscott and Van Os, 2010) as an inherited brain state ('schizotaxia') with problems in neurointegration and a particular personality type with a dimension with no clear demarcations between 'schizotypy' and schizophrenia.

A meta-analysis of studies of incidence and prevalence of psychotic experiences (PE) in the community found a *median* (not mean) annual incidence of 2.5% and a prevalence of 7.2% (Linscott and van Os, 2013). Social and demographic factors as well as methodology strongly influenced incidence and prevalence rates. About 20% of individuals with PE experience persistent PE and 7.4% go on to meet criteria for a psychosis diagnostic construct. A large worldwide survey of mental health problems of 31,261 participants in 18 countries reported mean lifetime prevalence of PEs of 5.8% with hallucinations (5.2%) much commoner than delusions (1.3%) and 72% of those experiencing PE reporting a single PE (McGrath et al., 2015).

In adolescents without a psychotic disorder, factors such as history of trauma and urbanicity (and to a lesser extent cannabis use) in combination with increased severity of non-psychotic symptoms was associated with psychotic experiences/symptoms being present (Guloksuz et al., 2015). Another study of adolescents found that psychotic symptoms tended to be associated with more severe anxiety and depressive symptoms (Stochl et al., 2015).

Van Os proposes that there is both an 'extended psychosis phenotype', that consists of a spectrum of unusual experiences that at the severe end would be regarded as hallucinations and delusions, and a 'transdiagnostic psychosis phenotype' in which psychotic symptoms can occur across diagnostic categories (Van Os and Reininghaus, 2016). The 'transdiagnostic dimension of psychosis' would be better represented by five dimensions.

Responses to the article include the earlier concern that apparent continuity between unusual experiences and psychotic symptoms may be a measurement error due to oversimplified criteria for defining psychotic symptoms that lose an important grasp of the whole nature of the experience and how it differs from more common unusual experiences (Parnas and Eriksen, 2016). They point out there is evidence of differences in the experience of auditory hallucinations between clinical and non-clinical populations (Stanghellini et al., 2012; Johns et al., 2014). This is consistent with arguments that psychotic-like experiences are different in important aspects such as distress and preoccupation from psychotic symptoms (David, 2010). Another reply to the article points out that the relationship between psychotic experiences predicting development of mood or anxiety problems more than a psychotic disorder is because mood and anxiety problems are more common than psychotic disorder (Yung and Lin, 2016).

A more recent paper points out that prevalence of psychotic or psychotic-like experiences may have been overestimated by including experiences as that were misunderstood (or wrongly classified) as psychotic experiences or were likely to be realistic experiences, and that these types of experiences were not more likely in relatives of people with a psychotic disorder compared to those without such relatives (Landin-Romero et al., 2016). This would suggest there may not be continuity between psychosis-like experiences and psychosis, but the sample size was relatively small.

A different approach to focusing on positive psychotic symptoms as the central element of schizophrenia has been taken by Professor Parnas and colleagues. They focus on 'anomalous self-experience' as a core feature of schizophrenia from the early descriptions of German and other European psychiatrists. Examples include distorted sense of passage of time or feeling as if one's external boundaries are merging with the environment (these anomalous self-experiences are described in greater detail in papers available from the website <http://www.easenet.dk>). Anomalous self-experiences are assessed using an interview schedule (Parnas et al., 2005) called EASE (Evaluation of Anomalous Self Experience) that has been shown to have acceptable inter-rater reliability (Møller et al., 2011).

Studies have shown that scores on the EASE are significantly much higher in people diagnosed with schizophrenia or at risk of psychosis or with schizotypal disorder (similar to schizotypy as described above) than healthy controls (Parnas and Henriksen, 2014). Direct comparisons of scores is difficult to achieve as different scoring methods are used in different studies, but there is clear evidence of discontinuity in scores between healthy controls and people meeting criteria for a 'schizophrenia spectrum' disorder. Not everyone with schizophrenia or related conditions reported anomalous experiences but if several are present it is a clear differentiating feature from healthy states and other conditions including bipolar disorder.

Difficulties related to long-standing patterns of thinking, behaviour, experience, or interpersonal relationships are often referred to as personality disorders; whether this is an appropriate term for difficulties that often arise after traumatic experiences will be discussed in Chapter 14. Current diagnostic constructs of personality disorder derive from nine personality types described by the German psychiatrist Kurt Schneider in 1923, based on his clinical experience (Tyrer et al., 2015).

These constructs continue to be used despite the frequent use of 'not otherwise specified' personality disorder diagnostic codes (as patients do not fit neatly into a single category) and as well as several personality disorder categories being used for the same patient (Tyrer et al., 2011). The use of several categories is because the difficulties used as diagnostic criteria seem to be present in multiple dimensions that cut across several diagnostic categories (Widiger and Simonsen, 2005).

There has been interest in determining if difficulties described under the personality disorder categories are extreme examples of personality traits found in the general population described under 'general population' personality models. Experts have tried to describe personality disorders using the Five Factor Model of personality (Lynam and Widiger, 2001) as well as other dimensional models of personality (Widiger and Simonsen, 2005). Some experts in personality disorder have criticized this model of continuity between the clinical prototypic descriptions of personality disorder features with general population personality traits (i.e. developed from research on non-clinical samples) pointing to lack of evidence for this, and that general population personality traits in return do not map well onto the clinically important features of personality disorder (Shedler et al., 2010). However other experts view the evidence as demonstrating a high correlation between features of personality disorder and general population personality traits (Widiger and Samuel, 2005).

The commonly used personality disorder categories have a dimensional distribution of their features in clinical populations; there is a range of number of diagnostic criteria found in populations studied not restricted only to those that met personality disorder criteria. This can be found for a specific category such as borderline personality disorder but a threshold effect on clinical utility is found once a certain number of diagnostic criteria are met (Asnaani et al., 2007; Zimmerman et al., 2013). This dimensional distribution of features of multiple DSM-IV personality disorder categories was also found to be present in clinical populations and to predict outcomes better than general population dimensional personality models (although the latter predicted some outcomes better) (Skodol et al., 2005). One large study following participants for ten years compared the predictive utility of DSM-IV personality disorder diagnostic constructs (both as categories and dimensions) with those of general population personality models (Morey et al., 2012). This study found that personality disorder diagnostic constructs and general population personality models contributed to different elements of predictive utility.

, A 'hybrid model' of classification was proposed for DSM-5. This included both several personality disorder prototypic categories as well as personality disorder diagnosed on the basis of troublesome personality traits based on the general population personality models. This was rejected for the main section (but was allowed to be used as an 'alternative model') due to concerns about practical usability for busy clinicians as well as lack of research evidence for the use of general population personality models in a clinical population (Zachar et al., 2016).

Taxometric studies have found that dimensional models more accurately reflect distribution of personality traits than categorical models (Haslam, 2003; Haslam et al., 2012). Earlier taxometric studies suggested that psychopathic personality may be better classified with a categorical model (Haslam, 2003), but a more recent review concluded that psychopathy is also distributed dimensionally in the population (Haslam et al., 2012). Schizotypal personality (the personality type associated with 'schizotypy') is best classified as a separate category (Haslam, 2003; Haslam et al., 2012). Schizotypal personality may be better classified as part of the spectrum of schizophrenia conditions (Meehl, 1962) rather than with personality disorders.

Psychiatric disorders commonly seen in adult psychiatry usually follow dimensional distributions, not discrete categorical models. Either there is a spectrum that is continuous with health (such as depressive and anxiety symptoms or ADHD; Asherson et al., 2016) or there may be a spectrum of condition that is separate from health on some measures (such as the schizoptyal–schizophrenia–psychosis spectrum). Sometimes conditions that appear to sit on a spectrum continuous with health may in fact be a syndrome (such as melancholia).

Diagnostic constructs have often been created by applying thresholds across a dimension to create a category (Goldberg, 2000; Kraemer et al., 2004). These categories may reflect the underlying dimensionality of psychopathology with titles indicating varying severity (e.g. mild, moderate, and severe depression). Categories are used to classify participants for research, to identify cases as eligible for care and treatment, to certify people as being eligible for welfare benefits, and, as part of administration and statistics, to assist in all the other functions of diagnosis (see Chapters 2 and 3).

General medical conditions and separation from normality

This section will mainly discuss some conditions—but not all—in general medicine that do not exhibit a 'zone of rarity' with the healthy population.

The National Institute for Health and Care Excellence (NICE) produced guidelines on obesity, justifying this being a condition of medical interest because of its association with many illnesses such as hypertension, its psychological consequences, and costs to society in general (NICE, 2014c). It used a definition based on body mass index calculated by dividing the body mass in kg by the height in metres squared

- healthy weight: 18.5–24.9
- overweight: 25–29.9
- obesity I: 30–34.9
- obesity II: 35–39.9
- obesity III: 40 or more

Different thresholds are used in different ethnic groups to trigger intervention and care is advised in certain body types such as people with high muscle mass. This definition defines large segments of the UK population as having a medical condition—obesity—24% of men and 26% of women (NICE, 2014c).

These thresholds do not identify 'zones of rarity' and there is little absolute difference in risk between people with an overweight body mass index (BMI) of 29.9 compared with people with an obesity I BMI of 30.0. These thresholds are defined to identify cases for offering interventions/treatment as well as identifying different groups for research and those at differing levels of risk. These thresholds are defined by expert committees interpreting the evidence. The measurements may be more objective than number and severity of mental health symptoms, but subjective judgement is still used in deciding the thresholds.

Thresholds for identifying hyperlipidaemia are applied to continuous values of lipids in the population based on risk of health consequences—mainly risk of cardiovascular disease (Chapter 16 in Walker et al., 2014). Hyperlipidaemia is usually caused by a complex mix of factors such as genetics and diet, but some cases are due to syndromes/ diseases such as familial hypercholesterolemia (Chapter 16 in Walker et al., 2014)

High blood pressure is also called hypertension. Blood pressure values exist as a continuum within the population. Hypertension is defined at a pragmatic threshold where treatment benefits are likely to outweigh the risks or adverse effects of treatment (Chapter 18 in Walker et al., 2014). Hypertension is usually asymptomatic—albeit associated with pathological changes—but is considered a medical condition due to the associated complications such as heart disease, stroke, or kidney disease. Sometimes hypertension is caused by an identifiable syndrome such as Cushing's syndrome (Chapter 20 in Walker et al., 2014), but it is usually caused by complex mix of factors such as genetics and lifestyle (Chapter 18 in Walker et al., 2014). Thresholds are again decided by expert committees based on evidence of harm caused by higher levels of blood pressure (Emdin et al., 2015b), not distress caused by symptoms, and benefits of medical interventions to reduce these risks (ALLHAT, 2002; NICE, 2011).

Type 2 diabetes is a heterogeneous diagnostic construct of *exclusion* made when diagnostic criteria for diabetes are met and known causes of diabetes, such as diabetes type 1, are shown to be absent. It usually has complex multifactorial causes. Diagnostic thresholds are applied to blood glucose values which are distributed continuously throughout the population. The thresholds are chosen to identify those at higher risk of complications due to microvascular pathology (e.g. diabetic retinopathy) but also associated with other complications such as large vessel disease (causing myocardial infarctions, for example). Impaired glucose tolerance is defined using a lower threshold to identify cases where there is a higher risk of developing diabetes in the future and large vessel disease (Chapter 21 in Walker et al., 2014).

Plasma glucose levels are used to divide the population into three groups—normal, impaired glucose tolerance (pre-diabetes), and diabetes—with no 'zone of rarity' between these three states. The latter two conditions are identified for the clinical utility of recognizing people at increased risk of complications despite the lack of validity as they are not clearly separated from normality.

The current diagnostic threshold for chronic kidney disease is controversial in elderly people; about 50% of people over 75 meet the criteria (Ellam et al., 2016). The diagnostic criteria are useful for epidemiological purposes; to identify people at increased risk, but for older people this threshold is not very predictive of the development of end-stage renal failure or risk of cardiovascular events (Ellam et al., 2016). There is a continuum of renal function in the population, and the diagnostic threshold when applied to the older age group experiencing normal age-related decrease in renal functioning leads to many people being given a diagnosis for little clinical utility.

Osteoporosis is the most common bone disease and affects 50% of women and 20% of men by their eighth decade (Chapter 25 in Walker et al., 2014). Osteoporosis and the milder form, osteopenia, can be diagnosed using bone scans to measure bone mineral density (BMD) which is then compared to age-matched controls. Osteoporosis is defined by BMD 2.5 standard deviations or more less than expected mean whereas osteopenia is diagnosed when the BMD is between −1.0 and −2.5 standard deviations below the expected mean. Again, we have populations divided into normal or a medical condition with experts setting thresholds on spectrums and no 'zones of rarity'.

Unfortunately, the thresholds identify many people who are healthy (especially those aged 50 or more) as having osteopaenia and some people who with osteoporosis have BMD vales in osteopaenic or even normal range, especially if other conditions such as aortic calcification or osteoarthritis are present (Chapter 25 in Walker et al., 2014). Even with objective measurements, subjective interpretation is needed, taking into account presence of other conditions. The major reason to treat osteoporosis is to prevent complications such as fractures of the hip and vertebrae. This diagnostic threshold was introduced in 1994 with the support of drug companies which shortly afterwards introduced drug therapies which were shown to prevent hip fractures (Jarvinen et al., 2015).

Osteoarthritis is the most common type of arthritis and affects up to 80% of people over the age of 75 (Chapter 25 in Walker et al., 2014). It is characterized by excessive wear-and-tear damage to the joints that exists on a continuum with normal wear-and-tear damage. There can also appear prominent signs of osteoarthritis on X-rays of joints without the patient complaining of symptoms (Bennell et al., 2012), meaning that objective changes do not always mean that a medical condition is present.

Gout is the commonest inflammatory arthritis and is caused by excessive uric acid which has a normal distribution in the population: hyperuricemia being defined as two standard deviations above the mean serum uric acid for the population (Chapter 25, Walker et al., 2014). This threshold does not perfectly identify cases of gout as there is little benefit from treating asymptomatic hyperuricemia. Slightly different therapeutic targets are set to lower serum uric acid to by different expert committees (Chapter 25 in Walker et al., 2014).

Acne vulgaris is a common condition that affects up to 90% of the population during adolescence (Chapter 28 in Walker et al., 2014). Even milder occurrences can be associated with low self-esteem, negative emotions, and bullying. It is regarded as a medical condition if the psychosocial consequences of acne are so severe that the patient wants medical help, such as antibiotics.

Even the presence of objective investigations can be unreliable, separating the healthy population (normality) from those with medical conditions without the addition of careful history taking and examination. The electroencephalogram (EEG) shows abnormal readings in about 5% of the normal population and shows normal readings in routine EEGs in up to 50% of patients with epilepsy (Chapter 25, Walker et al., 2014). In endocrine or autoimmune conditions, there can be an overlap in blood test results with healthy people. For example, 8–27% of the healthy population have antibodies to thyroid peroxidase and 5–20% antibodies to thyroglobulin (Chapter 20 in Walker et al., 2014), and 5% have anti-nuclear antibodies and 1.5% anti-smooth muscle antibodies (Chapter 23 in Walker et al., 2014), and 10% have 'rheumatoid factors', antibodies against IgG isotype form of antibodies (Mohan and Assassi, 2015).

An isolated raised thyrotropin score in the absence of signs, symptoms, or other lab tests suggestive of thyroid disease can be found in obese children but seems a consequence of obesity rather than a cause. This 'subclinical hypothyroidism' is best treated by measures to lose weight (Niranjan and Wright, 2016).

Chronic obstructive pulmonary disease (COPD)— sometimes called chronic obstructive airways disease (COAD)—is a common condition (Miller and Levy, 2015). There is a continuum of degree of airway resistance in the population and COPD is diagnosed based on exceeding a threshold of measured airway resistance. A relatively recent change in the diagnostic threshold from previously 'lower limit of normal' for someone based on age, gender, and other factors to the simpler 'GOLD' criteria has led to an increase in people being diagnosed with COPD. Moreover, these new 'milder' cases are actually at increased risk of cardiovascular mortality, possibly as a result of being treated for COPD (Miller and Levy, 2015).

In an article describing the chronic disease explosion, (McGrail et al., 2016), the Global Burden of Disease study (Vos et al., 2015) was discussed. It implied that only 4% of the global population do not have a diagnosable medical condition. Financial incentives to recognize and treat co-occurrence from third-party payers may be a factor in increasing rates of diagnosis. There was evidence that lower diagnostic thresholds were leading to more people being diagnosed with medical conditions. This merely emphasizes the conclusion from the above review of general medical conditions that identifying conditions clearly separate from health or normality is an issue across *all* medical specialties, not just psychiatry. It has been suggested that rather than rush to diagnose and treat people close to thresholds, a more holistic approach is warranted (Johannson et al., 2016).

'Overdiagnosis' in medicine is defined as 'when people without symptoms are diagnosed with a disease that ultimately will not cause them symptoms or early death' (Welch et al., 2011), which leads to concerns that 'too many people are being overdosed, overtreated, and overdiagnosed' (Moynihan et al., 2012). The term 'disease' is used here but could also be taken to mean 'condition'.

There is a concern that dropping thresholds for defining health states as conditions suitable for medical attention will lead to iatrogenic harm ('harm caused by doctors' actions'), waste of resources, and a false sense of tackling a complex situation (Treadwell and McCartney, 2016).

Setting thresholds across spectrums of human attributes (whether it is weight, blood pressure, or distressing emotions) measured by laboratory tests or assessing a patient's subjective experience in order to define conditions by committees of experts is common across medical specialties. There is concern across all medical specialties about whether the thresholds are set too low by these expert committees being influenced by drug companies to increase the numbers of people prescribed drugs (Le Fanu, 2012). Setting thresholds too low leads to high numbers of people being 'medicalized' and offered treatments that may be unnecessary at best and dangerous at worst. Setting thresholds too high may lead to denial of access to care to people that may be beneficial in reducing distress or preventing adverse outcomes. Some medical conditions, such as hypertension, are largely asymptomatic and treated to prevent adverse outcomes (such as heart disease). Arguably, conditions such as depression and anxiety, which are in themselves distressing and associated with impaired functioning as well as risk of adverse outcomes (such as suicide), are better examples of illness than conditions such as hypertension, even if their measurement and assessment is more subjective and more culturally influenced.

Alternative forms of classification and separation from normality

Psychological formulations do not need to set thresholds across a continuum when explaining how the client's current predicament has come about and why it continues. These formulations may use evidence based on classification systems that use thresholds. In self-paying services or if the service is open access, there may no administrative necessity to apply a threshold in order to justify access. In services with a third-party payment, someone will need to apply a threshold for the client to be permitted access to the service and for activity recording. For access to other societal benefits (e.g. welfare) a formulation will need to demonstrate a threshold has been exceeded. Sometimes an additional classification system (e.g. diagnosis) can be utilized, either by the 'formulating' professional or another member of the team to allow access to the service. If a formulation does not include thresholds it may not be suitable as a classification system for participants in research.

Symptom-based classification will often incorporate measurements of distress and/or impairment of functioning. They do not necessarily have to incorporate thresholds but it is necessary to do so in order to classify people for clinical, research, and administrative/statistical purposes (see Chapters 2 and 3) such as access to care in a third-party payer system. Use of symptoms alone as a basis of classification may be both administratively burdensome in terms of the sheer number of symptoms that are possible and make it more difficult to identify relationships *between* symptoms.

Dimension-based classification systems are ideally constituted to reflect the continuous nature of spectrums between health and illness that are commonly found in both mental and physical health. A dimension-based classification can therefore be useful to give a more accurate picture than subdividing the population into 'healthy' and 'diagnosis *x*'. If the attributes being measured are continuous then measuring them as a dimension is more useful for researchers as it allows them to better represent the data and thus test a hypothesis (Kraemer et al., 2004).

On the other hand, thresholds applied to dimensional ratings still need to be established ('lines in a fog'; Goldberg, 2010) for clinical, research, administrative, or statistical reasons (see Chapters 2 and 3). Often categorical decisions need to be made, such as which aspects of mental health to measure. Otherwise, a comprehensive dimensional classification of mental health would be very extensive in nature. Dimension-based classification, even when pruned down to areas of interest, uses more cognitive and time resources than a simpler categorical alternative (Goldberg, 2010), and so may be more useful to professionals who have more time than doctors to see their clients, such as researchers and psychotherapists.

Another potential issue is that using a purely dimensional approach may lead to conditions being classified that are actually syndromes but the clinical picture overlaps with conditions that are on a spectrum of health. Examples include subtypes of autism (Szatmari, 2011) as well as melancholia and identified causes of hypertension (such as Cushing's syndrome), or familial hyperlipidaemia described in this chapter.

All these alternative classification systems can be used in conjunction with each other and with a categorical diagnostic system. For example, a diagnosis may be used (e.g. 'depression') by a psychotherapist for administrative or statistical purposes but the professional works with the client using a psychological formulation.

Conclusion

Many psychiatric diagnostic constructs are used to classify human emotions, thoughts, and other experiences that often lie on a continuum with normality or healthy states in the population. This is also seen with many common general medical diagnostic constructs. Thresholds are set to identify cases of the diagnosis in the whole population for the practical purposes of classification (see Chapters 2 and 3). These thresholds are often decided by committees of experts who should base their recommendations on good quality evidence, not just their august opinion (Kendler and Solomon, 2016), acknowledging the lack of absolute difference between people on either side of the thresholds. Dangers of setting thresholds too low in terms of 'overdiagnosis', 'medicalization', and harmful treatment are recognized. Even within these conditions that lie on a spectrum of health there can exist other conditions with similar clinical features that are more like the classic syndromes described in Chapter 3.

Other forms of classification of mental health problems, such as psychological formulation, symptoms, or dimensions, may be used depending on the needs and roles of the person using them. They can also be used in combination with diagnosis, either to augment clinical decision-making/practice or to fulfil roles that diagnosis is better able to achieve. These alternative classifications in themselves may also need to set thresholds depending on their roles/functions.

Although medical conditions that are highly prevalent in the population, such as high blood pressure, exist on a spectrum of health, it is true that many more medical conditions are able to be separated from normality (these were not discussed in this chapter). For this reason, 'some' but not 'near total' overlap exists between diagnostic constructs used in psychiatry and those used in general medicine (see Table 9.1). Medical diagnostic constructs (sometimes) and psychiatric diagnostic constructs (often) exhibit fuzzy boundaries between states labelled as 'health' and condition' although extreme examples of states are less contentious, indicating some overlap between general medicine and psychiatry. It should also be noted that some psychiatric diagnostic constructs, such as the dementias, are more clearly separated from normality, but milder cases or those in the early stages the differences may not be so clear-cut.

Table 9.1 Psychiatric diagnostic constructs' and medical diagnostic constructs' separation of conditions from normality.

	No Overlap	Some Overlap	Near Total Overlap
Is the condition clearly separated from normality?		X	

Chapter 10

Variability of clinical picture

Box 10.1 Questions to compare diagnostic constructs of psychiatry with general medicine

- Is the condition associated with variable clinical pictures?
- Is the condition diagnosed with polythetic criteria?

The questions posed in Box 10.1 refer to variability of clinical pictures of people meeting criteria for the same diagnostic category (see Box 10.1). Can we really say that two people should be in the same diagnostic category if their symptoms or signs have little in common? Common sense suggests not, but many factors can affect the clinical picture apart from causes or differences in structure or process (see Chapter 4), such as the patient's and doctor's views as well as cultural factors. General medical conditions will be used for comparison. Often these have been shown to have common identifiable differences of structure/process or cause (see Chapter 4).

Polythetic diagnostic categories are a reason why diagnostic constructs may show variable clinical pictures (see Chapter 6). This is where a diagnostic criterion is neither necessary nor sufficient to be present for a patient to qualify for being diagnosed with the diagnostic construct. Some diagnostic constructs have some features that are essential whilst containing other criteria in the same construct that are polythetic. This results in people with the same diagnosis having different clinical pictures.

Another reason for variable clinical pictures existing between people with the same diagnosis is comorbidity or co-occurrence (Widiger and Samuel, 2005). Co-occurrence is discussed in Chapter 6 in more detail and refers to the situation where a patient can meet the criteria for more than one diagnostic construct (Dell Osso and Pini, 2012). If *all* people who meet criteria for diagnosis *x* also meet completely different criteria for diagnosis *y* then this does not lead to variable clinical pictures. On the other hand, if only *some* people who meet criteria for diagnosis *x*, say, 50%, also meet different criteria for diagnosis *y* then that indicates a variable clinical picture is present amongst people who meet criteria for diagnosis *x*.

This chapter will discuss variability of clinical pictures and the use of polythetic criteria in psychiatric diagnostic constructs followed by examining whether theses issues occur in general medical diagnostic constructs. A brief discussion of alternative systems of mental health classification concludes the chapter.

Variability of clinical pictures in psychiatric diagnostic constructs

The 'outputs' of the mind/brain (such as thoughts) are by far the most diverse produced by any bodily system. Arguably, the range of thoughts possible about just one topic, for instance the plays of Shakespeare, is similar to the range of variability possible in the outputs of any one bodily system such as the cardiovascular system (although measuring this may be difficult). Given this massive diversity in functioning/outputs of the mind/brain that is described as 'healthy' or within the ranges of 'normality', it is clear we can also expect massive heterogeneity of functioning/outputs regarded as outside the 'normal' range. There is a vast range of different types of thoughts and experiences classified under a single symptom label of 'persecutory delusion' compared to the experiences classified under 'chest pain'. Therefore, we can expect a large degree of variability in mental health clinical pictures compared to other health conditions. This is even before we consider the potentially greater effects of factors such as culture on the *expression* and *interpretation* of mental health clinical pictures (see Chapter 4).

One of the functions of the mind/brain is to control the actions and responses of a person to the outside environment. On a simple level this can mean responses to physical danger or seeking food. On a more complex level, this can involve resolving complicated social and cultural challenges such as the evaluation of one's social standing. If a person is within a harmful environment or culture (and experiences such as bullying) then the mind/brain can express distress as a result. In order to identify the best way to help the person, the doctor or health professional may classify the resultant distress. Although the person's distress is being classified, in this case the problem lies not within that person's mind/brain but within the *environment* that caused the distress.

There are a number of conditions contained within a single diagnostic construct—major depression—including melancholia, atypical depression, secondary to medical causes such as Cushing's Syndrome, as well as variants with different types of additional symptoms (e.g. anxiety, 'somatizing symptoms', cognitive impairment) or accompanying physical illness (Goldberg, 2011). These different conditions may have different clinical pictures resulting in people meeting criteria for major depression having variable clinical pictures.

Some of the diagnostic constructs of depression include symptomatic criteria that are opposites such as increased or reduced appetite and/or sleep (Goldberg, 2011). Even when this does not occur, the use of polythetic criteria results in people with variable clinical pictures meeting the same diagnostic criteria. The ICD-10 diagnostic criteria for a depressive episode F32 (WHO, 1992) requires two out of three of depressed mood, loss of interest, and enjoyment or reduced energy, and at least two more symptoms out of a list of seven. This can result in two people meeting criteria for depression having potentially only one symptom in common. (The ICD10 diagnostic guidelines are available at <http://www.who.int/classifications/icd/en/bluebook.pdf>)

The common mental disorders were historically referred to as *neurosis* or *neurotic disorders* but are now often split into anxiety and depressive disorders. Results of some of the research on co-occurring anxiety with depressive disorders amongst different types of participants are summarized below. Chapter 11 will examine whether these are actually separate conditions or an example of a spectrum of conditions (see Chapter 3). If *some* but not *all* people who meet the criteria for an anxiety or depressive disorder meet the criteria for another anxiety or depressive disorder, this indicates a variable clinical picture amongst people who meet the criteria for anxiety or depressive disorders (see Table 10.1).

Post-traumatic stress disorder has recently had its diagnostic criteria modified in DSM-5. Compared to the previous diagnostic criteria in DSM-IV, the numbers of different symptom combinations that are possible in patients with the same diagnosis has increased from 79,794 to 636,120 (Galatzer-Levy and Bryant, 2013)!

Schizophrenia is a diagnostic construct that has varied greatly in terms of its name and associated diagnostic criteria throughout history (Taylor et al., 2010; Parnas, 2011). In Europe, the tradition has been to base the diagnostic criteria on first-rank symptoms such as thought broadcasting or auditory hallucinations commenting on the person's actions. These first-rank symptoms, however, are not always present in people diagnosed with schizophrenia (Lewine et al., 1982). They can be found in people who meet the diagnostic criteria for other conditions, such as mania (Taylor et al., 2010). Even if first-rank symptoms are present in a patient they are found in varying numbers and types.

The heterogeneity of first-rank symptoms is just one aspect of the highly variable clinical pictures in different people given the same diagnosis of schizophrenia, even the same subtype of schizophrenia such as paranoid or hebephrenic/disorganized (Andreassen and Flaum, 1991; Taylor et al., 2010). This variability is increased by use of differing diagnostic criteria for schizophrenia which can lead to markedly

Table 10.1 Studies of co-occurrence of anxiety with depression.

Study	Participants (numbers)	Result
Kessler et al., 2005	9,282 US population	Anxiety or depressive disorder during previous 12 months' increases chance of meeting criteria for another anxiety or depressive disorder during previous 12 months
Coyne et al., 1994	1,928 US primary care attenders	28% of participants meeting major depressive disorder criteria also met criteria for current anxiety disorder
Sartorius et al., 1996	25,916 Primary care attenders in 15 international sites	Approximately 40% who met criteria for anxiety disorder also met criteria for current depressive disorder and vice versa
Brown et al., 2001	11,127 attending two specialised US university clinics (secondary care)	57% of participants who met criteria for an anxiety or depressive disorder also met criteria for at least one more anxiety or depressive disorder

different prevalence rates (Andreassen and Flaum, 1991) and has been blamed for the inability to find a common aetiological cause or abnormality of structure or process that could lead to a biological explanation or diagnostic test for schizophrenia (Taylor et al., 2010).

DSM and ICD-10 diagnostic systems prioritized diagnostic criteria that are reliable (Andreassen and Flaum, 1991), but in doing so have arguably created a diagnostic construct that is different from the prototype or 'gestalt' of schizophrenia, as it was initially described (Parnas, 2011). It has been proposed to reduce schizophrenia to a more homogenous entity of hebephrenia with positive symptoms (of certain delusions and experiences), negative symptoms (such as reduced facial expression), cognitive/motor deficits, and a typical prodrome (Taylor et al., 2010). This is likely to exclude some of the commoner types of presentation that are currently given the diagnosis of paranoid schizophrenia.

The ICD-10 diagnostic criteria for F20 schizophrenia (WHO, 1992) results in highly variable clinical pictures for this diagnostic construct. For example, Person A may have thought insertion and Person B may have neologisms and blunted affect not secondary to mood or medication. The diagnostic construct relies on a 'family resemblance' (Rosch and Mervin, 1975) that Persons A and B have similar qualities such as likelihood of outcomes and responses to treatment.

DSM-5 introduced an alternative or hybrid model for classifying mental health problems attributed to personality (Skodol et al., 2015). This hybrid model includes problems related to extremes of personality traits found throughout the general population and clinical featuresbased on personality disorder categories. It is obvious from our experience that personality traits found in the general population are highly variable amongst people.

What is the evidence of variability of clinical picture for the features comprising personality disorder diagnostic categories? These are often characterized using polythetic criteria. Borderline personality disorder in DSM-IV (APA, 1994) can be diagnosed if at least five out of nine criteria are met. This means it is possible for two people with this same diagnosis to have only one criterion in common. In fact, even the criteria are quite widely defined. For example, the ninth criterion is listed as 'transient, stress-related paranoid ideation or severe dissociative symptoms'. This means even people meeting the same criteria can differ from each other (so if two people had only the ninth criterion in common, one could have transient paranoia and the other dissociative symptoms resulting in *no* clinical features in common). Unsurprisingly, there are variable clinical pictures amongst people meeting the criteria for the same personality disorder diagnostic construct.

Further increasing variability is that people who meet the diagnostic criteria for a personality disorder diagnostic category often meet the criteria for another personality disorder category (Morey et al., 2015; Tyrer et al., 2015). The DSM system 'clustered' personality disorder categories together (such as paranoid, schizoid, and schizotypal personality disorder categories grouped together into 'Cluster A') so that if more than one set of diagnostic criteria were met then it would be for personality disorder categories within the same 'cluster'. This would suggest that the variability in clinical pictures was limited to a range of similar categories. In fact, research indicates that people who meet the diagnostic criteria for a personality disorder category have an increased,but not 100% chance of meeting diagnostic criteria for other personality disorder categories both *within* the same 'cluster' as well as *other* 'clusters' (Scott et al., 1998; Grant et al., 2005). This strongly suggests highly variable clinical pictures exist amongst people meeting personality disorder diagnostic criteria.

Even psychiatric diagnostic constructs based on demonstrated disease processes such as the different types of dementias can display mixed and variable clinical pictures within each diagnostic construct (e.g. Alzheimer's or vascular), as well as underlying mixed causative pathology (e.g. vascular pathology found in those with Alzheimer's disease), and use polythetic criteria for diagnostic constructs (Galasko et al., 1994; Bang et al., 2015; O'Brien and Thomas, 2015; Robinson et al., 2015; Walker et al., 2015b; Scheltens et al., 2016).

This brief overview has shown highly variable clinical pictures for psychiatric diagnostic constructs themselves. The reasons for this high degree of variability include the complex polymorphic outputs of the mind/brain, high degree of co-occurrence of other mental disorders and use of polythetic diagnostic criteria, and where disease processes have been demonstrated the frequent co-occurrence of disease processes associated with different diagnostic constructs.

Variable clinical pictures in general medical conditions

Some general medical conditions are associated with variable clinical pictures. Polythetic diagnostic constructs can also be found in general medicine. Co-occurrence will be mostly discussed when referring to spectrums of conditions with multiple aspects but is common in general medicine (Muth and Glasziou, 2015). This is not an exhaustive list of examples of variable clinical pictures, polythetic constructs, or co-occurrence in general medicine.

About half of all renal tumours are asymptomatic and detected incidentally through investigation for other reasons. For symptomatic presentations of renal tumour, only 10% present with the classic triad of pain, haematuria, and a renal mass; more commonly, only one of these features is present. There can be a great variety of additional features in the clinical picture such as fever, abnormal liver function tests, or increased coagulation of the blood (Chapter 13 in Walker et al., 2014).

Myocardial infarction can have a great variety of presentations. Breathlessness is common and may be the only feature. Pain may occur in several locations such as the central chest or radiating into the neck or left arm. Painless presentations (e.g. with nausea and feeling unwell) can occur in older patients or those with diabetes ('silent MI'), and sometimes there are no abnormalities detected on examination (Chapter 18 in Walker et al., 2014). Ethnic minorities (Barakat et al., 2003) and women (Elsaesser and Hamm, 2004) may present with atypical clinical pictures such as sharp, not crushing, chest pain.

Cystic fibrosis can present with a great variety of 'phenotypes'—what we can observe about an individual as a result of the interaction of genetic and environmental factors—with the diagnosis often missed in the rarer phenotypes (Chapter 19 in Walker et al.,

2014). Recurrent infections of the chest leading to bronchiectasis and progressive lung damage are classically associated with the diagnosis but other manifestations in the clinical picture can include gastrointestinal malabsorption and biliary cirrhosis with portal hypertension, male infertility, diabetes, arthropathy, and nasal polyps.

TB can present in a great variety of clinical presentations (Chapters 19 and 22 in Walker et al., 2014). This, along with syphilis, has led to it being called the 'great imitator' as it can frequently be confused for other conditions (Sievers, 1961).

Sarcoidosis is a multisystem disorder characterized by the presence of granulomas (a collection of histiocyte immune cells) that are 'non-caseating', that is they are distinct from caseating granulomas caused by TB. It is highly variable in its clinical picture (Chapter 19 in Walker et al., 2014). About 20% to 30% of the time it is detected in asymptomatic individuals through incidental findings in investigations such as chest X-rays or liver function tests. Roughly 20–30% of all patients present with respiratory and general constitutional symptoms such as lethargy. A similar proportion present with a skin condition (erythema nodosum) and joint pain. There are additional increasingly rare presentations of sarcoidosis such as hypercalcaemia or cardiac arrhythmias.

The clinical picture of endocrine disorders may be variable, ranging from classically described syndromes to non-specific symptoms or asymptomatic but with abnormalities detected in laboratory tests (Chapter 20 in Walker et al., 2014). Glucocorticoid excess leads to the diverse clinical pictures associated with Cushing syndrome, not all of which are present in every patient. Examples of such features include bruising, high blood pressure, central obesity, high blood glucose, osteoporosis, skin striae, or wasting of the thigh (Chapter 20 in Walker et al., 2014). This plethora of possible clinical features leads to a highly variable clinical picture for this diagnosis, and individual symptoms or signs have a low predictive value for the overall syndrome. Thyroid problems can show a great degree of variability as to the presence of a variety of related autoimmune antibodies (Chapter 20 in Walker et al., 2014).

Gastro-oesophageal reflux disease can present in atypical fashion in up to 50% of people with symptoms such as sore throat, chronic cough, or chest pain (Chapter 22 in Walker et al., 2014). Peptic ulcer disease can present with an atypical clinical picture in up to a third of patients, for example with minimal or no pain or sudden presentation with vomiting of blood (Chapter 22 in Walker et al., 2014). Individual symptoms often have poor predictive value for the diagnosis. Coeliac disease can have a highly variable clinical picture from obvious malabsorption to non-specific features (e.g. tiredness) to oral ulceration, and 10% of people have dermatitis herpetiformis (Chapter 22 in Walker et al., 2014).

The inflammatory bowel diseases, ulcerative colitis and Crohn's disease, can vary amongst cases of these diseases in the degree of intestinal involvement and presence of extra-intestinal features (Chapter 22 in Walker et al., 2014). Intestinal involvement can vary from only perianal lesions to partial or whole involvement of the large bowel and/or small intestine. There is a large range of extra-intestinal features that are associated with inflammatory bowel disease, both related to active phases of disease activity (such as mouth ulcers, inflammation of the cornea, fatty liver, venous thrombosis, and skin lesions) and unrelated to active phases of disease activity (such as amyloidosis, sacroiliitis, metabolic bone disease, and primary sclerosing cholangitis).

Hepatic cirrhosis has a highly variable clinical picture (Chapter 23 in Walker et al., 2014). Some cases are asymptomatic with incidental discovery of the diagnosis, for example on abdominal ultrasound. Some cases can present with enlarged liver or spleen, or the consequences of portal hypertension or signs of hepatic failure such as jaundice or poor clotting/multiple bruises. Symptoms may be non-specific such as lack of energy, poor appetite, vomiting, or even shortness of breath. Pyogenic liver abscess has a high frequency of unusual or atypical presentations leading to the diagnosis being frequently missed (Chapter 23 in Walker et al., 2014).

Chronic myeloid leukaemia can be asymptomatic in about a quarter of cases. Almost all cases have enlarged spleen (10% massively so) and half of all cases have an enlarged liver (Chapter 24 in Walker et al., 2014). The highly variable clinical picture of antiphospholipid syndrome includes one or more associated clinical conditions in conjunction with a persistently raised antiphospholipid antibody. Some of these associated clinical conditions are adverse pregnancy outcomes (such as more than three first trimester miscarriages or severe pre-eclampsia), thromboembolism in veins or arteries, and transverse myelitis (Chapter 24 in Walker et al., 2014).

Rheumatoid arthritis can have a highly variable mode of onset; acute, insidious, or fluctuating (palindromic), or resembling polymyalgia rheumatica (Chapter 25 in Walker et al., 2014). Rheumatoid arthritis is also associated with a wide range of extra-articular (non-joint related) manifestations usually found in those with longstanding disease with rheumatoid factor (an auto-antibody found in up to 80% of patients), or sometimes acute presentations in males. These include fever, fatigue, weight loss, musculoskeletal (e.g. bursitis, osteoporosis), haematological (e.g. anaemia), lymphatic (Felty's syndrome with splenomegaly and neutropaenia amongst other features), pulmonary (pleural effusion, pulmonary nodules), or peripheral neuropathy (Chapter 25 in Walker et al., 2014).

A group of similar diseases referred to as seronegative spondyloarthropathies (Chapter 25 in Walker et al., 2014), for example, ankylosing spondylitis and arthropathies associated with psoriasis or inflammatory bowel disease, have a wide range of articular and extra-articular features (these are different from those of rheumatoid arthritis) which can be variable in their presence in individual cases. They have highly variable clinical pictures which will be discussed later in the section on polythetic criteria in general medical conditions

Multiple sclerosis is a neurological disorder with a highly variable clinical picture with the commoner features including optic neuritis, fluctuating sensory symptoms, loss of function of the upper limb or sixth cranial nerve palsy, and rarer presentations such as trigeminal neuralgia or recurrent facial nerve palsy (Chapter 26 in Walker et al., 2014).

Diagnostic constructs used in dermatology such as eczema and psoriasis are highly variable in their clinical picture. Type of onset such as acute or chronic can vary. There is a great deal of variety in the size, colour, and three-dimensional shape, location, and associated features of the lesions. Additional features associated with eczema and psoriasis can also vary (Chapter 28 in Walker et al., 2014).

Lichen planus is another condition that can be highly variable in its clinical picture including sites of lesions such as mouth, skin, lesion, nail involvement. The more unusual types can be hard to identify as cases of lichen planus (Chapter 26 in Walker et al., 2014).

Tuberous sclerosis is a genetic condition that results in abnormal growths—hamartomas—in several areas of the body. This results in some common features—skin lesions, epilepsy, learning difficulties—but also a highly variable clinical picture depending on what area of the body is affected and subsequent clinical consequences such as kidneys, lungs, eyes, heart, or different areas of the brain (Chapter 28 in Walker et al., 2014).

General medical conditions can also have highly variable clinical pictures.

Use of polythetic diagnostic constructs in general medicine

This section will discuss how some medical conditions use polythetic diagnostic criteria which can result in two people with the same diagnosis varying as to how much in common they have in their clinical pictures.

Myocardial infarction (MI) is diagnosed in most clinical situations using polythetic criteria (different criteria apply to diagnosing MI as a complication of a medical or surgical procedure such as a coronary artery bypass graft). The most commonly used criteria (Chapter 18 in Walker et al., 2014) are changes in biomarkers associated with myocardial infarction, for example cardiac troponin beyond suitable threshold *and* at least one of:

- typical symptoms of cardiac ischaemia, for example crushing central chest pain
- acute ECG changes such as ST elevation
- onset of pathological Q-waves in the ECG
- dead cardiac muscle or abnormal cardiac regional wall movement seen on imaging
- confirmation of a clot in a coronary artery by angiography or at post-mortem

Modified Duke University criteria are used to diagnose infective endocarditis (Chapter 18 in Walker et al., 2014). Definite infective endocarditis is diagnosed if two major, or one major and three minor, or five minor criteria are present. Possible infective endocarditis is diagnosed if one major and one minor criteria, or three minor criteria are present. There are two major criteria possible (positive blood cultures of typical causative organisms and evidence of endocardial involvement on echocardiography). There are six minor criteria, for example, history of IV drug misuse, body temperature > 38 degrees Celsius, or suggestive echocardiographic findings

Acute rheumatic fever (ARF) is diagnosed according to polythetic criteria (the revised Jones criteria) that vary depending on whether the patient lives in a country with moderate to high incidence of the disease or a low incidence of the disease (Gewitz et al., 2015). If history of Group A streptococcal infection is confirmed, then three major *or* two major and two minor manifestations are needed to confirm diagnosis of ARF. For a recurrent case of ARF, then a lower standard of two major manifestations, or one major and two minor, or three minor manifestations are required. There are five to six possible major manifestations, and four possible minor manifestations. These manifestations may vary depending on rate of incidence in the patient's country. For example, fever is a minor manifestation in all countries but polyarthralgia is a minor manifestation in a low-incidence country but is a major manifestation in a moderate to high incidence country (Gewitz et al., 2015). It is possible for two people with a diagnosis of ARF to have nothing in common in their clinical pictures apart from evidence of past Group A streptococcal infection.

Churg–Strauss syndrome is identified if four or more out of six possible features is present (Chapter 19 in Walker et al 2014) such as asthma, peripheral blood eosinophilia, or pulmonary infiltrates. Polycystic ovarian syndrome is a common medical condition. The diagnosis requires the presence of at least two of irregular periods, androgen excess, or multiple ovarian cysts (Chapter 20 in Walker et al., 2014).

Irritable bowel syndrome is another common medical condition that is diagnosed using polythetic criteria created using a consensual 'Delphic process' involving international experts. The presence of recurrent abdominal pain and discomfort for three months with at least two out of three 'Rome II' criteria (e.g. symptoms relieved by defaecation) and the absence of 'alarm' features (e.g. weight loss, bleeding, or anaemia) are used to make the diagnosis (Chapter 22 in Walker et al., 2014). Other clinical features may increase confidence in the diagnosis (e.g. stress worsens symptoms).

Peutz–Jeghers syndrome is a genetic condition featuring polyps throughout the small and large intestine and pigmentation of the mouth and digits. The diagnosis requires the presence of two out of three of multiple small bowel polyps, pigmentation in the lips or mouth, or a family history fitting autosomal dominant pattern.

The diagnosis of multiple myeloma requires the presence of two out of three criteria: increased numbers of bone marrow malignant plasma cells in the bone marrow, M-protein in urine/serum, or skeletal lytic lesions (Chapter 24, Walker et al., 2014).

The rheumatic diseases have highly variable clinical pictures and as a result have polythetic diagnostic criteria set by expert committees. They often combine laboratory test results and clinical features (Mohan and Assassi, 2015). Rheumatoid arthritis is diagnosed on a standardized system of scoring sufficient points, with points given for number of joints involved, duration of illness, and the result of laboratory tests for rheumatoid factor and anti-cyclic citrullinated peptides auto-antibodies (Chapter 25 in Walker et al., 2014; Mohan and Assassi, 2015). Systemic lupus erythematosus (SLE) can be diagnosed on the presence of four or more out of eleven clinical features and lab test results (such as a butterfly rash), whilst another diagnostic system for SLE asks for four or more criteria including at least one clinical feature (out of eleven) and at least one positive laboratory test result (out of six tests) *or* a typical biopsy result plus ANA or anti-DNA auto-antibodies (Mohan and Assassi, 2015). Thus, two patients who meet diagnostic criteria for SLE may have nothing in common in their clinical pictures. Axial spondyloarthritis also has polythetic diagnostic criteria; there must be back pain of at least three months with onset before 45 years old and either HLA-B27 major histocompatibility surface antigen plus two or more clinical features or sacroiliitis on imaging plus one other clinical feature. There are 11 possible clinical features including symptoms, laboratory tests, family history, and associated diseases (Mohan and Assassi, 2015). It is therefore possible again for two people meeting diagnostic criteria for axial spondyloarthritis to have little in common in their clinical pictures. Ankylosing spondylitis is diagnosed if either bilateral sacroiliitis mild or more severe changes are present on X-ray *or* definite unilateral sacroiliitis on X-rays combined with a typical history of back pain and reduced lumbar movement and chest expansion to meet the diagnostic criteria (Chapter 25 in Walker et al., 2014).

The diagnosis of multiple sclerosis (MS) uses the polythetic revised MacDonald criteria decided upon by an expert committee (Polman et al., 2011; Chapter 26 in Walker et al., 2014). The diagnostic criteria vary according to whether this is a first episode of MS or at least two episodes have occurred previously. There are five clinical picture types that can meet criteria for MS diagnosis using a mixture of clinical and objective evidence. Objective evidence that can be used includes certain imaging results or oligoclonal bands detected in cerebrospinal fluid. The diagnosis of MS requires the presence of clinical history and findings as well as laboratory test results (Chapter 26 in Walker et al., 2014).

Atopic eczema is diagnosed on the presence of pruritus (itch) and at least three out of five features such as the presence of associated diseases including in first-degree relatives (e.g. asthma), onset before two years of life, and location/nature/associated symptoms of the eczema lesions (Chapter 28 in Walker et al., 2014).

Polythetic criteria are also used in general medical diagnostic constructs.

Alternative forms of classification and variable clinical pictures

Psychological formulations can sidestep the issue of variable clinical pictures. A psychological formulation involves professional and client jointly forming a 'plausible' explanation and understanding of how the current predicament came about and why it continues. This explanation does not have to be 'true' in the scientific sense, it just needs make sense to both parties. It can choose to focus on particular areas and as psychological formulations are used to explain the clinical picture in an individual not a group of people, it does not have to address why a variety of symptoms or signs is present.

A symptom-based classification can attempt to treat individual symptoms as initially unrelated which would allow such a classification system to ignore variability in clinical pictures. That is, it just analyses each symptom that is present, which can make it easier to determine cause in scientific research (Bentall, 2014) and in clinical practice to address each symptom in turn. The problem is that mental health symptoms seem to associate together into particular factors in the general population such as 'internalizing' (anxiety and depressive disorders), 'externalizing' (alcohol or drug problems and difficult behaviours), and a 'psychosis'/'thought disorder' factor (unusual experiences) (Wright et al., 2013). Others have measured a general '*p*' psychopathology factor as a single factor or in a hierarchy with a second order group of factors similar to 'internalizing', 'externalizing', and 'psychosis', or splitting 'internalizing' into 'fear' and 'distress' and retaining 'externalizing' (Lahey et al., 2012; Caspi et al., 2014;

Stochl et al., 2015). In primary care, mental health symptoms are seen in recognizable groups or syndromes as commonly as other medical problems (Fink et al., 2009), although these groups of symptoms may be more mixed than classical categorical diagnosis, for example, anxiety and depression are often found together (Sartorius et al., 1996). A more complicated five-factor model of symptoms was found in a sample of participants in secondary care (Kotov et al., 2011).

A symptom-based classification will eventually need to account for this tendency of symptoms to associate together in certain patterns. The explanation could be either common underlying processes or a description of a combination often found together. An underlying process (not necessarily a disease, it could be purely psychosocial) could lead to symptom *x* and symptom *y*. Another explanation could be that symptom *x* causes symptom *y*—sometimes referred to as a network explanation (Borsboom and Cramer, 2013; Borsboom, 2017). Additionally, each symptom may need to be separated, depending on cause: hallucinations whilst intoxicated with LSD should be classified and managed differently than hallucinations associated with sensory impairment or hallucinations with no identified biological cause.

Dimension-based classification can address the problem of variability in clinical pictures by offering a full description of the groups of different symptoms present in each patient. Of course, within each dimensional rating there may be variability between different people given identical ratings, but this would be less than a diagnostic category covering many different dimensions within a single category. On the other hand, categorical decisions will still need to be made as to which dimensions to measure and whether to include a symptom in a dimension (e.g. was it present only briefly or as a result of substance intoxication). Is a comprehensive description of *all* aspects of the clinical picture to be attempted with vast number of potential dimensions or will the description be limited to a focused area with a still potentially large number of dimensions? For anxiety and depressive symptoms, it has been suggested to have an 11-dimension classification system (Brown and Barlow, 2009). HiTOP is a hierarchical dimensional organization of symptoms based on research; the various levels of dimensions include six spectra and eleven syndromal groupings (Kotov et al., 2017). For research purposes and for clinicians seeing small numbers of clients for long periods during office hours, then a more cumbersome but more comprehensive dimensional descriptive system may be more useful than a simpler diagnostic system is to clinicians seeing large numbers of patients for brief periods and at all hours (Kraemer et al., 2004; Goldberg, 2010).

Conclusion

Humans are a combination of complex systems and sub-systems that not only interact with each other but also with complex potential causes of medical conditions, and are embodied in complex systems of culture, social interactions, community, politics, and environment (Chapter 5 in Walker et al., 2014). We should not be surprised that there exists variability in clinical pictures. It is also not surprising that the most complex system of the body, the mind/brain, produces outputs of greatest complexity. Problems associated with the mind/brain, even if they are a result of the interaction of society with the individual rather than a problem located *within* the mind/brain, can be expected to show great variability. Diagnostic criteria of these problems which use polythetic criteria increase the likelihood of variable clinical pictures.

There are also highly variable clinical pictures amongst general medical conditions as well as the use of polythetic criteria. Even amongst general medical conditions we can find diagnostic categories where two people with the same diagnosis share little in common with their clinical picture. Auto-immune and auto-inflammatory conditions seem to have the most variable clinical pictures, that is, this seems most likely when the system involved is very complex and the immune system is amongst the more complex bodily systems and is often involved in the interaction between the body and the environment.

Alternative classification systems can either ignore variable clinical pictures (psychological formulation) or handle the problem by simply listing every aspect of the clinical picture separately (symptom-based classification). However, the latter approach will still at some point need to address why some patterns of the clinical picture are more likely to occur. Dimension-based systems can capture variable clinical pictures accurately but may be too complex for brief appointments or emergencies seen outside of hours.

In summary, although psychiatric diagnostic constructs often show highly variable clinical pictures and polythetic diagnostic criteria, this also seems to be a feature of some general medical conditions. Psychiatric diagnostic constructs seem to display greater variability in their clinical pictures and more frequently use polythetic criteria. This indicates some overlap between general medicine and psychiatry (see Table 10.2).

Table 10.2 Variability of clinical pictures of psychiatric diagnostic constructs compared to general medical diagnostic constructs.

	No Overlap	**Some Overlap**	**Near Total Overlap**
Is the condition associated with variable Clinical Pictures?		X	
Is the condition diagnosed with polythetic criteria?		X	

Chapter 11

Spectrums of conditions

Box 11.1 Questions to compare diagnostic constructs of psychiatry with general medicine

- Is the condition described by a diagnosis clearly separated from other conditions in terms of clinical features?
- Is there little co-occurrence of conditions; that is, are they separate entities?

Many psychiatric diagnostic constructs rely on distinguishing between different elements of the clinical picture, the 'manifestations' (Scadding, 1967; Chapter 4 in Schoenberg and Rosamond, 2000; Chapter 4 of this book), rather than identifying common differences of structure/process or a common cause (see Chapter 4). This chapter will compare psychiatric and general medical diagnostic constructs regarding whether they clearly identify a 'zone of rarity' (Kendell and Jablensky, 2003) in the clinical picture between different diagnostic constructs (see Box 11.1). The other possibility is that the diagnostic constructs describe different areas of a spectrum of illness/condition or of a spectrum of illnesses/conditions (see Chapter 3).

There is recent interest in the biosocial concept of *syndemics*, defined as the clustering of two or more conditions within a population due to social and contextual factors, and this clustering leads to worse biopsychosocial outcomes and worsening health (Singer et al., 2017). Examples include a mixture of mental and physical health conditions such as diabetes, TB, HIV, and depression in the context of poverty (Mendenhall et al., 2017).

Spectrums of conditions in psychiatric diagnostic constructs

Many psychiatric diagnostic constructs are based on the clinical picture which may be caused by unknown underlying causes or mechanisms (Pincus et al., 2004) or to a network of relationships between symptoms (Borsboom and Cramer, 2013; Borsboom, 2017).

The clinical features of personality disorder diagnostic constructs are distributed dimensionally through the clinical population without 'zones of rarity' (Skodol et al., 2005). People who meet personality disorder diagnostic criteria often meet the criteria for other personality disorders. In addition, these co-occurring personality disorders do not always fit into a cluster of related personality disorders (Scott et al., 1998; Grant et al., 2005). Personality disorder constructs do not have 'zones of rarity' with each other and may not occur in spectrums of conditions (see Chapter 3).

The classification of depression has long been thought of as being in a state of confusion (Kendell, 1976) that continues today (Cole et al., 2008). Although the division of depression into the commoner unipolar depression and depression as part of bipolar disorder is still commonly used (Cole et al., 2008), there is still debate as to whether unipolar depression should itself be divided into two categories. There are several names used for these categories which can have subtly different meanings (Kendell, 1977). One category may be called 'psychotic', 'endogenous', or 'melancholia/melancholic' with the other being commonly named 'reactive' or 'neurotic'. If depression is divided into endogenous/melancholic depression and reactive/neurotic depression, then this latter category may lie on a continuum with depressive symptoms in the general population (see Chapter 10; Ruscio and Ruscio, 2000).

Some researchers have been able to divide patients attending clinical services with depression into psychotic/endogenous/melancholic depression or reactive/neurotic depression on the basis of distinctive features of the clinical picture (Carney et al., 1965; Matussek et al., 1981; Feinberg and Carroll, 1982), but other researchers were unable to separate psychotic from neurotic depression clearly (Kendell and Gourlay, 1970). It should be noted that this distinctive clinical picture does vary to some extent between different studies and that there may be a further

subdivision of melancholia into psychotic melancholia and non-psychotic melancholia (Parker et al., 1991). There may be a continuum of clinical pictures with archetypal psychotic depression and neurotic depression at either pole (Kendell and Gourlay, 1970; Kendell, 1976), or that melancholia is simply severe depression that is on a continuum with less severe depression (Cole et al., 2008).

Some distinctive features associated with endogenous/psychotic/melancholic depression have been identified apart from distinctive symptoms. A significant minority of episodes of endogenous depression occur in the absence of a stressful life event causing it, in contrast to reactive depression (Matussek et al., 1981). The first episode of both endogenous and reactive depressions tends to be caused by stressful life events but subsequent endogenous depressive episodes are more likely to occur in the absence of stressful life events than subsequent reactive depression episodes (Brown et al., 1994). Differences in the clinical picture were also said to be not related to severity of symptoms in one study (Feinberg and Carroll, 1982).

Treatment responses may differ between melancholia and other forms of depression (Carney et al., 1965; Fink and Taylor, 2007). Further, the dexamethasone suppression test is said to be relatively effective in separating melancholia/endogenous depression from reactive/neurotic depression (Fink and Taylor, 2007).

Whilst it may be possible in some cases to distinguish between melancholia/endogenous depression and reactive/neurotic depression, does this mean melancholia/endogenous depression and anxiety are always easily distinguished? The proposed diagnostic criteria for melancholia include 'unremitting apprehension' (Parker et al., 2010) or 'unremitting mood of apprehension' (Fink and Taylor, 2007). Apprehension is an emotion that belongs to the category of anxiety. Furthermore, examination of historical accounts of depression in the medical literature confirm that a variety of anxiety symptoms are regarded as part of the typical clinical picture of depression (Kendler, 2016). Even in this 'archetypal' depressive syndrome, anxiety symptoms are a key part of the diagnostic criteria and recognized as part of the typical clinical picture.

This two-category model of unipolar depression is only one method of subdividing depression. For example, as described in Chapter 10, Goldberg suggests six forms of depression: major depression; depression presenting with somatic symptoms; depression with panic attacks; depression in people with obsessional traits; depression accompanying known physical illness; and depression presenting as pseudo dementia (Goldberg, 2011). All these different models of depression tend to accept the close relationship between depression and anxiety (Kendler, 2016). Chapter 10 summarized the results of four studies (Sartorius et al., 1996; Coyne et al., 1994; Brown et al., 2001; Kessler et al., 2005) which showed high rates of co-occurrence between depression and anxiety disorders.

Several studies analysing a variety of participants (e.g. general adult population or a clinical population attending mental health outpatients) found that anxiety and depressive symptoms and diagnostic categories tend to associate with each other, forming an internalizing factor (Kotov et al., 2011; Caspi et al., 2014), although it may split into anxiety–misery (e.g. generalized anxiety and depression) and fear (e.g. phobias) subfactors (Krueger, 1999). One longitudinal study (Moffitt, 2007) showed that there was high co-occurrence of generalized anxiety disorder (GAD) and depression; 72% of participants with a lifetime history of anxiety also had a lifetime history of depression, and 48% of participants with a lifetime history of depression also had a lifetime history of anxiety. Approximately one-third of anxiety cases started at the same time or before depression developed and vice versa. This study further demonstrated the close relationship between GAD and depression. Anxiety disorders are also highly likely to co-occur in the same person with some combinations being particularly common such as panic disorder with agoraphobia (Kessler et al., 2005).

Other forms of neurotic symptoms also have a close relationship to anxiety and depression. Somatization, defined as the expression of distress in the form of physical symptoms such as pain, is also found to have high rates of co-occurrence with depression and anxiety but could also exist by itself in about half of cases (Lowe et al., 2008). Hypochondriasis, overconcern over one's health leading to distress, can be found by itself but also has high rates of co-occurrence with anxiety, depression, and somatoform disorders (where medically unexplained symptoms are assumed to be related to distress), with higher correlations with anxiety symptoms than with somatoform symptoms and little correlation with depressive symptoms (Scarella et al., 2016). (The judgment that symptoms labelled somatizing are expressions of distress and not biologically explained can be unreliable and can be contested by the patient).

This reflects the fact that distress expressed in the form of these internalizing, or emotional disorders display multiformity (Winokur, 1990). The diagnostic constructs describe 'prototype concepts' (see Chapters 3 and 4) developed by clinicians observing 'prototypes' of depression, generalized anxiety, panic attacks, hypochondriasis, and so forth in patients they see. People experiencing distress may display features of one or more of these prototype concepts; these different diagnostic constructs reflect different aspects of internalizing disorders and any number (including only one) may be found in the person presenting to services for help.

The commonest psychiatric diagnostic construct in the UK population is mixed anxiety depression found in 7.7–8.8% of adults representing roughly 50% or more of the common mental disorders (Jenkins et al., 1997; Singleton et al., 2001; McManus et al., 2009). This was defined as scoring 12 or more on the CIS-R (see Chapter 9), that is, having sufficient number and severity of mental health symptoms to meet the criteria for mental disorder but not fitting 'prototype concepts' of the diagnostic constructs used for depression and anxiety disorders.

Mixed anxiety–depression has been shown to have a stable clinical identity (Hettema et al., 2015), as well as being common but does not have a clearly defined diagnostic construct, highlighting the fallibility of relying purely on historical descriptions based on clinicians seeing the more severely ill patients as the sole description of what people may experience in the population as a whole. This most common of mental disorders does not resemble the prototype concepts used to create anxiety or depression diagnostic constructs.

A review of the similarities and differences between the internalizing or emotional disorders, including similarities in genetics, family history, experiences of environmental adversity, personality temperament, as part of a proposed meta-structure of classification of mental disorders concluded there were many common elements (e.g. emotional and cognitive processing), and even though different symptoms are used for different diagnostic constructs, they should not be separated into different chapters of the ICD and DSM systems (Goldberg et al., 2009).

Kraepelin divided patients with psychosis into two diagnostic categories based on the course of their condition: dementia praecox (currently called schizophrenia) and manic-depression (now split into unipolar depression and bipolar disorder) (Kendell and Gourlay, 1970). Dementia praecox was associated with gradual deterioration at a variable rate—though even on Kraepelin's own figures some patients did recover (Hoenig, 1983)—whilst manic-depression had a better outcome including more complete recovery between episodes.

A more recent model of psychosis (Van Os and Reininghaus, 2016) posits an 'extended psychosis phenotype' which extends from experiences similar to milder psychotic symptoms in the community to full-blown psychotic symptoms and a 'transdiagnostic dimension' in which psychotic symptoms occur across a variety of diagnostic constructs (such as bipolar disorder, schizophrenia, depression, or post-traumatic stress disorder (PTSD)), particularly in severe cases. Some of these diagnostic constructs are regarded as psychotic conditions and schizophrenia would represent the more severe 30% of cases of these (Van Os, 2015). Schizophrenia and cases of bipolar disorder with psychotic symptoms would be regarded as parts of this 'extended pswychosis phenotype' (spectrum of illness/condition as described in Chapter 3).

A great deal of research has occurred on whether it is possible to separate bipolar disorder with psychotic symptoms from schizophrenia or whether they form opposite ends of a spectrum. Bipolar disorder with psychotic symptoms is itself a diagnostic construct at the severe end of a spectrum of mood disorders, featuring both elated and depressed moods (bipolar I disorder without psychosis, bipolar II disorder with hypomania and cyclothymia).

Discriminant function analysis based on age, gender, and certain symptoms and signs (Kendell and Gourlay, 1970) was performed on 146 affective psychosis participants (bipolar disorder with psychotic symptoms and depressive psychosis) and 146 participants with schizophrenia or related conditions. Instead of finding a bimodal distribution suggesting two diagnostic categories, researchers found a trimodal distribution. This suggested three diagnostic categories: an affective psychosis category, a schizophrenia category, and an intermediate category, commonly called schizoaffective disorder. Later research using a similar technique and including data on the course of the disorder did demonstrate a bimodal distribution in scores in a 'general psychotic sample' (Brockington et al., 1979) but could not repeat this in a sample of participants with schizoaffective disorder and only partially succeeded in finding a bimodal distribution in further analysis of more participants (Brockington et al., 1991).

A more recent study (Dikeos et al., 2006) performed factor analysis on symptoms in participants with psychotic conditions that concluded a five-factor model was the optimum solution. The factors were mania, reality distortion (e.g. hallucinations/delusions), disorganization (e.g. thought disorder, bizarre delusions), depression, and negative symptoms (blunted and restricted affect). The distribution of these factor scores across 41 participants with bipolar disorder diagnosis and 128 participants with schizophrenia was displayed on charts. There was overlap in symptom factor scores between both diagnostic constructs.

Bipolar disorder participants' symptom factor scores were clustered more tightly together, with high mania and depression symptom factor scores and lower reality distortion, depression and disorganization factor scores. The schizophrenia participants had more broadly scattered scores throughout the symptom factor scores, indicating greater symptom heterogeneity and they were more likely to have higher reality distortion, negative symptom, and disorganization factor scores, and lower mania and depression scores. Therefore, whilst there was great deal of overlap in symptom presentation, schizophrenia and bipolar disorder were more likely to present with certain symptom patterns (but not significantly so), and bipolar disorder was more symptomatically homogenous than schizophrenia (or 'schizophrenias', as Bleuler put it (Hoenig, 1983)).

There do appear significant differences between bipolar disorder with psychosis and schizophrenia in several areas, even if they do not amount to 'zones of rarity', with some overlap between the two conditions. Examples includes greater average impairments on neuropsychological testing and cognitive impairment in participants meeting schizophrenia criteria (Keefe and Fenton, 2007; Carpenter et al., 2009; Hill., 2013; Tamminga et al., 2014; Bora and Pantelis, 2015), greater reduction in brain tissue in participants meeting schizophrenia criteria that is not wholly explained by medication (Carpenter et al., 2009; Cosgrove and Suppes, 2013; Ivleva et al., 2013), differences in clinical picture not amounting to a 'zone of rarity', that is, with some overlap (Carpenter et al., 2009; Tamminga et al., 2014), participants meeting bipolar disorder criteria tend to have higher educational attainment than expected compared to participants meeting schizophrenia criteria (Vreeker et al., 2016), and differences in response of the core symptoms of the condition to certain medications like lithium and sodium valproate (Cosgrove and Suppes, 2013).

When disorders of self/anomalous experiences are assessed, these are significantly commoner, but not universally present, in participants meeting schizophrenia criteria compared to participants meeting bipolar disorder criteria (Parnas et al., 2003). However, the genetic evidence and family history of patients point to an overlap between schizophrenia and bipolar disorder (Crow, 1990; Craddock and Owen, 2010; Owen, 2012; Cross-Disorder Group of the Psychiatric Genomics Consortium, 2013a, 2013b). There has also been preliminary evidence that expression of the *VRK2* gene may vary between bipolar disorder and schizophrenia as measured by mRNA levels found in peripheral blood samples (Tesli et al., 2016); this needs replicated before it can outweigh the other genetic evidence. A review of the meta-structure of mental disorders concluded that bipolar disorder should not be classified with psychotic conditions like schizophrenia, but this was before the Psychiatric Genomics Consortium results appeared (Carpenter et al., 2009).

Several studies noted good outcome schizophrenia cases presented with both psychotic and affective (mood) symptoms and with a family history of both schizophrenia and bipolar disorder in their relatives (Robin and Guze, 1970). This 'clinical reality' (Malaspina et al., 2013) of patients presenting with mixed features was confirmed in the study described earlier (Kendell and Gourlay, 1970) showing a trimodal distribution of symptoms. Unfortunately, attempts to create a diagnostic construct identifying patients in the middle ground between schizophrenia and bipolar disorder are often unreliable (Malaspina et al., 2013).

Further studies have confirmed that the clinical picture of schizoaffective disorder overlaps with both schizophrenia and bipolar disorder with psychosis (Tamminga et al., 2013; Tamminga et al., 2014), and in people meeting criteria for schizoaffective disorder there are high rates of both schizophrenia and bipolar disorder amongst their relatives (Kendler et al., 1998; Tamminga et al., 2013). For changes in sizes of regions of the brain, schizoaffective disorder has a more similar pattern to schizophrenia than bipolar disorder (Ivleva et al., 2013). Impairments in neuropsychological testing and cognitive impairment are intermediate in severity between bipolar disorder with psychosis and schizophrenia (Hill et al., 2013; Tamminga et al., 2014).

A systematic review placed schizoaffective disorder in the affective psychosis group and compared cognitive functioning with schizophrenia where some significant differences were found between affective psychosis and schizophrenia (Bora et al., 2009). However, one study of over 400 participants meeting several psychotic disorder diagnostic constructs followed up for up to ten years found that there were clear discontinuities in outcome; episodic mania was associated with better outcomes than chronic mania or no mania and ten or more days of psychosis without mood symptoms was associated with worse outcome (Kotov et al., 2013), and the authors felt this was evidence for a bipolar/schizophrenia split rather than a spectrum.

One study of participants meeting bipolar disorder criteria compared 213 participants with a history of both psychosis and mood symptoms and 168 participants with mood symptoms without psychosis symptoms (Burton et al., 2019, pre-published article). There were no differences between participants with mood symptoms without psychosis and participants with both mood and psychosis symptoms on demographics and neuropsychological functioning. Contrary to the common perception that bipolar disorder with psychosis has the worse prognosis, the mood symptoms without psychosis participants had worse clinical outcomes for chronicity of mood symptoms and frequency of rapid-cycling of mood episodes. If this study is representative of the wider population in clinical practice, this suggests for people meeting bipolar disorder criteria that psychosis symptoms are not associated with worse prognosis and that mood symptoms are more important. This would be a point of difference with people meeting schizophrenia criteria where both psychotic and mood symptoms are important in prognosis (see Chapter 14).

A systematic review of taxometric studies of the structure of psychosis identified several studies demonstrating variable numbers of classes that seemed to match psychosis diagnostic constructs but there were several methodological shortcomings that reduced confidence in these findings (Linscott et al., 2009).

For psychotic conditions, there is some evidence both for and against a spectrum model of bipolar disorder, with psychosis and schizophrenia at opposite ends of this spectrum and schizoaffective disorder in the middle without a 'zone of rarity' between these constructs. This is similar to the spectrum of illness/condition discussed in Chapter 3. This spectrum may be because diagnostic constructs are based on the clinical picture rather than common differences in structure/process or causes. It should also be noted that there are many cases of psychosis that do not fit any of these three diagnostic constructs (Van Os, 2015).

Mixed pathological pictures can be found in a substantial minority of people with dementia (Galasko et al., 1994; Holmes et al., 1999) with lack of 'zones of rarity' between different dementia pathological processes (e.g. Alzheimer's, vascular, and Lewy body). One study found multiple disease process was common and cognitive impairment related to the sum amount of these co-occurring diseases processes (White et al., 2016). If Lewy bodies are found in the substantia nigra (as expected in Parkinson's disease with or without dementia), they can often also be found in the cerebral cortex (Galasko et al., 1994), which is associated with dementia with Lewy bodies. The beta amyloid plaques and tau fibrillary tangles associated with Alzheimer's disease can also be found in Parkinson's disease with dementia and particularly with dementia with Lewy bodies, which may in part be explained by some common genetic risk factors (Walker et al., 2015b). Features of vascular dementia are also commonly found in people with Alzheimer's disease; this may be because of common risk factors (e.g. high blood pressure or high serum cholesterol) or because vascular related damage contributes to the development of Alzheimer's pathology (Stewart, 2002).

Parkinson's disease (with or without dementia) and dementia with Lewy bodies are part of a spectrum of illnesses/conditions called the synucleinopathies (Chapter 26 in Walker et al., 2014). The location of where the characteristic lesions (Lewy bodies) first occur and then spread influences the clinical picture and thus the diagnosis the patient is given (McKeith, 2007). Similarly, frontotemporal dementia and motor neurone disease are said to form a continuum (Burrell et al., 2016) along with amyotrophic lateral sclerosis (Chapter 26 in Walker et al., 2014). People can display features of any or all these different diagnostic constructs in different time sequences, which may be due to common genetic vulnerabilities (Burrell et al., 2016).

Many psychiatric diagnostic constructs do not represent conditions that are clearly separated from each other and describe areas of spectrums as described in Chapter 3.

Spectrums of conditions in general medical diagnostic constructs

This section will discuss general medical diagnostic constructs that exist in spectrums, both a single spectrum of illness/condition as well those that exist as part of a spectrum of illnesses/conditions (see Chapter 3).

Acute coronary syndromes are caused by a ruptured coronary arterial plaque triggering a thrombotic response. If this results in a partially obstructed major or completely obstructed minor artery then the diagnosis is unstable angina or non-ST elevation (partial thickness or subendocardial) myocardial infarction (NSTEMI), and an obstructed major artery would lead to a diagnosis of ST elevation myocardial infarction (STEMI) (Chapter 18 in Walker et al., 2014; Timmis, 2015). NSTEMI is usually distinguished from unstable angina by the presence of raised cardiac troponin and from STEMI by the absence of ST wave changes on the ECG. There is a clear spectrum of severity from unstable angina to NSTEMI to STEMI without natural 'zones of rarity' between these diagnostic constructs; the troponin and ST elevation on ECG are both dimensional with thresholds applied to identify 'pathological' change and to differentiate diagnostic constructs.

Dilated cardiomyopathy is a diagnostic construct that shows great heterogeneity of causative factors such as alcohol, multiple genetic conditions, or autoimmune diseases. This results in a high degree of variability of pathological findings (Chapter 18 in Walker et al., 2014).

Doctors are taught to recognize 'pink puffers' and 'blue bloaters' in chronic obstructive pulmonary disease that are described as 'prototypical concepts'. It is recognized that in clinical practice, features of 'blue bloaters' and 'pink puffers' overlap in patients with no 'zone of rarity'; that is, patients with COPD can have features of both prototypes (Chapter 19 in Walker et al., 2014).

COPD is a diagnostic construct of limited airflow and chronic inflammatory response in the respiratory system to noxious particles that shows great heterogeneity amongst patients given this diagnosis. It is a 'group of conditions' (Conway et al., 2015) that were formerly diagnosed separately until the realization that given the high degree of comorbidity it was best diagnosed under this broader diagnostic construct. The major components are increased airway reactivity, fibrosis of the lung tissue, disease of the small airways (bronchitis) and of the air sacs called alveoli (emphysema). Varying degrees of these components exist amongst different patients which share common causes such as smoking (Chapter 19 in Walker et al., 2014).

Infection of the lungs by the aspergillus fungus is often a complication of other lung diseases and can take several forms—chronic necrotizing pulmonary aspergillosis and 'subacute' and 'semi-invasive' aspergillosis—that form a spectrum of illnesses/

conditions with indistinct boundaries, along with fibrosing aspergillossis (Chapter 19 in Walker et al., 2014).

Endocrine problems caused by autoimmune conditions frequently co-occur; for example, autoimmune thyroid disease may present with several types of auto-antibodies producing mixed clinical pictures (Chapter 20 in Walker et al., 2014).

Multiple endocrine neoplasia (MEN) is a genetic condition that presents with two main forms of comorbid endocrine tumours: MEN type 1 and type 2. MEN type 1 consists of primary hyperparathyroidism, pituitary tumours, and pancreatic insulinomas or gastromas. MEN type 2 consists of primary hyperparathyroidism, medullary carcinoma of thyroid, and phaechromocytoma. A MEN variant, type 2b, also includes features similar to Marfan syndrome and skeletal/dental abnormalities (Chapter 20 in Walker et al., 2014).

Inflammatory bowel disease has been suggested to be a continuum of three main and two intermediate subphenotypes partly due to genetic factors: ulcerative colitis, inflammatory bowel disease—unspecified (intermediate), colonic Crohn's disease, ileocolonic Crohn's disease (intermediate), and ileal Crohn's disease (Cleynen et al., 2016).

Others suggest Crohn's disease and ulcerative colitis are separate entities (but with overlapping features) that are themselves heterogeneous composites of multiple conditions (Sachar and Walfish, 2013)

Although type 1 (insulin-dependent) and type 2 (non-insulin-dependent) diabetes are described as two separate clinical entities, they may be opposite ends of a spectrum with no 'zone of rarity' between them (Gale, 2006). A diabetic complication—diabetic ketoacidosis—is a clinical problem that can be found on a spectrum with hyperglycaemic hyperosmolar state; cases can present with mixed features, features of only diabetic ketoacidosis, or hyperglycaemic hyperosmolar state (Chapter 21 in Walker et al., 2014).

Psoriasis has been shown to be more common in people with a raised BMI and/or type 2 diabetes. The risk is partly related to increased BMI and partly due to common genetic causes (Lonnberg et al., 2016). The onset of epilepsy has been shown to be significantly commoner in people with type 1 diabetes compared to people without type 1 diabetes (Chou et al., 2016a).

Gastro-oesophageal reflux co-occurs with several conditions, most notably asthma (for unclear reasons) and recurrent cough, chest infections, and chest pain that may mimic angina (Chapter 22 in Walker et al., 2014).

H. Pylori infection of the upper GI tract is common with a prevalence of 50–90% in different populations (Chapter 22 in Walker et al., 2014). It can present with a spectrum of conditions without intervening 'zones of rarity', from healthy/asymptomatic infection to gastritis to duodenal or gastric ulcer to gastric cancer, depending on when the condition presents, characteristics of the bacteria itself, 'host' factors such as nature of the immune response, and external factors, for example NSAID painkiller use or smoking (Chapter 22 in Walker et al., 2014).

Coeliac disease is associated with many auto-immune conditions (such as type 1 diabetes or primary biliary cirrhosis). Coeliac disease can exist on a spectrum of severity with prevalence in the United Kingdom of 1%; approximately half are asymptomatic and the rest have varying degrees of resultant symptoms. Some of the asymptomatic cases are latent and will display symptoms later (Chapter 22 in Walker et al., 2014).

TB infection exists in a spectrum from completely successful immune response with eradication to partially successful immune response but continuing infection (and infectiousness) and occasional flare-ups to a rapidly progressive illness which is 'imperfectly represented' by the current categorical classification (Rangaka et al., 2015).

Coeliac disease exists on a spectrum with dermatitis herpetiformis. Patients who present with dermatitis herpetiformis invariably have the characteristic intestinal pathological evidence of coeliac disease (but often without gastrointestinal symptoms) and share the same histocompatibility antigen groups as coeliac disease. By contrast, fewer than 10% of patients who present with coeliac disease have signs of dermatitis herpetiformis (Chapter 22 in Walker et al., 2014).

Alcohol causes a broad spectrum of damage to the liver with alcoholic liver disease being subdivided into three overlapping pathological types and associated clinical pictures: fatty liver, hepatitis, and cirrhosis. Pathology of alcoholic liver disease can overlap with other conditions such as non-alcoholic steatohepatitis (Chapter 23 in Walker et al., 2014).

Non-alcoholic fatty liver disease is associated with diet and sedentary lifestyle and is regarded as the hepatic aspect of the metabolic syndrome (Chapter 23 in Walker et al., 2014). It has a spectrum of severity without 'zones of rarity' between different stages (Glen et al., 2016). The mildest form, steatosis, is often asymptomatic and not associated with morbidity but is commonly found in people with the metabolic syndrome (Chapter 23 in Walker et al., 2014). More severe forms can be symptomatic and carry an increased risk of cirrhosis and liver cancer (Anstee et al., 2011).

Autoimmune hepatitis has great heterogeneity of immunomarkers but similar pathology and treatment (Chapter 23 in Walker et al 2014). Autoimmune hepatitis also exists on a spectrum with primary biliary cirrhosis (PBC) with overlapping features. PBC also tends to co-occur with autoimmune or connective tissue diseases, for example, systemic sclerosis and coeliac disease (Chapter 23 in Walker et al., 2014). Primary sclerosing cholangitis (PSC) is associated with the presence of many other conditions particularly ulcerative colitis. About two out of three people with PSC also have ulcerative colitis and 3–10% of people with ulcerative colitis have PSC, but only 1% of cases of Crohn's disease also have PSC (Chapter 23 in Walker et al 2014).

Antibodies associated with autoimmune disorders often do not segregate neatly into separate disease categories (Chapter 25 in Walker et al 2014). Rheumatoid factor is found in rheumatoid arthritis, mixed essential cryoglobulinaemia, infective endocarditis, tuberculosis, and even in healthy people aged over 65 years. Antinuclear antibody is commonly found in different connective tissue diseases (e.g. systemic lupus erythematosus or systemic sclerosis), other autoimmune diseases such as rheumatoid arthritis, autoimmune thyroid disease, and autoimmune hepatitis, as well as some malignancies and infections.

Rheumatoid arthritis has known co-occurrence with other autoimmune disorders and has associated systemic features such as pulmonary nodules, fibrosing alveolitis, peripheral neuropathy, or inflammation of the heart, and vasculitis (Chapter 25 in

Walker et al., 2014). It has also been shown to be comorbid with high blood pressure, diabetes, and cardiovascular disease (Siebert et al., 2016).

The division of neurological deficits caused by ischaemia into transient ischaemic attacks if duration is less than 24 hours or strokes if duration greater than 24 hours is described as 'arbitrary' (Chapter 27 in Walker et al., 2014). The division indicates that if more than 24 hours there is a greater likelihood of haemorrhage or extensive cell death (infarction) but the threshold is not based on a natural zone of rarity.

Connective tissue diseases are a broad range of autoimmune disorders. Examples include systemic lupus erythematosus (SLE), systemic sclerosis, polymyositis, and dermatomyositis (Chapter 25 in Walker et al., 2014). They share many common features and are best regarded as an overlapping spectrum of illnesses/conditions (see Chapter 3). There is a diagnostic category of mixed connective tissue disease for patients who display characteristics of at least two of systemic sclerosis, myositis, and lupus. Polymyositis and dermatomyositis exist on a spectrum with each other; dermatomyositis is similar to polymyositis (muscle weakness and other systemic features) with the addition of skin lesions (Chapter 25 in Walker et al., 2014).

Seronegative spondyloarthropathies are a group of related autoimmune joint diseases such as ankylosing spondylitis, reactive arthritis (including Reiter's syndrome), psoriatic arthritis, and arthropathy associated with inflammatory bowel disease (Chapter 25 in Walker et al., 2014). They share an association with HLA-B27 antigen and are called seronegative as they do not test positive for rheumatoid factor or ANCAP auto-antibodies. There are often several clinical features in common such as pattern of joint involvement, sacroiliitis, and inflammatory spondylitis, mucosal ulceration, bowel lesions, anterior uveitis, and nail pitting. They are separated on the basis of differences in the clinical picture or if a cause has been identified. Psoriasis and inflammatory bowel disease can be regarded as part of a complicated spectrum of autoimmune conditions that are linked in this case by spondyloarthropathic features.

Many of the conditions described above—the autoimmune disorders including type 1 diabetes, psoriasis, and multiple sclerosis—can be thought of as a spectrum of illnesses/conditions that include inflammatory disorders including asthma and atopic disorders (Becker, 2001). They differ in the site of pathology (sometimes one primary site such as the insulin-producing cells in type 1 diabetes or multiple sites such as in SLE) and environmental triggers even though these are not always known but are presumed. They share similarities of involvement of the different elements of the immune system and common genetic factors (Becker, 2001).

Abnormalities in tumour necrosis factor may either lead to tissue destruction or even protection of tissue in rheumatoid arthritis, multiple sclerosis, and inflammatory bowel disease (Kollias et al., 1999). Crohn's disease and ulcerative colitis have several common gene regions in common that are likely to be associated with cause, but Crohn's has some associated unique genes which may explain the similarities and differences between the two diagnostic constructs (Cho, 2008). The major histocompatibility complex (MHC) plays a key role in the immune system distinguishing between 'self' and 'non-self' molecules and is linked to autoimmune disorders. A pooled analysis of research into MHC haplotypes (or group of genes) and six autoimmune disorders found several commonalities between SLE, type 1 diabetes, ulcerative colitis,

Crohn's disease, multiple sclerosis, and rheumatoid arthritis (Fernando et al., 2008). Degree of commonality varied between conditions—five between SLE and multiple sclerosis to one between ulcerative colitis and Crohn's disease. This is intriguing as the overlap in clinical features between Crohn's disease and ulcerative colitis is much greater than between SLE and MS. Crohn's disease had several unique MHC haplotypes and ulcerative colitis had one unique MHC haplotype.

A study examining families where at least two of nine autoimmune disorders were present ('multiplex families') found a single nucleotide polymorphism was linked to type 1 diabetes, SLE, rheumatoid arthritis, and Hashimoto's thyroiditis but not to the other autoimmune conditions such as inflammatory bowel disease and multiple sclerosis (Criswell et al., 2005). In the wider population, genetic risk for autoimmune disorders is likely to be due to several genes combining their (possibly individually small) effects similar to metabolic syndrome conditions, bipolar disorder, and schizophrenia (Becker, 2001). The site of action varies depending on individual genetic variability and exposure to environmental triggers leading to one or more autoimmune conditions developing as part of a spectrum of illnesses/conditions (see Chapter 3).

Myeloproliferative disorders are a spectrum of chronic conditions including chronic myeloid leukaemia, myelofibrosis, or polycythaemia rubra vera that have overlapping clinical pictures, and people with a myeloproliferative disorder can change from one condition to another condition within this group of disorders. They are characterized by overgrowth of a 'cell line' in the bone marrow (Chapter 24 in Walker et al., 2014).

Hypertension is a common condition with two-thirds of cases having co-occurring conditions (Kennard and O'Shaunessy, 2016). Type 2 diabetes mellitus (T2DM) is also common and associated with co-occurring conditions; one study found about 20% of people aged between 65 and 74 have diabetes (96% of them have T2DM), 60% have at least one co-occurring condition, and nearly 40% have four co-occurring conditions (Huang, 2016). The reason for high rates of co-occurrence is threefold. First, they tend to be associated with other conditions as part of the metabolic syndrome (Chapter 21 in Walker et al 2014). Second, they often increase the risk of developing other conditions such as ischaemic heart disease. Third, they often arise in people who have risk factors for poor health in general who are therefore likely to develop multiple health conditions.

Variable definitions and constituent conditions of the metabolic syndrome have been proposed ever since it was first identified as syndrome X (Reaven, 1998) comprising lipid abnormalities, insulin resistance, high blood sugars, and high blood pressure. Insulin resistance was proposed as the common causative factor, which also led to the common consequence of coronary arterial disease and myocardial infarctions. The hyperlipidaemias along with T2DM and hypertension are often a consequence of polygenic factors (many genes of small effect) interacting with environmental factors such as diet, alcohol intake, or lack of exercise to produce states that are associated with poor health (Chapters 16, 18, and 21 in Walker et al., 2014). Familial combined hyerlipidaemias are common and likely to form a heterogeneous spectrum overlapping with insulin resistance (Chapter 16 in Walker et al., 2014).

Conditions commonly regarded as part of the metabolic syndrome are high blood pressure, T2DM, hyperlipidaemia, non-alcoholic fatty liver disease, and polycystic ovarian syndrome in women (Chapter 21 in Walker et al., 2014), but there are many suggested definitions of metabolic syndrome in which obesity is also included (Reaven, 1998; Bloomgarden, 2004; Grundy et al., 2004; Alberti et al., 2009; Kassi et al., 2011).

Obesity and insulin resistance are two common (but not universal) factors associated with increased risk for developing metabolic syndrome but other factors are recognized; for example, immunological molecules and proinflammatory/prothrombotic factors (Kassi et al., 2011) and changes in adrenal function (Chapter 20 in Walker et al., 2014). The major risks from metabolic syndrome (e.g. vascular events such as myocardial infarction or strokes) are from the individual components with no greater risk prediction given by the overarching metabolic syndrome category (Grundy et al., 2004). If diabetes is not already present then the risk of developing T2DM is due to individual components such as obesity or high blood pressure (Emdin et al., 2015a).

Metabolic syndrome and its components arise out of an interaction between many genes and the environment (Bloomgarden, 2004). How obesity is defined varies per ethnic group (Alberti et al., 2009). Given the common causative factors, the interaction of multiple genes with the environment, and the frequent co-occurrence of conditions, the individual component conditions are best regarded as a spectrum of illnesses/conditions that are also spectrums with health (see Chapters 3, 4, and 9). Many of the conditions comprising metabolic syndrome share common elements of treatment such as improved diet, increased exercise, and reduced alcohol consumption.

Many general medical conditions exist as part of spectrums. General medical diagnostic constructs are used to describe areas in spectrums of illness/condition and/or spectrums of illnesses/conditions (see Chapter 3).

Alternative forms of mental health classification

Psychological formulation has two approaches to deal with the issue of co-occurrence: explaining common causal factors using existing knowledge of causative mechanisms or not having an explanatory formulation based on the evidence. Causative psychological models have been described for several conditions and other clinical problems; for example, Beck's cognitive model of depression (Beck, 2008). Other causative psychological models are incomplete; for example, the link between traumatic experiences and psychosis (Gibson et al., 2016a). Many of the causative mechanisms cross diagnostic boundaries which allows a 'transdiagnostic' approach to psychological formulation and interventions in therapy (Mansell et al., 2009). These common causative mechanisms would show that co-occurrence of diagnostic constructs/clinical pictures are caused by different manifestations of common psychological mechanisms. This can allow creation of diagnostic constructs or other classification on the basis of similarities of processes and/or causes (see Chapter 4).

The other solution of not using an evidence-based solution to explain co-occurrence of different patterns of clinical picture in a person is reasonable if there is an absence of evidence of explanatory psychological mechanisms. As long as the proposed formulation is jointly agreed by the therapist and the client, that it 'makes sense' and allows progress in therapy, then that is 'good enough' on the grounds of clinical utility.

A symptom-based classification would sidestep the issue of co-occurrence (see Chapter 11). Very few people will be seen who have a single symptom, and as the discussion of co-occurrence in mental health earlier in this chapter shows, many people will present with a great diversity of symptoms. One can proceed without making any assumptions about relationships between symptoms that occur in diagnostic categories. One can work on the basis of what symptoms are present and then examine for potential relationships between these symptoms, perhaps in the form of a network of relationships between symptoms (Borsboom and Cramer, 2013; Borsboom, 2017).

This type of system works best for research (Bentall, 2014) or if you are working with the person for long periods in office hours rather than in brief appointments or in emergencies. It requires recording of a great deal of data—every symptom—so is unlikely to be useful for administrative or social purposes (see Chapter 2). It also ignores the fact that in the community and in clinical practice there are mental health symptoms tend to be associated in certain patterns or dimensions in people (Sartorius et al., 1996; Fink et al., 2009; Kotov et al., 2011; Lahey et al., 2012; Caspi et al., 2014; Stochl et al., 2015). In addition, there may be clinically important relationships such as duration of psychotic symptoms without significant mood symptoms (Kotov et al., 2013).

For professionals who can spend long periods of time with their clients, the improvement in precision of a symptoms dimension-based classification may be worth the extra complication of using multiple 'bits' of information compared to using simpler categorical systems. For depression and anxiety problems, a model involving 11 dimensions has been proposed (Brown and Barlow, 2009), and for psychosis a five-factor model (Van der Gaag et al., 2006b) or bifactor model comprising a general psychosis factor and five specific factors (Reininghaus et al., 2013) has been suggested. It has been argued that current psychosis diagnostic categories just describe different areas of multiple dimensions of psychosis (Reininghaus et al., 2013); that is, diagnostic categories simplify an existing multidimensional psychosis spectrum, thus categorical and dimensional psychosis classifications may be different ways of describing the same phenomenon (Kraemer et al., 2004). The HiTOP system proposes six spectra of 11 syndromal groupings of all symptoms (Kotov et al., 2017).

Dimensional systems must deal with the issue of cross-sectional versus lifetime psychopathology. When people improve, their symptoms may lessen so that a cross-sectional dimensional rating of their symptoms may be similar to people who have never experienced mental health problems. Diagnostic systems manage this, for example by having a category of 'diagnosis *x*, improved'. Dimensional systems can add another set of dimensions such as 'symptoms at worst' and 'symptoms currently experienced' to take this into account (Van Os et al., 1996, 1999). The presence of syndromes—as opposed to spectrums—and cases where psychotic symptoms are present in the absence of significant mood symptoms (Kotov et al., 2013) can also be measured using additional dimensions, yet this merely makes an already complicated system even more complex. Such a detailed system may be useful in research (Kraemer et al., 2004).

For clinical practice, a brief dimensional system along with other important clinical information, such as presence of syndromes, included as part of a formulation may be better. Diagnostic categories can summarize a lot of this information within a category (e.g. presence of a syndrome) so would be more useful in brief appointments or emergency work. A dimensional formulation would suit professionals who have long periods of time to spend with their clients or who are undertaking research using lengthy assessments. Conversely, a diagnostic system can be improved in descriptive accuracy by the addition of brief dimensions in a diagnostic formulation.

Conclusion

The review of the evidence on psychiatric diagnostic constructs demonstrates that there are often no zones of rarity between different diagnostic constructs and that they often co-occur. This happens even where clear disease processes are involved, such as the dementias. They may represent different areas of a spectrum of illness/condition and/or be part of a spectrum of illnesses/conditions (see Chapter 3). However, they share both these characteristics with many general medical diagnostic constructs. For spectrums, this may be because there are no natural boundaries but that it is important or seems obvious to recognize different areas of the spectrum for reasons of clinical utility (such as different prognostic implications or treatments) or different clinical pictures. For spectrum of illnesses/conditions, the reason for co-occurrence may be because different diagnostic constructs have similar causes/mechanisms (such as environmental factors or biological factors such as genetics or similar underlying processes). However, these problems of lack of boundaries are not present as commonly in general medical diagnostic constructs (general medical conditions with clear boundaries were not discussed in this chapter).

Alternative forms of classification may be useful. Psychological formulations may be able to identify common processes if evidence for these have been demonstrated. Symptoms and dimensions may ignore the co-occurrence issue by only describing what is present. All these classifications are not likely to be useful in brief appointments or emergencies or for social/administrative purposes.

The lack of clear boundaries is a commoner problem in psychiatric diagnostic constructs than in general medicine, and co-occurrence may be commoner in psychiatric diagnostic constructs, but there is still some overlap between the two types of diagnostic constructs (see Table 11.1).

Table 11.1 Zones of rarity and comorbidity of psychiatric diagnostic constructs compared to general medical diagnostic constructs.

	No Overlap	Some Overlap	Near Total Overlap
Is the condition described by a diagnosis clearly separated from other conditions in terms of clinical features?		X	
Is there little co-occurrence of conditions; i.e. they are separate entities?		X	

Chapter 12

Biological factors and health

Box 12.1 Questions to compare diagnostic constructs of psychiatry with general medicine

- Is the condition clearly identified with a causal mechanism (aetiology)?
- Is the condition clearly associated with a proven and detectable difference in structure or process? This difference acts as a proof of the diagnosis and can be identified with some sort of test such as biochemical or radiology tests.

This chapter will focus on biological factors that are part of the biopsychosocial model (Engel, 1981). It discusses whether biological causative factors and/or differences of structure or functions/processes common to all people who meet the criteria for a diagnostic construct (including the presence of biomarkers) have been identified (see Box 12.1). Establishing causality is complex and one suggested method is to weigh up factors such as strength of relationship, specificity, and plausibility (see Chapter 4). There will be an abbreviated summary of the evidence for psychiatric diagnostic constructs then discussion of general medical diagnostic constructs with gaps in the knowledge of causation or differences of structure or process. The information in this chapter is necessarily a brief, non-comprehensive summary of a large field of knowledge.

The strength of relationship between factors thought to be involved in causation (or prevention) of a condition is often measured using case-control or cohort studies. The prevalence of a given factor is compared between participants who meet the criteria for a condition and those who do not. If this factor is found to be much commoner in participants who meet criteria for a condition then this may indicate a causative relationship, and if it is much less common compared to people without the condition then this may indicate a protective role preventing the condition. This relationship between being exposed to the factor and chances of developing the condition compared to those not exposed to a factor is often expressed in terms of a relative risk or an odds ratio (Chapter 7 in Schoenbach and Rosamond, 2000).

Relative risk for these purposes is the incidence of the condition in those exposed to the factor divided by the incidence of the condition in those not exposed. The odds ratio in this scenario is the probability of meeting the criteria in those exposed to the factor divided by the probability of meeting the criteria in those not exposed to the factor. The relative risk and odds ratio can be regarded as roughly equivalent in conditions that are 'rare' in the population, with less than 10% incident in the population being used as the yardstick for rare. In commoner conditions, the odds ratio tends to overstate the relationship and the relative risk is preferred (Chapter 7 in Schoenbach and Rosamond. 2000; Sedgwick, 2014).

The magnitude of relative risk for a condition can be summarized using terms such as 'weak', 'moderate', and 'very strong'. A guide to the meaning of these terms and how they correlate with relative risk is given below (Chapter 9 in Schoenbach and Rosamond, 2000).

1.1–1.3	Weak
1.4–1.7	Modest
1.8–3.0	Moderate
3–8	Strong
8–16	Very strong
16–40	Dramatic
40+	Overwhelming

Population attributable fraction (PAF)—also known as population attributable risk proportion/percent—describes the proportion of people who meet the criteria for a condition in a population attributed to exposure to a risk factor for that condition (Chapter 7 in Schoenbach and Rosamund, 2000). It indicates the percentage of cases of the condition that would be prevented if the specified risk factor was eliminated from the population. For example, worldwide the PAF for smoking and deaths due to tracheal, bronchial, and lung cancers is 70% (Danaei et al., 2005), but in the United States the PAF for smoking and lung cancer is 82–87% depending on whether the effects of passive smoking are included or not (US Department of Health and Human Services, 2014) due to different prevalence of risk factors in different populations.

'Attributed' implies an established causal relationship but this is not always the case. Many conditions have several causes with complex relationships (see Chapter 4; Rothman, 1976) so the PAFs for a condition often add up to greater than 100%. The PAF in a population depends on the strength of the relationship between the risk factor and the condition as well as how prevalent the risk factor is in a population.

Biological factors and mental health

This section discusses 'organic' mental conditions where there has been a biological factor (e.g. general medical condition) identified as the cause. It then briefly reviews the evidence in other mental conditions for associations with biological factors causing them or changes in biological structure/processes.

For the ICD10 schizophrenia diagnostic construct (WHO, 1992), once a known biological cause that explains the clinical picture is identified then the diagnosis cannot be schizophrenia but is transformed into an aetiological diagnosis listing this cause of 'organic psychosis' instead. From a logical or linguistic point of view, we can never identify a biological cause of schizophrenia as a diagnostic construct because the diagnosis becomes 'organic psychosis' instead. Similar criteria occur in other 'functional' psychiatric diagnostic constructs.

The usual methodology linking cause to subsequent differences in structure/process and then production of clinical picture (see Chapters 3 and 4) using criteria such as plausibility and coherence (Hill, 1965) is difficult when our understanding of the functioning of the mind/brain is poor; for example, how nerve activity transforms into thoughts (or vice versa) (Tononi and Koch, 2015). We may identify biological causes (e.g. amphetamines leading to increased paranoia) but we do not know all the links in the chain producing the clinical picture. We may never solve the 'hard problem of consciousness' but perhaps in 50 years' time we might have a good understanding of the brain changes and causes associated with mental health problems (Adolphs, 2015); however, the same has been said over 50 years ago.

In functional psychiatric diagnostic constructs there may be evidence of differences in structure or process in some or many individuals (McGorry et al., 2014), but this has produced little in terms of useful tests for biomarkers in functional psychiatric diagnostic constructs (Kapur et al., 2012). Reframing diagnostic constructs onto subtypes based on common structure/process differences or causes rather than similar clinical pictures would be better (Kapur et al., 2012), and these changes in structure/process should also include psychological and social factors. Biological causes/differences in structure or process can be used as biomarkers which have several roles in medicine e.g. confirming a diagnosis, measuring treatment response and estimating prognosis (Davis et al., 2015). Examples exist in psychiatry but far less than in other medical specialties where an estimated 60–70% of important clinical decisions are made using investigations (Chapter 16 in Walker et al., 2014).

Lishman's textbook, *Organic Psychiatry*, is the authoritative source on the 'psychological consequences of cerebral disorder' (Lishman, 1997). Table 12.1 summarizes biological factors identified as having causal roles in some mental health problems. This causal relationship is more direct than the increased risk of mental health problems in people with chronic medical illness such as depression (Katon, 2011; Chapter 10 in Walker et al., 2014) where the medical illness can be viewed as a psychosocial stressor. Recognizing a causative biological factor in a patient has several implications. If the biological factor is recognized and eliminated, then the mental health problems will improve. Next, sometimes disease presents initially as mental health problem to doctors and is missed, leading to progression of the disease process and missed opportunities for prompt treatment. Even when medical disease is recognized as directly causing mental health problems, there are usually gaps in our knowledge of the entire pathway from cause to clinical picture, and some parts of the pathway—including vulnerability or mediating factors—may be due to psychosocial processes, for example, psychological interpretations of disease symptoms (Katon, 2011).

There are close links between some diseases, especially disease affecting the brain and mental health problems beyond that of a psychosocial stressor. Most people with mental health problems in clinical practice (let alone those in the community not seeking care) will not have a disease process identified as a cause. Dementia is obviously different: the focus is on identifying the cause, particularly if reversible and not degenerative (e.g. hypothyroidism), or distinguishing from 'pseudo dementia' caused

Table 12.1 Diseases or other biological factors causing psychiatric symptoms.

	Type of Psychiatric Symptom			
Type of disease/ Biological factor	**Mood symptoms (depression, mania)**	**Anxiety symptoms**	**Psychosis**	**Major Cognitive Impairment/ Dementia**
Neurological	Strokes (CVAs), MS, Parkinson's' disease, Alzheimer's disease, epilepsy Head injuries (Chapter 5 in Lishman, 1997) Intra-cranial space-occupying lesions, e.g. tumours, Head injuries (Chapter 6 in Lishman, 1997)	Temporal lobe epilepsy, head injuries (Chapter 5 in Lishman, 1997)	Temporal lobe epilepsy, Huntingdon's disease, Dementia Head injuries (Chapter 5 in Lishman, 1997) Intra-cranial space-occupying lesions, e.g. tumours, Head injuries (Chapter 6 in Lishman, 1997)	Cerebrovascular disease, e.g. as result of CVA, Inherited or degenerative disease, e.g. Alzheimer's or Parkinson's. Progressive supranuclear palsy. MS, Head injury, Chronic subdural haematoma, Hydrocephalus
Infectious	Infectious mononucleosis, brucellosis, toxoplasmosis, herpes simplex			Syphilis HIV Post-encephalitis, Subacute sclerosing pan-encephalitis Prion diseases–CJD, Kuru
Connective tissue / Inflammatory disease	SLE		SLE (Chapter 25 in Walker et al., 2014)	Sarcoidosis

(continued)

Table 12.1 Continued

	Type of Psychiatric Symptom			
Type of disease/ Biological factor	**Mood symptoms (depression, mania)**	**Anxiety symptoms**	**Psychosis**	**Major Cognitive Impairment/ Dementia**
Endocrine/Metabolic	Cushing's syndrome Hypothyroidism, Hyperthyroidism, Hyperparathyroidism, Addison's disease	Hyperthyroidism, Phaechromocytoma, Hypoglycaemia	Hypothyroidism (Chapter 11 in Lishman, 1997)	Hypothyroidism (Chapter 11 in Lishman, 1997)
Cancer	Space occupying lesion in brain or as part of cancer's systemic effects		Space-occupying lesions in brain such as tumours	Primary tumour in brain or secondary spread to brain or Para- neoplastic syndrome
Nutritional/Toxic	Pellagra (niacin deficiency) (Chapter 12 in Lishman, 1997)		Vitamin B12 deficiency (Chapter 24 in Walker et al., 2014)	Thiamine/ Vitamin B12 deficiency Anoxia, carbon monoxide poisoning, Heavy metal poisoning
Medication	Corticosteroids, oral contraceptive pill, interferon, phenothiazines		L-dopa and methyl-dopa, anti-malarial drugs, corticosteroids	
Drugs of abuse	Alcohol	Alcohol and benzodiazepine withdrawal	Cocaine and amphetamine (Chapter 13 in Lishman, 1997) Cannabis in 'especially predisposed' (Chapter 13 in Lishman, 1997) Alcohol withdrawal, alcoholic hallucinosis after prolonged alcohol abuse	Alcohol
Other		Paroxysmal arrhythmia	Delirium	Delirium

Source: data from (Walker et al., 2014) and (Lishman, 1997)

by a depressive condition, although this diagnostic construct is still controversial (Jolley, 2015). Further examples of diseases and biological factors will be described later in this section.

Delirium is a transient condition but can last up to 12 months or more (McCusker et al., 2003). It is characterized by acute onset of fluctuating attentional and cognitive impairment, sleep disturbance, psychotic symptoms, and over- or underactivity (Young and Inouye, 2007). It is caused by factors such as acute medical illness or medication and is commoner in people who already have dementia; 50% of cases of delirium in a hospital also have dementia (Ryan et al., 2013). All the steps from causes to the production of symptoms and signs in delirium are not fully understood (McCusker et al., 2003). It is common in medical and surgical inpatients, from 20% of acute admissions to the general hospital (Ryan et al., 2013) to 30% of older inpatients (Chapter 7 in Walker et al., 2014). In absolute numbers there are often more people with psychotic symptoms (due to delirium) in the medical and surgical wards than in the acute adult psychiatric wards (due to functional mental health conditions).

Genetic factors causing mental health problems have been extensively researched. For general medical conditions, these are often associated with classic Mendelian genetics where single dominant genes or pairs of recessive genes or single X-linked recessive genes in males are clearly causative. This type of pattern is rarely found in people with functional mental health problems, hence the frequent failure of 'candidate gen studies' in psychiatry (Flint and Kendler, 2014).

A recent review of genetics and psychology (Plomin et al., 2016) listed ten important findings that have been replicated in multiple studies (and thus more likely to be true). Those relevant for mental health are listed here:

- Genetic factors substantially influence all psychological traits including mental health symptoms.
- Environmental factors including culture and individual experience also affect psychological traits.
- Many genes of small effect contribute to this heritability of psychological traits.
- Psychological traits correlate with each other in large part due to genetic mediation (so that the identified genetic risk factors often do not map neatly onto separate diagnostic categories but *across* several diagnostic categories).
- Continuity of psychological traits including mental health symptoms through time is related to genetics as opposed to fluctuating mental health problems where the fluctuations are usually caused by environmental effects like life events.
- Genetics also has a significant effect on measured environmental factors—our neat division of nature/nurture is often false.
- Genetics has a significant effect on the relationship between environmental factors and psychological traits.
- Environmental effects are often divided into shared/common or non-shared/individual and even children growing up in the same family have greatly differing experiences.

- Most experiences we label as mental health symptoms and signs are often at the extreme end of a spectrum distributed throughout the population (see Chapter 10) and it is better to talk about *diverse* psychology not *abnormal* psychology.

The contribution of genetics to the expression of a trait or chance of developing a condition is often expressed as 'heritability'. This measures how much of a difference for risk of developing a condition/value of a trait *between* individuals is due to genetic differences and not the contribution of genetics towards the whole value of the difference/trait. This is different from the PAF. Some traits like height are highly heritable but an individual's adult height is greatly affected by environmental factors such as diet, poverty, and exposure to severe or recurrent illness. A high heritability statistic does not therefore mean that the level of expressed trait or condition is almost always due to genetics not environment.

Conditions with a high level of heritability do not necessarily have all the specific contributing genetic factors known. Another issue is where the methods of classifying a participant as meeting the criteria for a condition have reliability concerns which make it harder to identify the contributing genetic factors.

Heritability is often measured by comparing differences in traits or prevalence of conditions between monozygotic twins (genetically identical) and dizygotic twins (who share 50% of their genes). It is either expressed as a percentage of variance or as a fraction (0.2 would be equivalent to 20% of variance). This type of twin study often divides causative factors into genetic and environmental factors, which are further split into common/shared (amongst all offspring such as family environment, economic, culture) and individual/non-shared (such as life events or trauma) factors. The use of twins tries to control for shared environmental factors whilst attributing differences between dizygotic and monozygotic twins to genetics—the Equal Environment Assumption (EEA)—and differences between monozygotic twins are attributed to non-shared environmental effects. The review by Plomin and colleagues (Plomin et al., 2016) noted that non-shared environmental factors have more effects than shared environmental factors.

A review of studies of several traits where twins were misclassified as monozygotic or dizygotic (Conley et al., 2013) assessed whether the EEA still held in these cases; it seemed to do so (but not for depression, in my reading of the paper). Another review (Fosse et al., 2015) concluded that rates of childhood trauma were commoner in monozygotic compared to dizygotic twins, which may explain some of the apparently high rates of heritability of schizophrenia (and other mental health problems). The authors included evidence that some of this higher rate of adverse childhood environments may be partly attributed to genetics, and the authors imply that no conclusions about heritability can be drawn from twin studies on schizophrenia (and this could also be extended to other mental health problems). A more evidence-based conclusion is that heritability estimates from such twin studies are at the upper limit of the potential figure and may be overestimates, but heritability cannot be dismissed. One study tested the EEA amongst twins for five common mental disorders—such as major depression or alcoholism—and found it was a reasonably valid assumption in these disorders (Kendler et al., 1993).

Genome Wide Association Studies (GWAS) measures frequency of common single nucleotide polymorphisms (SNPs)—variations of possible nucleotides at a specific location in the genome—amongst participants who meet the criteria for a specified condition compared to participants who do not (Bush and Moore, 2012). Very large numbers of participants allow for detection of genetic markers that are only present slightly more frequently in participants with conditions (the genes of small effect referred to earlier). GWAS can also be used for traits on a dimension/spectrum. They often identify genetic loci genomic regions, rather than genes and often do not directly code proteins but may affect regulation of gene activity or just be a marker close to the location that is actually causative (Harrison, 2015).

Copy number variants (CNVs) affect more than 1,000 DNA base pairs in the form of deletions, duplications, inversions, or translocations of portions of a chromosome; they tend to have large effects if associated with a condition (Kirov et al., 2015).

Further complicating genetic analysis is that mutations in the same gene or region of genes can be associated with the development of different and related neuropsychiatric conditions (Zhu et al., 2014). Even where causative genetic factors have been identified, the sequence of events from genetic factors to clinical picture is often not wholly established (Chapter 1 in Mitchell, 2015).

Another commonly used technique in researching biological factors and mental health is the use of imaging techniques on the structure and function of the brain (see Martinelli and Shergill, 2015, for a brief review). Computer tomography (CT) and magnetic resonance imaging (MRI) scan assess the structure of the brain, such as size of different regions or intra-cerebral changes such as damage due to ischaemia. Positron emission tomography (PET), single-photon emission computed tomography (SPECT), and functional MRI (fMRI) can be used to measure aspects of functioning such as increased blood flow to a region indicating increased activity or the reverse indicating reduced activity in brain regions or connections between different brain regions during specified activities. Other measurements that are possible using PET/SPECT/fMRI include number of receptors for neurotransmitters and level of activity of neurotransmitters. Electroencephalogram (EEGs) can measure electrical activity of the brain and magnetoencephalographies (MEGs) can measure magnetic activity. Imaging techniques allow measurement of activity whilst performing tasks to allow correlation between brain activity and psychological functions. A meta-analysis of various classification methods of brain scans to separate participants meeting schizophrenia criteria from healthy controls found an average approximately 80% sensitivity and specificity to identify participants meeting schizophrenia criteria (Kambeitz et al., 2015), but this is not accurate enough for clinical practice due to high rates of false positives and false negatives.

Caution should be applied to biological research in mental health. For example, researchers have found evidence of bias in unbalanced reporting of 'positive' findings for peripheral biomarkers in bipolar disorder (Carvalho et al., 2016). Other types of bias include unbalanced citing of research, for example tending to cite studies that positively linked serotonin transporter gene status as a mediating factor between life events and depression rather than the more numerous negative studies (De Vries et al., 2016a). There has also been concern that until recently, fMRI results may have been returning 'false positives' due to use of faulty statistical results (Eklund et al., 2016), although this problem may be mitigated by meta-analytic studies combining multiple studies and, more recently, use of better statistical methods. Many biological factors identified below are common across several diagnostic constructs. One meta-analysis concluded that there were few differences in structural changes between different diagnostic constructs but they had in common grey matter volume reductions in the dorsal anterior cingulate, right insula, and left insula which formed a connected network, and that this loss in grey matter volume would result in reduced executive functioning across several diagnostic constructs such as depression or schizophrenia (Goodkind et al., 2015).

In most cases, our knowledge of the biology of mind/brain is insufficient to explain the whole clinical picture; there is still a need for insights from psychology and sociology.

Estimates of heritability of mental disorders have been made through a variety of methods including twin studies and GWAS and other techniques using electronic healthcare records or national databases have identified common genetic factors, usually a *polygenic* effect involving many genes of individually small effect, associated with several different psychiatric diagnostic constructs (Antilla et al., 2016; Pettersson et al., 2016). Heritability of psychiatric conditions is in the middle of the range of different types of medical conditions (Polubriaginof et al., 2016). Other large studies have suggested that there are often two broad types of genetic factors linked to vulnerability for broad groups of mental health problems (Kendler et al., 2003. 2011a). One study identified a common genetic factor with two genetic subfactors for psychotic problems and non-psychotic problems which included crime (Peterson et al., 2015). Other studies (Kendler et al., 2003, 2011a) have identified broad genetic vulnerability factors for 'internalizing disorders' (e.g. depression or anxiety) and 'externalizing disorders' (e.g. antisocial personality disorder or drug dependency). These two studies agreed that shared environmental factors had little effect (except for conduct disorder) and that genetic and individual environmental factors had major effects, though the balance varied per disorder and within studies, with combined genetic factors contributing approximately 33–67% in variance to liability to developing the condition.

Within these broad internalizing and externalizing genetic factors there can be further subdivisions, for example internalizing genetic factor may split into anxious–misery (such as generalized anxiety and depression) and fear subfactors (such as phobias) (Kendler et al., 2003), or internalizing and external factors may split into two genetic subfactors in both factors (Kendler et al., 2011a).

This pattern of broad polygenic vulnerability factors splitting into more specific polygenic factors is also repeated in twin studies for related diagnostic constructs such as anxiety conditions in general using dimensional measures (Tambs et al., 2009), and of obsessive–compulsive disorder and related diagnostic constructs such as body dysmorphic disorder (Monzani et al., 2014). These show multilevel polygenic factors increasing liability for any anxiety condition, then polygenic factors with increasing specificity for related conditions, and then for specific diagnostic constructs. On average, variation in liability for these diagnostic constructs was split 50:50 between genetic factors and individual experience.

Polygenic factors increasing risk for anxiety in general also increase risk for phobia, but four genetic factors for types or groups of phobias exist that also correlate with each other (Loken et al., 2014). Variations in heritability are large between individual phobias (from 0.06 to 0.57) but are, again, split roughly 50:50 between genetics and individual experiences. All these twin studies carry caveats of being carried out in largely homogenous ethnic groups and in only female twins in one study (Monzani et al., 2014).

There is extensive evidence that personality traits in particular excessive neuroticism—'the propensity to experience negative emotions' (Jeronimus et al., 2016)—increases the risk of developing mental health problems such as depression or anxiety even when other risk factors are controlled for (Kotov et al., 2010; Hengartner et al., 2016; Jeronimus et al., 2016). There is a substantial genetic contribution to personality traits (Turkheimer et al., 2014; Plomin et al., 2016); theories that children learn neurotic attitudes from their parents may be explained by genetically determined neurotic parental traits having multiple effects on their offspring, including modelling of neurotic behaviour to their offspring (Turkheimer et al., 2014). Genetic risk factors for neuroticism may cause increased risk of mental health problems either via psychosocial mechanisms (such as greater tendency to develop depression in response to adversity (Kendler et al., 2004)) or genetic factors may be common to both neuroticism and mental health problems like depression (De Moor et al., 2015; Smith et al., 2016). GWAS has identified a tiny proportion of these many genetic risk factors for neuroticism and they seem to be related to brain function (Smith et al., 2016). The shared genetic factors increasing risk for both depression and alcohol problems affect traits of negative emotionality and lack of control of behaviour (Ellingson et al., 2016).

Anxiety conditions are amongst the commonest of mental health conditions (Tye et al., 2011), thus there is extensive research (often using rodents) on the role of different brain regions in the generation of anxiety. The amygdala plays an important role in anxiety (Maren and Quirk, 2004) at the hub of neuronal circuits communicating with the bed nucleus of the stria terminalis, hippocampus, cortex, and nucleus accumbens (Tye et al., 2011), the prefrontal cortex (Adhikari et al., 2011), and brainstem (Herry et al., 2010). A circuit of neurons (using glutamate excitatory or GABA inhibitory neurotransmitters; Yates, 2013) in the bed nucleus of the stria terminalis, basal amygdala, ventral tegmental area, parabrachial nucleus, and hypothalamus, modulate anxiety behaviour and responses (Johansen, 2013). Others have suggested this subcortical neural circuitry controls defensive behaviours and that fear and anxiety are conscious experiences generated by prefrontal and parietal areas of the brain that link to the subcortical defensive circuitry centred on the amygdala (Ledoux and Pine, 2016).

Several differences in structure or process, including those located in the brain, have been associated with anxiety. Some, such as non-suppression of cortisol in dexamethasone suppression test or increased amygdala activity, do not distinguish between different anxiety diagnostic constructs or depression (Bandelow et al., 2016a, 2016b). Some may be found in both obsessive–compulsive disorder (OCD) and depression such as reduced serum brain-derived neutropic factor (BDNF) (Suliman et al., 2013). Some may be specific to diagnostic constructs, such as participants meeting panic disorder criteria more likely to have panic attacks on carbon dioxide provocation (Bandelow et al., 2016a, 2016b). The biomarkers associated with anxiety conditions are not suitable for use as diagnostic tests as there is overlap between people who meet criteria for the condition and those who do not. A possible exception is the presence of anti-basal ganglia antibodies found in 64% of paediatric autoimmune neuropsychiatric disorder associated with streptococcus (PANDAS) but only 9% of controls with a proven streptococcal infection but no neuropsychiatric symptoms (Bandelow et al., 2016A, 2016B), but this is an organic psychiatric condition.

A paper discussing the complex 'dappled' multifactorial aetiology of psychiatric conditions summarized the evidence for depression (Kendler, 2012). The difference in liability for developing depression between individuals was about 30% for combined genetic factors, 15% for traumatic experiences, 15% for social/political/cultural factors, and 15% for cognitive/personality factors. This is different from PAF (the PAF for traumatic experiences causing depression is far higher (see Chapter 13), and a Swedish twin study on depressive symptoms found genetic factors contributed 30% to variability of symptoms between individuals but that individual experiences contributed 70% (Kendler et al., 2013). Genetic factors may contribute to cognitive vulnerability factors for depression like hopelessness (Wasczuk et al., 2016).

A review of the genetics of depression came to several conclusions (Flint and Kendler, 2014). Depression is a heterogeneous condition. One study identified two genetic factors associated with different types of symptoms and clinical features such as co-occurrence (Kendler et al., 2013). Genetic factors for depression overlapped for males and females but showed some gender differences such as a greater heritability in females than males (Kendler et al., 2001, 2006). This may be the cause of greater vulnerability to depression in females in the absence of adversity (Kendler et al., 2004). The genetic vulnerability factors for generalized anxiety disorder were almost the same as those for depression. It was hard to identify separate genetic factors for melancholia as a subtype of depression or to separate depression from bipolar disorder. GWAS studies would need tens of thousands of participants to be likely to identify genes associated with depression, and that thousands of genetic loci, mostly having small effects, are probably involved (Flint and Kendler, 2014). Given this high proportion of 18,000 genes involved in brain expression, it was further predicted that there would probably be overlap of genetic factors with other mental disorders such as anxiety disorders, bipolar disorder, and schizophrenia (Flint and Kendler, 2014). There may be rare genes that have a large effect on increasing risk for depression but it would be very hard to find them.

Recent GWAS studies identified several genetic loci associated with depression (but most likely a tiny fraction of all causative genetic loci), often, as predicted, shared with other psychiatric diagnostic constructs (Hyde et al., 2016; Wray and Sullivan, 2017) like schizophrenia, bipolar disorder, or autism (Cross-Disorder Group of the Psychiatric Genomics Consortium, 2013B; Wray and Sullivan, 2017), shared genetic architecture with neuroticism (Smith et al., 2016), or body mass and educational attainment (Wray and Sullivan, 2017). Many of these genetic loci are implicated in brain function.

In a study comparing effects of genetics, life events, and childhood trauma on depression risk, life events had a far greater effect than (the small proportion) of known genes on risk of depression, and childhood trauma had an increased risk of depression in participants with lower amounts of genetic risk factors (Mullins et al., 2016). These life events were described as 'dependent', that is, they could have been caused by depression or the prodromal symptoms of depression, which complicates the comparison suggesting life events do have a greater contribution than other factors such as genetics, but maybe less than the paper suggests. Early reports that variations in the serotonin transporter gene increased risk of depression when stressful life events were experienced were not confirmed in subsequent meta-analysis, except if favourable assumptions to the hypothesis are made (Taylor and Munafo, 2016).

Table 12.2 summarizes differences in brain structure or activity as well as other differences found in association with depression such as differences in inflammatory

Table 12.2 Differences in brain structure or activity or other biological factors associated with depression.

Brain Structure	Reduced grey-matter volumes in areas of the orbital and medial PFC, ventral striatum, and hippocampus, and enlargement of the third ventricle in individuals with mood disorders. Hippocampal volume may show some reduction after depression. Small reductions in fractional anisotropy in corpus callosum and anterior corona radiata (unclear if medicated or not) (Kelly et al., 2016).
Brain Function	Increased in the amygdala, orbital cortex, and medial thalamus, and decreased in the dorsomedial/dorsal anterolateral PFC and anterior cingulate cortex (ACC) ventral to the genu of the corpus callosum (subgenual PFC). Increased activity in subcallosal cingulum part of ACC (note contrast to the above) (Hamani et al., 2011). Default mode network or DMN—(ventromedial prefrontal cortex (vmPFC) and posterior cingulate cortex (PCC) are regions most involved) activity associated with increased depressive rumination; Increased connectivity between DMN and subgenual PFC, right medial dorsal thalamus, left dorsal ACC, right posterior lateral parietal cortex in depression. However, only increased activity of subgenual PFC (not DMN) in depression. Suggested link between DMN via medial dorsal thalamus that increases activity in subgenual PFC—depressive rumination in DMN causing affect-laden behavioural withdrawal associated with subgenual PFC activity (Hamilton et al., 2015). Differing responses in DMN comparing melancholic to non-melancholic depression (Guo et al., 2016); differing patterns of reduced connectivity comparing melancholic to non-melancholic depression and comparing melancholic depression to healthy controls (Guo et al., 2016; Hyett et al., 2015) both are small studies < 20 participants in each subgroup. However, a conceptual meta-analysis could not identify any convergent results suggesting previously identified patterns may be spurious (Müller et al., 2017)

(continued)

Table 12.2 Continued

Neurotransmitters	Reduced platelet imipramine binding—suggests may be lower amounts of high-affinity serotonin transporter binding but unclear if this applies to brain serotonin transporter binding. Reduced 5HT1A receptor binding in cortex and raphe nuclei. Reduced prolactin release in unmedicated depressed patients in response to SSRIs suggesting reduced serotonergic brain function (Cowen, 2008). Depletion of tryptophan (serotonin precursor) or depletion of catecholamines (such as noradrenaline or dopamine) triggers brief depressive symptoms in those with *prior* history of depression and currently unmedicated but not in those without prior depression, so is unlikely to be a cause but may be a sign of a compensating mechanism that prevents recurrence of depression (Cowen and Browning, 2015).
Inflammation	Increased levels of interleukin-6 and tumour necrosis factor-alpha in depressed patients; increased levels of c-reactive protein *precedes* development of depressive symptoms (Mondelli et al., 2015). Childhood trauma has a small effect—size increasing c-reactive protein, interleukin-6, and tumour necrosis factor-alpha in adults but further analysis showed only increase in c-reactive protein significant for all types of trauma; physical or sexual abuse increases interleukin-6 and tumour necrosis factor (Baumeister et al., 2016). Inflammation and depression have bidirectional effects in a *subset* of depressed patients increasing each other. Inflammation increased by diet, obesity, childhood adversity (Kiecolt-Glaser et al., 2015)—note links with metabolic syndrome.
Other	Reduced BDNF (Brain-Derived Neurotrophic Factor) levels in brain, e.g. from post mortem human studies and evidence from mouse models but implication controversial (Groves, 2007); reduced serum BDNF levels in unmedicated participants with depression compared to healthy controls—large effect size but overlap in values with healthy controls (Sen et al., 2008). Low blood folate levels associated with depression. Low cholesterol levels associated with depression. Non-suppression in the DST indicating excessive cortisol production but poor sensitivity—many cases of depression will show suppression—and poor specificity—also occurs in other mental health conditions, e.g. psychosis or mania (Arana et al., 1985). Non-suppression DST and/or high night time cortisol in melancholia (Fink and Taylor, 2007) Reduced latency to REM sleep in melancholia (Fink and Taylor, 2007).

PFC = prefrontal cortex

5HT1A = serotonin receptor Type 1A

DST= dexamethasone suppression test

Source: data from (Mössner et al., 2007) and other sources listed

markers. This will be based on a review of biomarkers for depression (Mössner et al., 2007), and other sources of information will be referenced. As is the case with all functional psychiatric conditions, differences in structure or process may be secondary to other causes and not a cause. No suitable biomarkers are known that can be used as diagnostic tests and any differences listed below often do not clearly separate people meeting depression criteria from healthy controls. Changes due to medication are not listed.

Schizophrenia does not follow single-gene Mendelian inheritance and a family history of schizophrenia is uncommon in people who meet the diagnostic criteria (about 10% is a commonly quoted figure; Pope et al., 1980), but still commoner in their relatives than the general population (i.e. a strong to very strong relationship) (Taylor and Abrams, 1975). A meta-analysis of twin studies estimated heritability of schizophrenia at 81% (consistent amongst studies of varying quality), with shared environmental effects contributing 11% of the variability of risk *between* individuals to developing the disorder (Sullivan et al., 2003). Bipolar disorder has a similar estimated heritability of 0.75, equivalent to 75% (Sullivan et al., 2012). Population-based studies of relatives found heritability of 58–59% for bipolar disorder and 64–76% for schizophrenia (Lichtenstein et al., 2009; Song et al., 2015), with contribution of non-shared environmental experiences accounting for most of the rest of variability between individuals. These heritability figures for schizophrenia and bipolar disorder are greater than for common mental disorders including depression described earlier (Kendler, 2012), indicating the greater role of genetic factors for bipolar disorder and schizophrenia than for depression.

Twin and population studies have indicated genetic factors common to both schizophrenia and bipolar disorder have equal to or greater contribution to variability of risk between individuals than genetic factors unique to these diagnostic constructs (Cardno et al., 2002; Lichtenstein et al., 2009; Song et al., 2015). Genetic risk factors for schizoaffective disorder were common to both bipolar disorder and schizophrenia without any unique genetic factors for schizoaffective disorders (Cardno et al., 2002). Heritability for milder psychotic experiences in the community varies per type of experience and is less than heritability for psychotic illness with a greater contribution by non-shared environmental experiences for these milder experiences (Zavos et al., 2014). The association between stressful life events and psychotic experiences in adolescents is partly due to genetics (Shakoor et al., 2016). Genetic risk factors increasing risk for schizophrenia are also associated with living in economically deprived neighbourhoods (Sariaslan et al., 2016).

Copy number variants (CNVs) are commoner in people meeting schizophrenia criteria (Costain et al., 2013) but they are usually estimated to be present in under 1% of people meeting schizophrenia criteria (Marshall et al., 2016), but higher estimates of 2.5% (Rees et al., 2014) to 5% of cases (Costain et al., 2013) exist. The classic CNV associated with schizophrenia is a deletion of approximately 3 million base pairs on chromosome 22q11.2 causing velocardiofacial syndrome which has a high incidence rate of schizophrenia (Kirov et al., 2015). CNVs linked to schizophrenia greatly increase the chances of developing the condition, but the penetrance—or how often a CNV is associated with meeting schizophrenia criteria—varies from 2–7.5% to 55%

(i.e. from moderate to overwhelming strength of relationship), with about 11 CNVs linked to increased risk for schizophrenia at levels of statistical significance (Kirov et al., 2015).

Identified effects of CNVs associated with schizophrenia include on neuregulin (Harrison, 2015), a presynaptic cell adhesion protein that affects neurotransmitter functions (Rees et al., 2014), and on excitatory (glutamate) and inhibitory (GABA) neurotransmitter functioning (Pocklington et al., 2015). CNVs associated with schizophrenia are also associated with other early onset neurodevelopmental disorders like autism spectrum disorder or attention deficit hyperactivity disorder (ADHD) (Kirov et al., 2015).

The Psychiatric Genetics Consortium has completed GWAS in large international samples and identified over 100 genetic loci increasing the risk of meeting schizophrenia criteria (Ripke et al 2014), some of which have been replicated in the Han Chinese population (Li et al., 2015). The increase in odds ratio for meeting schizophrenia criteria for each SNP is usually tiny—about 1.1–1.2 (Harrison, 2015). A great many risk-associated SNPs are needed to increase the risk of schizophrenia by a moderate degree and these SNPs are common amongst non-affected individuals with 8,300 genes likely to be implicated in schizophrenia (Ripke et al., 2013)—a *polygenic* inheritance pattern. This is in contrast to CNVs which are rarer but have large effects on risk. Like CNVs, SNPs that increase the risk for schizophrenia are also implicated in other disorders such as bipolar disorder, ADHD, autism spectrum disorder, and depression (Cross-Disorder Group of the Psychiatric Genomics Consortium, 2013A, 2013B; Bulik-Sullivan, 2015); that is, they have *pleiotropic* effects (a gene affecting more than one trait and/or increasing risk of developing multiple disorders). The identified SNPs include those thought to alter brain function through actions on calcium ion channels, dopamine receptor type 2, and glutamate receptors (Ripke et al., 2014; Harrison, 2015).

SNPs with effects on the immune system have also been associated with increased risk for meeting schizophrenia criteria including those associated with the major histocompatibility complex (MHC) (Ripke et al., 2014) which may also affect neurodevelopment and glutamate function (Harrison, 2015). One study showed that MHC genetic loci that increased multiple sclerosis risk also decreased the schizophrenia risk but with no association with bipolar disorder (Andreassen et al., 2015). Genetic loci associated with increased risk for schizophrenia have been discovered near the gene increasing expression of C4 component of the immune complement system, which increases synaptic pruning in the brain (Sekar et al., 2016). This may happen by increasing microglial cell activity (associated with synaptic pruning; Hughes, 2012) which a systematic review including four studies suggested may be increased in brain white matter in schizophrenia (Najjar and Pearlman, 2015). A study too recent to be included in this review suggested that microglial activity was increased in schizophrenia (Bloomfield et al., 2015), but this was not replicated in unmedicated participants who met criteria for schizophrenia (Holmes et al., 2016), or in a study with mostly unmedicated participants (Hafizi et al., 2016).

Single gene/environmental interactions that may increase the risk of psychosis have been possibly identified for cannabis (Di Forti et al., 2012), childhood trauma (Colip et al., 2013; Alemany et al., 2016), and serious obstetric complications (Nicodemus et al., 2008).

Approximately 25% of genetic factors contributing to heritability may have been identified but this did not include recent GWAS research (Owen, 2012). Three contributory factors toward this 'missing heritability' were suggested: that more genetic factors will be identified in future; unidentified gene–gene interactions (epistasis) may contribute to heritability; and the effect of external factors on genes (epigenetics) such as DNA methylation (Harrison, 2015). It could also be that heritability has been overestimated.

Several identified genetic loci increase risk for both bipolar disorder and schizophrenia. In a case-control study, it was impossible to identify genetic loci that were significantly more common in bipolar disorder than schizophrenia (or vice versa) but a polygenic risk score, based on genetic loci that tended to be more common in one diagnostic construct than the other, was able to significantly differentiate between bipolar disorder and schizophrenia. Participants with schizophrenia diagnosis but who also tended to have manic symptoms tended to correlate with bipolar polygenic risk scores suggesting clinical heterogeneity of schizophrenia may have a genetic basis (Ruderfer et al., 2014).

It is likely that further genetic research will lead to change in psychosis diagnostic constructs to those based on biological pathways (Owen, 2012). Genetic research based on identifying *endophenotypes* (based on structural or process differences, not diagnosis, and present also in people who do not meet diagnostic criteria but may be either vulnerable to developing the illness or inherited some of the features of it) associated with genes may be more fruitful than diagnostic-based research (Owen, 2012). Examples of endophenotypes include brain structure (e.g. cortical folding and thickness) and process (e.g. theory-of-mind tasks) (Gurung and Prata, 2015), including neuropsychological functioning (Greenwood et al., 2013). Linking endophenotypes to genetic loci increasing risk for schizophrenia has so far had none to suggestive only success in demonstrating a significant association (Greenwood et al., 2013; Liu et al., 2017b). No pathway from gene to clinical picture with all intervening stages known has been identified.

Table 12.3 lists differences in brain structure and/or activity as well as other biological factors that have been associated with psychosis or schizophrenia. Usual caveats apply about whether they represent causation, and that overlaps in values occur between healthy controls and people who meet schizophrenia diagnosis. They are based on reviews of evidence on schizophrenia including biomarkers and endophenotypes for schizophrenia as well as other sources referenced in the table ((Matheson et al., 2014; Thibuat et al., 2015; Schmitt et al., 2016a, 2016b), chosen because they seem reliable or have been replicated, for example, from meta-analysis. No biomarker has been identified that is diagnostic of schizophrenia.

Biological factors associated with mental health problems described by the personality disorder diagnostic construct have been identified, although none can be used as diagnostic biomarkers. Two of the most important in clinical practice—antisocial personality disorder/psychopathy and borderline personality disorder—share both common and condition-specific genetic factors; the genetic factors produce temporally

Table 12.3 Differences in brain structure or activity and other biological factors associated with schizophrenia/psychosis.

Brain Structure	Increases in volume of basal ganglia, lateral, and third ventricle (may be caused by antipsychotics). Reductions in whole brain volume, grey matter volume in the frontal lobe, superior temporal gyrus, medial temporal lobe, and multiple brain regions, especially left fronto-temporal and limbic regions. Meta-analysis of AP-naïve (i.e. never had antipsychotics) participants showed large effect size grey matter volume reduction in brains of participants meeting criteria for psychosis overall compared to HC. Participants meeting FEP criteria, grey matter reductions particularly right temporal gyrus, left insular cortex, and left cerebellum (Fusar-Poli et al., 2011). Older never-medicated participants meeting schizophrenia criteria in India and China compared to healthy controls showed evidence of brain volume loss globally and in certain areas, e.g. thinner cortex in bilateral ventromedial prefrontal cortex and left superior temporal gyrus and increase in size of certain brain areas, e.g. basal ganglia (McCreadie et al., 2002a; Zhang et al., 2015).
Brain Function	Medium—large effect sizes in participants meeting schizophrenia criteria for deficits in Smooth Pursuit Eye Movement task, P50 neuropsychological paradigm, fMRI activation during a two-back task, oculomotor delayed response, and Continuous Performance Test. Can be used as endophenotype as present to lesser degree in relatives. During executive functioning, working memory, and emotion-related tasks multiple areas of brain show reduced activity, e.g. frontal, parietal and temporal lobes, hippocampus, amygdala, and other limbic system and subcortical areas as well as increased activity in similar areas. (Similar patterns seen in bipolar disorder but some differences with schizophrenia (Tamminga et al., 2014). Smaller changes in similar areas can be seen in relatives of participants who meet criteria for schizophrenia. Reduced white matter integrity in multiple areas of brain such as frontal, parietal, occipital and temporal lobes, limbic system such as amygdala, corpus callosum, and cerebellum.
Neurotransmitters	Large effect size increase in presynaptic dopamine function in participants who meet criteria for schizophrenia compared to HC (Howes et al., 2012)—in one study approximately 50% unmedicated participants meeting schizophrenia criteria had greater dopamine release in response to amphetamines than all HC (Laruelle and Abi-Dargham, 1999). On average 14% increase in striatal dopamine synthesis capacity in participants who meet schizophrenia criteria compared to HC (Fusar-Poli and Meyer-Lindenberg, 2013b) No differences in Dopamine Active Transporter (Fusar-Poli and Meyer-Lindenberg, 2013a; Howes et al., 2012) and no changes in dopamine type 2/3 receptor density (Howes et al., 2012; Kambeitz et al., 2014) compared to HC.

Table 12.3 Continued

	Increased presynaptic dopamine activity may cause psychosis by causing aberrant salience leading to hallucinations and delusions (Kapur, 2003). Presynaptic dopamine dysfunction is final stage in a common pathway caused by multiple 'hits' leading to psychosis in schizophrenia or mania (Howes and Kapur, 2009). Some evidence for normal dopamine functioning in some people who meet schizophrenia criteria whose psychotic symptoms are unresponsive to antipsychotics (Demjaha et al., 2012; Demjaha et al., 2014). Possibility of hyperdopaminergic and normal dopamine subtypes of schizophrenia (Howes and Kapur, 2014). Some evidence for changes in levels of glutamate, glycine (glutamate precursor), and Glx (mix of both glutamate and glutamine) in several brain areas including in unmedicated participants, e.g. increased Glx in thalamus, medial prefrontal cortex, and cingulate gyrus. Increased glutamate levels in medial prefrontal cortex (Poels et al., 2014). Hypothesized that NMDA-type glutamate receptor hypofunction causes deregulated glutamate function including increased glutamate transmission at non-NMDA glutamate receptors in, for example, prefrontal cortex leading to symptoms, cognitive deficits, and neurophysiological indices of schizophrenia (Moghaddam and Javitt, 2012). There is insufficient evidence of glutamate abnormality in all who meet criteria for schizophrenia.
Inflammation	Autoimmune encephalitis caused by antiNMDA receptor antibodies—significantly associated with IgG antibodies (in 1.46% of cases of psychosis and for all classes of antibodies in FEP; Pollak et al., 2014) though effect of antibodies may be minimized by one large study with high rates of non-IgG antiNMDA receptor antibodies in HC. Autoimmune encephalitis associated with distinctive clinical picture: marked neurological and cognitive deficits and can also be associated with other autoimmune antibodies (Rickards et al., 2014). One paper suggested antiNMDA receptor antibodies are rare but can be found across several psychiatric diagnostic construct classes (Schou et al., 2016). Elevation of peripheral inflammatory markers such as Il-6 and sIL-2R in schizophrenia. Elevated serum CRP also found but inconsistent association with clinical features and recovery. Similar findings in bipolar disorder (Mondelli et al., 2015). Higher serum Il-6 levels in participants with chronic stabilized schizophrenia compared to euthymic bipolar patients may be due to levels of activity of mental disorder (greater in those with persistent symptoms than those who are currently well)—Il-10 levels elevated in both groups compared to HC (Kunz et al., 2011). Moderately increased schizophrenia risk of schizophrenia if toxoplasmosis gondii antibodies present (odds ratio 2.73) (Torrey et al., 2012). A more recent meta-analysis concluded toxoplasmosis gondii antibodies was associated with increased risk for bipolar disorder and OCD as well with an odds ratio 1.43 for schizophrenia (Sutterland et al., 2015).

(*continued*)

Table 12.3 Continued

Cognition	Seven areas of cognitive deficits: processing speed, attention/vigilance, working memory, verbal learning and memory, visual learning and memory, reasoning and problem solving, and verbal comprehension. Medium-large effect sizes in meta-analysis of cognitive deficits in studies of AP-naïve participants meeting schizophrenia criteria (Fatouros-Bergman et al., 2014). Similar findings from meta-analysis of cognitive deficits in FEP (may not be all AP-naïve and includes people who do not meet criteria for schizophrenia including, for example, manic psychosis)—large effect size deficits in variety of cognitive domains including IQ, executive functioning, memory impairment, processing, and motor speed (Aas et al., 2014). Possibly two types of cognitive impairment in schizophrenia—no/minimal impairment and greater impairment (Chiang et al., 2016). Negative and disorganization symptoms associated with executive impairment and lower IQ (Dibben et al., 2009). Small effect size greater cognitive impairment in participants meeting schizophrenia criteria compared to participants meeting bipolar disorder criteria. Bipolar disorder cognitive impairment may show three patterns—none, selective (processing speed) or more global impairment (Jensen et al., 2016)
Other	Medium effect sizes of reduced BDNF (Brain-Derived Neurotrophic Factor) levels in blood and brain in schizophrenia and disruption of association between BDNF blood levels and brain activity in schizophrenia (Skilleter et al., 2015). Increased rates of minor physical abnormalities and neurological 'soft signs'. Stimulant drugs—e.g. amphetamines or cocaine—increase dopamine release and increase risk of psychosis. Ketamine and PCP cause psychotic type symptoms by NMDA receptor antagonism. Cannabis associated with strongly increased risk of meeting criteria of psychosis disorder but with a dose-related increase in risk associated with severity of use (odds ratio of about 2 for any use and 3.9 for heavy use) (Marconi et al., 2016). Longitudinal study in the Netherlands calculated PAF for 'any use' cannabis of 50.4% for needs-based diagnosis of psychotic illness (Van Os et al. 2002). PAFs in South London PAF of 24% for first episode psychosis caused by potent cannabis, 6.2–13.3% in Germany, New Zealand, and the Netherlands respectively. Variations probably due to different prevalence of heavy cannabis use and strength of cannabis (Di Forti et al., 2015). To prevent one case of schizophrenia would need several thousand people stopping smoking cannabis (Hickman et al., 2009). Cannabis relationship with psychosis likely to be complex interaction with other causes (Hamilton, 2017). Circulating specific microRNA levels may be a promising biomarker for schizophrenia but more evidence needs gathered to prove this (Carins, 2015).

AP = antipsychotics FEP= First Episode Psychosis HC = Healthy controls

Source: data from (Matheson et al., 2014), (Thibaut et al., 2015), (Schmitt et al 2016A, 2016B), and other sources listed

stable psychological traits with fluctuations due to environmental causes (Reichborn-Kjennerud et al., 2015).

Heritability has been estimated at 40% for borderline personality disorder but with (unidentified) genes interacting with environmental causes such as childhood trauma to increase the risk of meeting the diagnostic criteria with the involved genes best thought of as being part of a 'plasticity' rather than a 'vulnerability' process (Amand et al., 2014). A review of biological factors associated with borderline personality disorder focused on younger people but also discussed adults noted evidence for structural changes in fronto-limbic circuits (including amygdala and hippocampus); reduced recruitment of regulatory processes in the anterior cingulate cortex and prefrontal cortex; alterations of serotonin, glutamate and GABA neurotransmitter systems; and poorer neuropsychological functioning (Winsper et al., 2016). These biological factors may be a result of causative processes including psychosocial causes such as childhood trauma.

Psychopathy (which overlaps with antisocial personality disorder) has been associated with grey matter reduction and functioning abnormalities in ventromedial prefrontal cortex and anterior cingulate cortex, although there are methodological caveats (Koenigs, 2012). A review of evidence of biological factors for antisocial and violent *behaviour* identified reductions in structure and function within the orbitofrontal cortex, anterior cingulate cortex, and dorsolateral prefrontal cortex; heritability for antisocial and aggressive behaviour of 40–60% (but no identified causative genes); low levels of cerebrospinal fluid serotonin associated with increased risk for impulsive aggression; low resting heart rate as a correlate of aggression and antisocial behaviour in children and adolescents; and reduced amygdala volumes in participants meeting psychopathy criteria (Glenn and Raine, 2014).

Dementia caused by Alzheimer's disease is a psychiatric diagnostic construct identified with a disease process which has identified causative genetic factors such as APOE4 (Scheltens et al., 2016). There exist useful diagnostic biomarkers that can improve diagnosis made on clinical picture alone such as cerebrospinal fluid beta amyloid or phosphorylated tau (Scheltens et al., 2016), or beta amyloid PET imaging to identify fibrillar plaques (Ossenkoppele et al., 2015). Despite this clear identification of a disease process, treatments targeted at amyloid build up have been largely unsuccessful at improving symptoms (e.g. reducing cognitive impairment) and functioning (Scheltens et al., 2016). This has led to some questioning that beta amyloid deposition is the *cause* of Alzheimer's disease. It may instead be a product of the real cause and have little effect on the development of the clinical picture (Harrison and Owen, 2016). Similarly, treatment aimed at reducing aggregations of tau protein to prevent formation of neurofibrillary tangles, another pathological hallmark of Alzheimer's disease, has so far proven ineffective in improving symptoms and functioning (Gauthier et al., 2016).

Some causative biological factors have been identified for mental health conditions and biological factors that may be either causal or related to upstream causative factors, including psychosocial factors, have also been identified, but there may be methodological caveats. Some general medical conditions cause mental health conditions; this means doctors will always be involved to some degree in mental health. The commonest type of genetic contribution to mental health conditions is *polygenic*—many genes of small effect—interacting with the environment to increase the risk of meeting the criteria for the diagnostic construct. These are split into genetic factors common across several diagnostic constructs as well as genetic factors more specific to certain diagnostic constructs. There is also evidence for genetic vulnerability factors operating across multiple diagnostic constructs rather than specific to diagnostic constructs such as those for schizophrenia, bipolar disorder, and other mental/neurodevelopmental conditions. Heritability for psychiatric diagnostic constructs may be average compared to medical illnesses as a whole. The lack of knowledge of the mind/brain means there is incomplete information about links between biological factors and the clinical picture.

Uncertainty of biological factors in general medical conditions

For many general medical conditions, we know a great deal about causes and resultant differences in structure or process and relationship to clinical picture (Walker et al., 2014). This section will discuss medical conditions where there is uncertainty over biological factors for causation or changes in structure or processes.

The previous section discussed how many psychiatric diagnostic constructs had complex aetiologies—often polygenic interactions with environmental factors—that are not completely understood. Table 12.4 will list some (not all) general medical conditions that have similar complex, partially understood aetiologies. The range of conditions listed below will overlap with Table 12.5, which lists poorly understood or unknown aetiology.

It is said that 90% of diagnosis in neurology can be made based on the history if the doctor is experienced enough; investigations are often less useful in identifying accurately causative pathology (Chapter 26 in Walker et al., 2014). Epilepsy is an example of a clinical diagnosis based on recognizing seizures either from description or observation; this diagnosis is often supplemented by using EEGs to detect spike and wave discharges, but EEGs can be abnormal in people who do not experience epileptic fits thus clinical history is important (Chapter 26 in Walker et al., 2014). Several general medical conditions have recognizable common differences in structure or process but poorly understood causes in some or most cases seen in clinical practice, and can be called idiopathic if aetiology is unknown. The distinction between partially understood, poorly understood, or unknown is on a spectrum and I have used my judgement as to where to draw the threshold.

'Medically unexplained symptoms' (MUS) in research are usually defined as physical symptoms in an individual for which the doctor cannot identify a cause such as a disease or pathophysiological abnormality (Steinbrecher et al., 2011). This definition is problematic. Doctors may disagree between themselves as to whether there are medical explanations, the doctor may be mistaken, the medical cause may become apparent later in the fullness of time, the doctor may not have carried out sufficient investigations to come to this view, or have no access to investigations. This latter objection has some evidence. Rates of MUS are higher in less well-developed countries,

Table 12.4 Medical conditions with complex partially understood aetiology.

General Medical Condition	Aetiology
Ischaemic Heart Disease (Chapter 5)	Complex multi-level PGxE causation including polygenic effects e.g. causing hypercholesterolaemia, social effects such as employment and poverty, diet, smoking, access to exercise.
Hyperlipidaemias (Chapter 16)	Some single gene causes but most cases are PGxE: environmental effects include diet, exercise. Genetic factors overlap with other metabolic syndrome conditions.
Porphyrias (Chapter 16)	PGxE for many of the porphyrias, often reliant on environmental factors for disease expression such as alcohol, iron, chemicals.
Atherosclerosis (Chapter 18)	PGxE 40% of variance in risk between individuals due to unknown risk factors. Metabolic syndrome risk factors are PGxE. Environmental factors include diet lifestyle, social class.
Asthma (Chapter 19)	PGxE Genetic factors important, e.g. for course if illness and risk of developing illness but rise in prevalence due to environmental factors (e.g. atmospheric pollutants), not all clearly identified.
Type 2 diabetes (Chapter 21)	PGxE Environmental factors such as diet, overeating, obesity, lack of exercise. Minority of obese people meet type 2 diabetes criteria. Overlap with genetic risk factors for psoriasis (Lonnberg et al., 2016)) and other metabolic syndrome conditions.
H. pylori infection (Chapter 22) and resultant GI disease (e.g. peptic ulcer) or no disease	Factors related to strain of infecting *H. pylori* (e.g. presence of cytotoxin-associated gene), host immune factors, e.g. tumour necrosis factor-alpha polymorphism, and environmental factors, e.g. diet and smoking interact to determine if disease present (in addition to infection) and type of disease.
Inflammatory Bowel Diseases (IBD) (Chapter 22) (Crohn's disease and ulcerative colitis)	PGxE. Genes predisposing to IBD may protect against infectious disease, e.g. TB. IBD thought to occur when genetically mediated abnormal immune response occurs with environmental trigger, e.g. intestinal bacteria.
Non-Alcoholic Steatohepatitis (NASH) and Hepatic Fibrosis (Chapter 23)	> 50% of metabolic syndrome have hepatic steatosis but only minority develop NASH or hepatic fibrosis—likely complex PGxE process is reason for liver disease progression in minority.
Osteoarthritis (Chapter 25)	Combination of personal susceptibility (e.g. polygenetic, high bone mineral density) and mechanical factors (e.g. trauma to joint, load factors).
Rheumatoid Arthritis (Chapter 25)	PGxE including epigenetic factor, environmental factors include smoking or exposure to certain viruses. Trigger for onset of rheumatoid arthritis unknown. Implicated genes vary per ethnic group.

(*continued*)

Table 12.4 Continued

General Medical Condition	**Aetiology**
Multiple Sclerosis (Chapter 26)	PGxE Genes involve immune system; environmental factors include sunlight exposure and exposure to Epstein Barr Virus. Causation unclear.
Psoriasis (Chapter 28)	PGxE but almost 50% of heritability due to one gene PSORS1; environmental factors include skin trauma, infections, drugs, anxiety/stress. Causation unclear. Genetic overlap with metabolic syndrome conditions like obesity and type 2 diabetes (Lonnberg et al., 2016).
Pityriaisis rosea (Chapter 28)	Uncertain cause but an infection thought to be the trigger possibly herpes virus 6 and 7 (Eisman and Sinclair, 2015).

PGxE Polygenic interaction with Environment causation

Source: data from (Walker et al., 2014) and other sources listed

Table 12.5 Medical conditions that have poorly understood or unknown ('idiopathic') aetiology.

General Medical Condition	**Aetiology**
End-Stage Renal Failure (Chapter 17)	5–20% Unknown Cause
Hypertension (Chapter 18)	95% of cases no specific cause found—often unknown what processes lead to the high blood pressure; PGxE causation; environmental factors include diet, lack of exercise, alcohol.
Atrial Fibrillation (Chapter 18)	20% of persistent or permanent AF and 50% of paroxysmal AF cases are idiopathic in nature with structurally normal hearts.
Dilated Cardiomyopathy (Chapter 18)	Diverse group of conditions with unclear pathogenesis.
Idiopathic Interstitial Pneumonias (Chapter 19)	Unknown cause, subdivided into diagnostic constructs based on similarity of pathological appearances.
Sarcoidosis (Chapter 19)	Idiopathic multisystem disorder with characteristic lesion of non-caseating granulomas. Genetic susceptibility, environmental factors—variation in geographic distribution, smoking associated with reduced incidence of disorder,
Pulmonary Eosophinilias (Chapter 19)	Diverse group of disorders—including Churg–Strauss syndrome—often 'intrinsic' (i.e. idiopathic) cause.
Polycystic Ovarian Syndrome (Chapter 20)	Common—about 10% of women in reproductive age range—and often as part of metabolic syndrome. Causation is uncertain with genetic factors and obesity important.
Type 1 diabetes (Chapter 21)	PGxE but largely different genes than type 2 diabetes. Trigger for onset of disease process unknown with several unproven theories.

Table 12.5 Continued

General Medical Condition	Aetiology
Recurrent oral apthous ulcers (Chapter 22)	Common—up to 30% of population. Often idiopathic, in some women occur before menstruation but pathogenesis otherwise unclear.
Acute and chronic pancreatitis (Chapter 22)	Both acute and chronic pancreatitis can be idiopathic.
Chronic liver injury/ hepatic cirrhosis (Chapter 23)	5–10% of cases of chronic liver injury have unidentified causes ('cryptogenic'). About 15% of cases of hepatic cirrhosis cryptogenic causes.
Primary sclerosing cholangitis (Chapter 23)	Aetiology not clearly established but suspected to be immune response to infectious agents in genetically vulnerable individuals.
Aplastic anaemia (Chapter 24)	Causation can be idiopathic.
Leukaemias (Chapter 24)	Initiating cause unknown in > 50% of patients but risk factors include radiation or cytotoxic drugs.
Idiopathic thrombocytopenic purpura (Chapter 24)	Often found in association with other immune system problems like connective tissue disorders.
Systemic juvenile idiopathic arthritis (Still's disease) and adult onset Still's disease (Chapter 25)	Systemic inflammatory disorder, negative for autoantibodies, unknown cause.
Seronegative spondyloarthropathies (Chapter 25), e.g. ankylosing spondylitis; psoriatic arthritis	Similar inflammatory joint disorders with strong association with HLAB27; thought to be triggered by immune response—sometimes environmental trigger is obvious, e.g. reactive arthritis after infection; other times unknown or suspected but unproven.
Systemic lupus erythematosus (Chapter 25)	Autoimmune disorder; aetiology not completely understood but includes genetic vulnerability.
Sjogren's syndrome, poliomyositis, dermatomyositis	Related autoimmune disorders; cause unknown; genetic contribution.
Tension headache (Chapter 26)	Commonest type of headache; cause unknown; strong emotions can initiate headaches by unknown mechanism but associated muscle spasm can worsen symptoms
Cluster headache (Chapter 26)	Cause unknown—genetics/hormones/diet plays no role.
Restless legs syndrome (Chapter 26)	Common—up to 10% of population; cause can be idiopathic.

(*continued*)

Table 12.5 Continued

General Medical Condition	Aetiology
Parkinson's disease and related diseases (Chapter 26)	Often idiopathic cause but genetic vulnerability factors probably contribute but causative genes only identified in a small percentage of cases (Lewis, 2016).
Motor Neurone Disease (Chapter 26)	Often idiopathic, up to 10% may be familial indicating genetic cause.
Lichen planus (Chapter 28)	Cause unknown but suggested to be autoimmune disorder, unproven viral trigger, genetic component.
Vitiligo (Chapter 28)	Affects 1% of population, family history is a risk factor, may be autoimmune but usually idiopathic.

Source: data from (Walker et al., 2014) and other sources listed

perhaps because doctors are less able to order investigation due to their costs (Kisely et al., 1997). There is also evidence that doctors are more likely to describe symptoms as 'medically unexplained' if they have a poor relationship with the patient (Nimnuan et al., 2000). Patients often prefer the term 'functional' (Stone et al., 2002) and MUS terminology promotes mind–body dualism (Creed and Oreje, 2012).

Remembering these caveats, research has shown that the frequency of MUS in primary care is staggering. They may be more common than medically explained physical symptoms and can be present in over 50% of primary care patients (Kisely et al., 1997; Katon and Walker, 1998; Steinbrecher et al., 2011). More than half of all people with MUS do not meet the criteria for psychiatric conditions such as anxiety or depression, excluding diagnostic constructs defined by the presence of MUS such as somatoform disorder (Kisely et al., 1997; Steinbrecher et al., 2011).

MUS are associated with a higher risk for meeting criteria for a mental disorder especially if the person experiences high numbers of MUS (Kisely et al., 1997; Katon and Walker, 1998). MUS are also relatively common in secondary care, despite greater use of intensive investigations. One study found 20% of outpatient appointments for frequent attenders were for MUS (Reid et al., 2001). Another study found about 50% of secondary care new referrals to seven specialties (including dental and gynaecology) had MUS, and an equal level of psychiatric symptoms between participants with medically explained symptoms and MUS (but bear in mind people with medically explained health problems are likely to have more psychiatric symptoms than the healthy population), and that only multiple MUS were associated with psychiatric symptoms (Nimnuan et al., 2001).

An expert review suggested combining total numbers of symptoms together (medically explained and unexplained) to decide if people meet criteria for the somatoform disorder diagnostic construct (Creed and Oreje, 2012) and to move away from the contentiousness of medically unexplained. Doctors often presume MUS have psychological explanations, find them frustrating to deal with (their sapiental authority of knowledge of bodily system dysfunction causing symptoms is challenged), with a negative effect on their relationship with the patient (Wileman et al., 2002). Despite doctors' belief that MUS are psychogenic in origin, a review of the evidence in neurological MUS, and by extension other types of MUS, found little support for this assumption (Wilshire and Ward, 2016).

MUS may present in recognizable patterns or syndromes referred to as 'functional disorders' because the medical problem has little to variable explanation by pathological or pathophysiological changes (Ivbijaro and Goldberg, 2013). They are commonly seen by doctors in all specialties in primary and secondary care (Chapter 10 in Walker et al., 2014). Rather than focusing on MUS, assessing total number of somatic symptoms in conjunction with raised anxiety and focusing on psychological factors as mediators affecting health processes and outcomes not necessarily as suggested causes may improve the clinical utility of somatoform disorders (Creed and Oreje, 2012).

An incomplete list of functional medical disorders is given in Table 12.6 as an example of medical conditions with poor knowledge of cause and/or changes in structure/processes. There is a lack of diagnostic biomarkers. Treatment often includes addressing psychosocial aspects that affect all medical conditions.

Even in general medical conditions with identified pathology or pathophysiology there can be gaps in understanding how this produces the clinical picture. Examples include the duration and nature of episodic attacks in porphyria or the mechanism causing persistent microalbuminuria and the reason for associated higher risk of atherosclerosis/cardiovascular disease (Chapter 16 in Walker et al., 2014). Peripheral arterial disease is common in middle-aged people but only 25% are symptomatic for unclear reasons (Chapter 18, Walker et al 2014). The same pathology can produce markedly different syndromes in ion channel 'channelopathies' (Chapter 26 in Walker et al., 2014).

Some people possess clear biological abnormalities but are not regarded as medically ill and requiring treatment, due to the absence of distress or impairment of functioning. They may need monitoring in case an illness develops, depending on the level of risk. Some examples are listed in Table 12.7.

Our knowledge of most medical conditions is extensive for causation and pathological mechanisms and the use of biomarkers is common. Some medical conditions have complex aetiology often involving polygenetic interactions with the environment, as is the case for mental disorder and for other medical conditions whose aetiology we either do not or only partially understand. Sometimes there are unclear relationships between demonstrated pathology and clinical picture. MUS are very common in primary and medical care and are often not associated with psychiatric conditions. Functional disorders, with an absence of biomarkers, are commonly seen in medical practice. Clear biological abnormalities do not always result in a medical condition requiring treatment.

Conclusion

The review of the evidence shows that there is often a lack of identified causal biological mechanisms or biological abnormalities of structure or process for many psychiatric diagnostic constructs. There is a lack of useful biomarkers common to all people

Table 12.6 Functional medical conditions.

General Medical Condition	Aetiology
Irritable Bowel Syndrome (Chapter 22)	10-15% of population affected at times but only 1 in 10 present to doctors. Higher rates of anxiety/depression in those seen by doctors. Unclear causation but biopsychosocial factors, e.g. childhood trauma, and bowel factors, e.g. gut microbial population and diet are implicated. Self-reported anxiety or depression may double the risk of onset of irritable bowel syndrome (Sibelli et al., 2016). No structural abnormality present. Different subtypes may have altered serotonin function in bowel such as diarrhoea predominant subtype with increased serotonin release and constipation subtype having reduced serotonin release.
Functional dyspepsia and gallbladder dyspepsia (Chapter 22)	Related conditions where symptoms are experienced but no medical cause for them can be discovered.
Fibromyalgia (Chapter 25)	2–3% of population. Risk factors include life events/childhood trauma. Two factors may be important—sleep disturbance (different from that in depression) causing non-restorative sleep and altered central and peripheral pain processing.
Atypical or non-cardiac chest pain (Chapters 10 and 18)	Chest pain when investigations are negative for coronary artery disease that would explain it. Sometimes caused by gastro-oesophageal reflux disease (Chapter 22).
Non-epileptic seizures (Chapter 26)	Seizures that are not caused by epileptic activity, the clinical picture often differs from epileptic seizures. Associated with emotional distress/traumatic life events. Non-epileptic seizures commoner in people with epilepsy (Chapter 10).
Idiopathic facial pain (Chapter 26)	Persistent facial pain with no causative abnormalities detected.
Wide variety of functional neurological problems (Chapter 26)	Patients can present with wide variety of neurological symptoms e.g. weakness, movement problems, sensory deficits and cognitive impairment present to neurologists for which no causative disease process can be identified. Sometimes disease becomes apparent later.
Chronic Fatigue Syndrome/ME/Post Viral Syndrome/SEID (Chapter 10)	Heterogeneous disorder without an established name; likely to be many different conditions; sometimes a clear viral trigger is identified; many different symptoms. Widely different diagnostic criteria make research difficult to interpret. Institute of Medicine report suggests core diagnostic features are substantial six month or longer history of impairment and fatigue; post-exertional malaise; cognitive impairment and/or orthostatic intolerance (Clayton, 2015)
Food allergies (Chapter 22)	1–2% of adults, 5–7% children have proven food allergies but up to 20% of public report that they have food allergies
Temporomandibular syndrome (Chapter 10)	Complex range of conditions with causation thought to be combination of biopsychosocial factors. One of commonest types of mouth/facial pain with prevalence of 2–5% (Durham et al., 2015)

Source: data from (Walker et al., 2014) and other sources listed

Table 12.7 Biological abnormalities but no or low risk of developing medical illness.

General Medical Condition	Aetiology
Orthostatic proteinuria (Chapter 17)	Benign condition with presence of protein in urine after upright posture during the day but no renal disease; < 1 gram protein in urine daily
Asymptomatic bacteriuria (Chapter 17)	Healthy and no symptoms but > 100,000 bacteria/ml of urine (the usual threshold for diagnosing urinary tract infection). Found in 3% of women—more commonly in elderly or pregnant women. Up to 30% go on to develop symptomatic urinary tract infection. Often benign outcome but treated in vulnerable groups, e.g. pregnant women
Asymptomatic diverticula (Chapter 22)	Asymptomatic diverticula in the large bowel are common, particularly in the elderly (over 50% of those aged 70 or more).
Antigen reactions but no hypersensitivity pneumonitis (Chapter 19)	Identifying immune reactions to antigens by serum precipitin tests reveals that far more farmers and pigeon fanciers have positive tests than develop hypersensitivity pneumonitis
'Incidentaloma' lesions	'Incidentalomas' are abnormalities detected on CT scans or other medical imaging that were not expected and often benign; e.g. 'incidentalomas' in the adrenal gland are detected in up to 10% of population—85% of these cause no ill-effects as they are non-functioning adrenal adenomas (Chapter 20)
Benign glycosuria (Chapter 21)	Benign condition causing glucose in urine. Not associated with diabetes. Caused by low renal threshold for excreting glucose, e.g. in pregnancy
Hiatus Hernia (Chapter 22)	Common abnormality (e.g. in 30% of people over 50 years old) but often asymptomatic
Gilbert syndrome (Chapter 23)	Transient mild jaundice/transiently raised serum bilirubin but no hepatic injury as a result. Benign prognosis and no treatment—the biggest risk is getting diagnosis wrong and mistaking for a more serious condition
Simple steatosis (Chapter 23)	Fatty infiltration of liver, the mildest form of non-alcoholic fatty liver disease—not associated with increased morbidity related to liver disease. Often asymptomatic
Monoclonal gammopathy of uncertain significance (MGUS) (Chapter 24)	Monoclonal paraprotein present in 1% of >50 year olds, increasing with age to 5% of >80 year olds in the absence of myeloma or other related conditions. Usually asymptomatic with the paraprotein detected incidentally whilst investigating other condition. About 1% annually develop myeloma or similar condition—by 20 years' duration, 75% will not have developed a serious illness.

Source: data from (Walker et al., 2014) and other sources listed

who meet criteria for a psychiatric diagnostic construct that differentiates them from the healthy population. This can also be the case for general medical conditions for both aetiology and pathology/pathophysiology and a lack of useful biomarkers, but this to a lesser extent. There are also occasions when medical conditions directly cause mental health problems. For this reason, doctors will always be involved in mental health to some degree and will use diagnostic constructs to describe these conditions as they are familiar with diagnosis in their medical practice.

Given the incredible complexity of, and resultant lack of knowledge about, the mind/brain, the prospects for gaining missing information on causes or differences in structure or process is greater for general medical conditions than psychiatric conditions. This highlights the importance of researching psychosocial factors in mental health as they may be easier to measure than complex and often unknown biological factors.

There are examples of clear biological abnormalities that are often detected accidentally that do not require treatment. Medically unexplained or functional symptoms/syndromes are commonly seen in general medicine although the term 'medically unexplained' is contentious. Many diagnostic constructs—medical or psychiatric—involve complex polygenetic interactions with the environment.

Given this evidence, there is some overlap between psychiatric and general medical diagnostic constructs (see Table 12.8).

Table 12.8 Knowledge of biological aetiology and pathology/pathophysiology of psychiatric diagnostic constructs compared to general medical diagnostic constructs.

	No Overlap	Some Overlap	Near Total Overlap
Is the condition clearly identified with a causal mechanism (aetiology)?		X	
Is the condition clearly associated with a proven and detectable difference in structure or process?		X	

Chapter 13

Social factors and health

Box 13.1 Questions to compare diagnostic constructs of psychiatry with general medicine

- Is the condition caused by social difficulties and/or traumatic events?
- Is the diagnosis associated with stigma?
- Is the diagnosis associated with a restriction of liberty?

This chapter will examine the role of social factors in the causation of health problems. It will then briefly discuss the negative social consequences of diagnostic constructs such as stigma and admission or treatment without consent (see Box 13.1). For reasons of brevity. this review will not discuss all social factors but will focus on socioeconomic difficulties, ethnicity, life events, and past childhood maltreatment/trauma.

Social factors and mental health conditions

The bodily system most in contact with factors causing adverse consequences is most likely to suffer subsequent health conditions. Atmospheric poisons/micro-organisms are often associated with pulmonary disease, for instance. Since it is the mind/brain that is responsible for dealing with society, its demands and the difficulties it presents the individual, as well as interacting with other people, then it is unsurprising that social factors are associated with mental health conditions.

Data from the WHO World Health Survey in 2002–2003 from 187,496 individuals from 53 countries included an assessment of depression (Rai et al., 2013). Prevalence of depression varied greatly from 0.4% to 15.7% across different countries, and was commoner in females. This variation may be partly explained by criteria used to define depression (see Chapter 11) may not fit how distress is experienced, expressed, and described in different cultures (Marsella, 1978; Kleinman, 1987; Kleinman, 2004). Culture strongly influences how people think about themselves, others, the world and how it works, so it will also strongly influence the type of thoughts people have when they have mental health problems, and the subsequent clinical picture (see Chapter 4). The variation in prevalence also partly reflects how social/environmental causes of depression vary between countries, not necessarily measured at the countrywide statistics level but in the immediate environment and experience of individuals. Incidence and prevalence of schizophrenia both show wide variation in different populations which indicates the likely role of social/environmental factors in causation of schizophrenia (Saha et al., 2005; McGrath et al., 2008; McGrath et al., 2014,).

Broad socioeconomic adversities or 'socioeconomic position' are a complex group of factors that can refer to class, income, poverty, debt, material possessions, or housing tenure, or the degree of control people have over their lives (Muntaner et al., 2004). These are often defined in different ways in different studies (Fitch, 2011). They are also common; poverty (defined as living on a household budget below 60% of the median national income, with insufficient resources to meet minimum needs) occurs in 20% of the UK population (Boardman et al., 2015). The relationship between socioeconomic position and mental health is complex and may affect women more than men (Muntaner et al., 2004). Increased social inequality has been associated with increased rates of mental illness in developed countries (Pickett et al., 2006). Assuming the relationships are causal (and not markers of association with other underlying causative factors) then adverse socioeconomic position may cause mental health problems or mental health problems may cause adverse socioeconomic position or they may have a bidirectional relationship.

For common mental disorders such as anxiety or depression, reviews of evidence from Western countries noted that most studies are cross-sectional which make it difficult to confirm causation (Fryers et al., 2003; Muntaner et al., 2004; Fryers et al., 2005; Fitch et al., 2011). Adverse socioeconomic factors can cause common mental disorders both immediately in the short term but they can also have long-lasting effects if experienced in childhood (Muntaner et al., 2004)). These reviews show adverse socioeconomic factors have mostly weak to moderate associations with mental disorders, though with some exceptions such as a German study with odds ratios of 5.42 for mood disorder if unemployment was experienced within the past 12 months (Muntaner et al., 2004), or people with six or more debts had odds ratios of 6 for a common mental disorder adjusting for income (Jenkins et al., 2008). A systematic review of the health effects of the recent economic crisis in Europe found strongest evidence for increased male suicide rates and mental health problems for men (Parmar et al., 2016).

In the cross-sectional second British National Survey of Psychiatric Morbidity conducted in 2000, several economic questions were asked. People on low incomes had an odds ratio of 2.09 for common mental disorder compared to those on higher incomes (but this became much more attenuated after controlling for variables such as debt), and 23% of people in debt met criteria for common mental disorder and only 8% of those not in debt (Jenkins et al., 2008). An 18-month follow-up of participants who met criteria for common mental disorder at baseline and 20% of participants who did not meet criteria found that subjective financial difficulties at baseline was associated with higher risk of depression at 18 months (but not anxiety disorders or common mental disorders as a whole). This association was greater for cases at baseline with an odds ratio of 4.20, a strong association, and for cases who were at baseline non-cases, the odds ratio was 2.05 (Skapinakis et al., 2006), a moderate association. In this survey, past psychiatric history was not measured therefore some of the baseline non-cases may have developed depression due to a recurrent depressive episode precipitated by financial difficulties rather than these difficulties causing a completely new mental disorder. Using cross-sectional data from the WHO World Mental Health Survey Consortium there is a threefold difference in prevalence of mental illness between countries with high and low social inequality (Pickett and Wilkinson, 2010).

Socioeconomic position effects are complex. Income deprivation increases risk of common mental disorders at neighbourhood levels more than income inequality, but income inequality at regional levels increases common mental disorders in Wales (Fone et al., 2013). Occupational social class may not independently increase rates of common mental disorders (Meltzer et al., 2003). Different types of debt, such as borrowing for investment, may not increase rates of common mental disorders (Fitch et al., 2011). The WHO World Health Survey reported prevalence of depression varied mostly due to individual factors (fewer material assets, lower education, female gender, economic inactivity, and being divorced or widowed had modest to moderate associations), rather than country-level income or inequality (Rai et al., 2013). Less education is associated with higher rates of mental disorder (Meltzer et al., 2003; Jenkins et al., 2008).

Reviews of studies from low and medium income (LAMI) countries show consistent associations between poverty and common mental disorders (Lund et al., 2010; Patel and Kleinman, 2013). Associations between factors and common mental disorders range from modest to moderate and sometimes strong for less education, food and financial insecurity, housing, social class, hopelessness, rapid social change, physical illness, or violence. There is often a vicious circle with mental health problems worsening financial problems which then exacerbate mental health problems.

Adversities in socioeconomic position have a mostly moderate association with common mental disorders. On balance, there is likely to be a causal relationship in both directions. Although the association is moderate because socioeconomic adversities are common, they are likely to contribute greatly to the amount of mental health problems in the community. The moderate association means that socioeconomic factors combine with other factors, such as other social, psychological, or biological factors, for an individual to exceed thresholds to meet criteria for a diagnostic construct, and this interaction also affects the form of clinical picture in the patient presents. It may be, for example, that psychological processes mediate the relationship between social stressors and mental health conditions (Kinderman et al., 2013). A large study including data on 2.4 million Swedish people based on various population registries found that links between deprivation and depression were confounded by unobserved familial factors (Sariaslan et al., 2015), such as genetic factors.

Socioeconomic factors may have a greater impact on females, which may partially explain the higher prevalence of common mental disorders in females. Strength of association for socioeconomic factors is often measured using odds ratios, which may overestimate the strength of the relationship with conditions such as common mental disorders as a group that occur in more than 10% of the population (Chapter 7; Schoenbach and Rosamond, 2000; Sedgwick, 2014). Measures targeting social adversity to prevent mental health conditions may fail to gain backing for two reasons: only moderate association, and public antipathy to those in poverty who are often regarded negatively and responsible for their predicament (Chapter 3 in Fell and Hewstone, 2015).

Evidence for socioeconomic position and schizophrenia is more mixed. It may be that higher prevalence of schizophrenia in people with socioeconomic adversity reflects the effects of schizophrenia causing this adversity—the 'social drift hypothesis'—including effects caused by the prodrome of the illness before psychosis becomes apparent (Muntaner et al., 2004). Higher rates of schizophrenia in several studies have been associated with neighbourhood factors such as social deprivation (O'Donoghue et al., 2016). A review of international studies measuring incidence rates of schizophrenia correlated with measures of social inequality found a significant moderate association between social inequality and schizophrenia incidence rates (Burns et al., 2014). A study comparing incidence rates of first-episode psychosis over five years in South Dublin and Co. Wicklow found a 3.4× difference for incidence rates between least and most deprived areas (O'Donoghue et al., 2016). These incidence studies can still be explained by social drift in the schizophrenia prodrome and presenting to services after deprivation caused by the condition has occurred. Furthermore, a study combined data from multiple Swedish population registers on 2.4 million individuals found that effects of deprivation on incidence of schizophrenia disappeared after effects of familial risk factors were accounted for (Sariaslan et al., 2015). Further analysis using additional twin study data and genetic testing confirmed that the link with deprivation was mostly due to genetics (Sariaslan et al., 2016).

A meta-analysis of urban/rural differences in prevalence of all mental health conditions, anxiety, depression, and substance misuse problems found a weak to modest association with urban environments (Peen et al., 2010). A Danish large population cohort study found weak to modest associations with being born in Copenhagen and increased incidence of a broad range of mental health conditions (except 'intellectual disability' and behavioural and emotional conditions with onset in childhood) compared to being born in a rural area (Vassos et al., 2016). Meta-analysis of the risk for schizophrenia and a broader non-affective psychosis diagnostic construct found moderate association with 2.37 times higher incidence rate ratio for schizophrenia in the most urban environments compared to the most rural environments and a similar figure for non-affective psychosis (Vassos et al., 2012). Suggested factors linking urbanicity to schizophrenia include social fragmentation, social deprivation, population density, or loss of social capital (O'Donoghue et al., 2016). For schizophrenia, it has been suggested that these associations, similarly to deprivation, are a result of unobserved familial factors (Sariaslan et al., 2015) such as genetics (Sariaslan et al., 2016).

Ethnicity has been researched as a risk factor for mental health problems. The prevalence of common mental disorders as a whole was equivalent between White Europeans and African-Caribbean residents in central Manchester (although the relative balance of anxiety and depressive disorders varied) (Shaw et al., 1999). A study of older adults in north-west London found that depressive symptoms were often linked to physical health problems in South Asians and socioeconomic factors in black Caribbean people, but even controlling for these there were still weak-modest association with increased number of depressive symptoms compared to white Europeans (William et al., 2015).

A large longitudinal study (40,000 households including 4,000 ethnic minority households) with data from four timepoints in the United Kingdom using the mental health section of 12-item short-form measurement of health functioning found that experience of racism negatively affected the mental health component, with more frequent experiences leading to greater effects, and this combined with socioeconomic factors helped explain ethnic differences for the scores in this item (Wallace et al., 2016). A US study of black adults (Rodriguez-Seijas, et al., 2015) found that the link between perceived racial discrimination and mental health problems may be due to psychobiological vulnerabilities to 'internalizing disorders' (see Chapter 12). A meta-analysis of research of ethnic minority status compared to ethnic majorities found weak associations with depression (relative risk 1.21) for ethnic minorities but no association with anxiety; there was significant heterogeneity of results, probably due to methodological differences (Tarricone et al., 2012); a meta-analysis risk for depression and/or anxiety in first- or second-generation immigrants also found weak associations with relative risks of 1.16–1.25 (Mindis and Boffetta, 2017).

There is evidence of a large increased risk of schizophrenia in some migrant populations, including second or further generation migrants (Cantor-Graae et al., 2005). In the United Kingdom, a meta-analysis of incidence rates of schizophrenia in Caribbean-born migrants and their descendants found an average increased incidence rate ratio for 4.7 for this population—a strong risk factor (Tortelli et al., 2015). This risk is not associated with an increased risk in the parents of first-generation Afro-Caribbean participants who met criteria for schizophrenia, suggesting genetics is not the reason (Sugarman and Craufurd, 1994; Hutchinson et al., 1996), and it persists after controlling for socioeconomic factors (Kirkbride et al., 2008). The risk seems greater in African and Caribbean participants than in South Asians; both experience racism but other aspects of their social experience may differ (Thomas et al., 1993; Bhugra et al., 1997), although one study found an increased rate of psychosis amongst Bangladeshis and Pakistanis but this disappeared after controlling for socioeconomic factors (Kirkbride et al., 2008).

This increased risk in migrants for schizophrenia has been found in several countries such as the Netherlands, Denmark, and Sweden (McGrath et al., 2004). Meta-analysis of incidence and prevalence of worldwide studies of schizophrenia comparing migrant populations with native-born populations show increased incidence rates of 4.6 and prevalence increased rates of 1.8 (Saha et al., 2005; McGrath et al., 2008; McGrath et al., 2014). It is likely that the increased risk is for the broader psychosis spectrum including affective psychosis (Harrison et al., 1997), and psychiatrists may be confusing manic psychosis for schizophrenia in people from ethnic minorities (Zandi et al., 2016).

This consistently strong risk factor for increased incidence of psychosis across several countries is selective for certain migrant populations and not apparently related to genetics suggests social environmental causes (Kirkbride, 2017). Suggestions for the mechanism include increased suspicion, vigilance, and mistrust leading to paranoia (Cromby and Harper, 2009), and race-based rejection sensitivity has been shown to be linked to a distress measure associated with attenuated psychosis spectrum experiences (Anglin et al., 2016). These seem to describe links with the milder end of the psychosis spectrum and do not explain all the symptoms associated with schizophrenia such as negative symptoms or cognitive impairment. Analysis of the large AESOP study found moderate association with separation from a parent before 16 years old and psychosis which was commoner in black Caribbean participants, and this may explain part of the increased risk (Morgan et al., 2007). The increased risk for schizophrenia in some migrant groups is evidence for a strong social causative factor, but what exactly this is and the mechanism by which it operates are not clear. Incidentally, the difference between ethnic minority status and much higher risk for schizophrenia/psychosis compared to common mental disorders is a discriminating factor that demonstrates the value of these separate diagnostic constructs.

There has been extensive research into the effect that life difficulties that people face have on mental health problems. These can be divided into life events (such as losing a job or getting married) or hassles, mini-events that require behavioural adjustment, or chronic stress (reviewed in Lloyd, 1980; Paykel, 1994; Kessler, 1997; Kraaji et al., 2002). Life events are described as independent if they are not related to mental health problems, and dependent if could be possibly affected by a mental health problem or its prodrome (Brown and Harris, 1978).

There does seem to be a relationship between increasing number of negative life events and depression and anxiety (Finlay-Jones and Brown, 1981; Kessler, 1997; Kraaji et al., 2002). There is also a relationship between life events and onset of psychosis with just over threefold increased odds of a life event in those with psychosis or psychosis-like experiences compared to healthy controls; this is in the lower end of the strong association range (Beards et al., 2013).

The relationship may be stronger between hassles and depression than for life events (Kraaji et al., 2002). Only a minority of people experiencing negative life events develop depression (Kessler, 1997) In one study of women, one in five experiencing severe negative life events went on to meet depression criteria (Brown et al., 1987), and a minority of people who meet criteria for depression have experienced a precipitating life event (Lloyd, 1980). In the systematic review of life events and psychosis, the prevalence of life events in the psychosis group appeared to be 50% or less averaged over the studies, thus indicating the fact that life events do not explain psychosis in a large proportion (Beards et al., 2013).

There appear to be some specificity effects. Threatening life events tend to cause anxiety and loss life events tend to cause depression, whereas events that are both losses and threats (such as losing a job) tend to cause both anxiety and depression (Finlay-Jones and Brown, 1981) (the latter effect may explain some co-occurrence of anxiety/depression). Intrusive life events, such as being assaulted, may be more closely linked to psychosis (Beards et al., 2013). These intrusive life events may cause post-traumatic stress disorder, which strongly increases the risk of later meeting criteria for schizophrenia or bipolar disorder by approximately fourfold (Okkels et al., 2017). Life event research has some methodological concerns such as recall bias and there is also likely to be a two-way relationship between life events/chronic stress/hassles and mental health problems (Kessler, 1997). There is often an interaction between these social experiences and other social factors, for example, absence of social support (Paykel, 1994) or psychobiological factors such as coping strategies, appraisal of experience, and family history of depression/genetic vulnerability that produces mental health problems (Kessler, 1997; Kraaji et al., 2002). Although the effect of life events may not be strong and dependent on other factors, the population attributable fraction (PAF) has been calculated to be about 40% for depression (quoted in Paykel, 1994).

Maltreatment of children—often referred to as child abuse—including abusive acts or neglect, is tragically common. Childhood adversity or childhood trauma is a broader concept that includes childhood maltreatment and other risk factors such as parental loss including parental death. Accurate measurement of maltreatment is difficult for several reasons including differences between various methodologies of measuring rates and reluctance of some people to disclose maltreatment. Another issue is that maltreatment exists on a spectrum and for 'counting purposes' in research, a threshold has to be drawn, but exactly where it should lie can be debatable. A recent systematic review of worldwide studies provided the following average prevalence figures (Stoltenborgh et al., 2011) summarized in Table 13.1.

Amongst children experiencing maltreatment, it is common to experience more than one type. According to the Crime Survey for England & Wales, 42% of adults who experienced abuse during childhood suffered two or more types of abuse (Office of National Statistics, 2016). This co-occurrence of several different types of abuse makes it difficult to identify relationships between specific types of abuse and mental health problems accurately (Vachon et al., 2015).

A meta-analysis found that there was moderate association between individual types of childhood maltreatment and the risk for developing depression or anxiety disorders; the pooled odds ratio for all types of childhood maltreatment was 2.03 for depression and 2.70 for anxiety disorders (Li et al., 2016), ranging from increased odds ratio from neglect of 1.74 to 2.66 for sexual abuse. Pooled PAF for childhood maltreatment was calculated—58.59% of depression and anxiety—but this is an overestimate created by adding up the PAFs for individual types of childhood maltreatment but because maltreatment frequently co-occurs this will inflate the figure. For depression, a meta-analysis reported odds ratios varying from type of childhood maltreatment from 2.45–3.73 (any childhood maltreatment 2.81) and multiple childhood maltreatment odds ratio 3.61 (Nelson et al., 2017b). A similar odds ratio range was identified in another meta-analysis between childhood abuse and depression, drug use, suicide attempts, and other mental health problems with evidence of a dose–response

Table 13.1 Worldwide prevalence of childhood maltreatment in self-report studies.

Type of Abuse	Prevalence of Abuse
Sexual Abuse	127/1,000 average both sexes (76/1,000 among boys and 180/1,000 among girls)
Physical Abuse	226/1,000
Emotional Abuse	363/1,000
Physical Neglect	163/1,000
Emotional Neglect	184/1,000

Source: data from (Stoltenborgh et al., 2011)

relationship for severity of abuse (Norman et al., 2012). Childhood trauma may have a greater association with depression in those with a lower genetic risk for depression (Mullins et al., 2016).

An 18-year follow-up of a community sample of 639 youths found a strong association (odds ratio 7.94) with documented child abuse, and meeting criteria for cluster B personality disorder diagnostic constructs (e.g. antisocial or borderline personality disorder) in young adulthood (Johnson et al., 1999). A review of the evidence for aetiology of borderline personality disorder (Zanarini, 2000) identified four important strongly associated factors: sexual abuse by male non-caregiver, female gender, emotional denial by male caregiver, and inconsistent treatment by a female caregiver; 40–71% had a history of sexual abuse, and about 90% had a history of any child maltreatment. This condition clearly has a strong relationship with childhood adversity but other risk factors include family history of neurotic conditions (Bandelow et al., 2005), so there seems to be a combination of childhood maltreatment in combination with psychobiological factors that results in people meeting criteria for the condition (Zanarini, 2000). Males are more likely to be exposed to violent events and develop antisocial personality disorder (Ballard et al., 2015).

For psychotic symptoms and illnesses including schizophrenia, one meta-analysis (Varese et al., 2012) found mostly moderate associations between individual types of childhood adversity and psychosis (pooled odds ratio for any adversity was 2.78) and ranging from 1.70 for parental death to 3.40 for emotional abuse, and the PAF was calculated at 35%. Another meta-analysis (Matheson et al., 2013) found a strong association between childhood adversities and schizophrenia of approximately 4 pooled odds ratio depending on which studies were included. There was little difference between the strength of association for schizophrenia compared to depression and personality disorders but less strong association compared to dissociative and post-traumatic stress disorders in this study. This suggested that the link between childhood trauma and subsequent psychosis was not specific; that is, childhood trauma is associated with multiple types of mental health problems (Cannon and Coughlan, 2017).

An analysis of data from 23,998 adults in the WHO World Mental Health Surveys (McGrath et al., 2017) found moderate associations between childhood adversity and psychotic experiences apart from a strong relationship (odds ratio 8.5) between childhood sexual abuse and childhood-onset psychotic experiences (which differs from schizophrenia which has typical onset in late teens to the mid-30s), and the PAF for psychotic experiences caused by childhood adversity was 31%. There are similar mostly moderate associations between childhood maltreatment and bipolar disorder: 2.63 times more likely to have occurred in bipolar disorder compared with non-clinical controls, varying from 4.04 times for emotional abuse (a strong association) to 1.16 times for parental loss (Palmier-Claus et al., 2016).

There is a dose–response relationship with a history of experiencing multiple types of childhood adversity resulting in a very strong association with psychosis, and some types of adversity are more strongly linked to certain types of psychotic symptoms than others (Bentall et al., 2012; Coughlan and Cannon, 2017). Childhood trauma often has a significant effect on the content of symptoms in psychosis (Coughlan and Cannon, 2017).

However, one study examining links between childhood adversity and dimensions of psychotic symptoms identified relationships with positive and excited dimensions but not negative or disorganized/concrete dimensions (Ajnakina et al., 2016), suggesting childhood adversity is only associated with some aspects of psychosis. A review demonstrated that childhood trauma is neither sufficient nor necessary to cause psychosis, and the mechanisms linking trauma to psychosis are not specific to psychosis and are incomplete explanations (Gibson et al., 2016a). Pathways between childhood trauma and psychosis are likely to involve other complex biopsychosocial factors (Coughlan and Cannon, 2017) rather than a simplistic trauma-causes-psychosis mechanism. The PAF figures of around a third for childhood adversity as a causal factor for psychosis also indicates that majority of cases of psychosis are not related to childhood adversity—a conclusion which agrees with an assessment of the role of trauma in causes of first episode psychosis (Fisher, 2010).

Childhood maltreatment increases the chances of developing mental health problems but this is often not specific to any type of mental health problems (Bulik et al., 2001; Vachon et al., 2015) and is associated with adverse clinical features such as increased risk of suicide, poorer response to treatment, and greater co-occurrence of conditions (Teicher and Samson, 2013) which may include a mix of anxiety, mood, and psychotic symptoms (van Nierop et al., 2015). The effect of childhood trauma may vary, depending on gender (Ballard et al., 2015).

Traumatic events experienced during adulthood are also associated with mental health problems. Mass conflict and displacement is globally common with a systematic review showing high rates of post-traumatic stress disorder and depression, particularly amongst torture victims (with moderate to strong association) and/or those exposed to high numbers of potentially traumatic events (Steel et al., 2009). Victims of sexual assault also have high rates of mental health problems such as a strong association with depression or substance misuse (Burnam et al., 1988). In a community sample in the United States for post-traumatic stress disorder, exposure to combat situations was the commonest cause in men and sexual assault in women (Kessler et al., 1995). The large WHO World Mental Health Survey with 34,676 respondents reported an odds ratio of 2.7 for sexual violence and PTSD and 4.2 for witnessing atrocities and PTSD, moderate to strong associations (Liu et al., 2017a).

Apart from the nature of the trauma, other biopsychosocial factors associated with development of post-traumatic stress disorder include past history of mental health problems, family history of mental health problems, history of childhood trauma, and psychological responses to the trauma such as disassociation and degree of emotional response (Brewin et al., 2000; Ozer et al., 2008).

Vulnerability to mental health problems is strongly associated with social factors such as childhood adversity, war, torture, persecution, financial hardships or poverty, unemployment, lack of education, social inequality, and social isolation (Priebe, 2015). These social factors also have a powerful effect on outcomes (Priebe, 2016). The most obvious major omissions from that list of social factors include stressful life events, especially sexual assaults. Mostly the associations are moderate and non-specific. Psychobiological factors interaction with social factors are important to determine if people exposed to these social factors develop sufficient symptoms and impairment of functioning to meet criteria for a psychiatric diagnosis. Culture combines with other social and psychobiological factors to determine the type of clinical picture they present with and hence their diagnosis.

Social factors and general medical conditions

This section will describe the effects of socioeconomic factors on health before discussing effects of social factors on various general medical conditions before ending with a brief review of childhood maltreatment's effects on health.

Health is a product of complex interactions of biological systems with their environment which is impacted by psychosocial factors including effects on several levels from local—such as family—to national or global factors such as economics (Chapter 5 in Walker et al., 2014). The life course, beginning in childhood, can impact on how people behave, which then affects their health (Chapter 5 in Walker et al., 2014). Culture has a central place in how people conceptualize their health and illness and cannot be ignored in medical practice (Napier et al., 2014).

Several socioeconomic factors have been shown to have moderate strength associations (usually odds ratios of 1.5–2.0) with increased all-cause mortality: poor education, measures of low income, occupational class, unemployment, worse living conditions, social deprivation, and increased income inequality (Kaplan and Keil, 1993). A systematic review of the effects of loneliness on physical health found an association with increased mortality from cardiovascular disease and increased risk of prevalence and mortality from stroke (Petitte et al., 2015).

Income inequality may have more effect than average income in rich countries on several health outcomes: life expectancy, health and social problems, child well-being, and infant mortality rates (Wilkinson and Pickett, 2010). The association of income inequality with life expectancy operates on all sectors of society: the richest live longer than those who are merely well-off who live longer than the poor (Marmot and Allen, 2014). There is evidence of narrowing in the mortality gap (especially in men) associated with social inequality in Europe, mostly due to behavioural change (e.g. reduced smoking with resultant falls in deaths due to heart disease and other smoking-related illnesses), improved health prevention, and medical care (Mackenbach et al., 2016). Whilst there seems ample evidence of these associations, the linking mechanisms between income inequality and health outcomes are not clear and they may be confounded with other factors such as the welfare and social policies found in countries with high income inequalities (Coburn, 2015).

Main contributors to the health population have been said to be 'genetic predispositions, social circumstances, gestational endowments, environmental conditions, behavioural patterns, and medical care' (McGinnis et al., 2002). There is often a focus on behavioural causes of ill-health such as smoking, diet, alcohol, and drugs, without acknowledging the causes of these behaviours, for example, social inequalities (Marmot and Allen, 2014). A summary of contributions to population health from three sources (Marmot and Allen, 2014) is presented in Table 13.2. Social factors appear the biggest contributors toward the health of the population.

Table 13.2 Determinants of population health.

Reference	Contributions Towards Health
McGinnis et al., 2002	Social circumstances and environmental exposures—45% Health behaviour patterns—40% Health care—up to 15%
Canadian Institute for Advanced Research in Kuznetsova 2012	Socio-economic—50% Health care—up to 25% Genetics—up to 15% Environmental—10%
Bunker et al., 1995	Health care—43% Other factors—57%

Source: data from (Marmot and Allen, 2014) and other sources listed

An expert review identified social factors that lead to increased risk of cardiovascular disease (Kaplan and Keil, 1993). Worse socioeconomic status, worse education, occupational class such as being a manual worker, and type of housing tenure have mostly moderate associations with cardiovascular disease and related mortality. The relationship with worse socioeconomic status and cardiovascular disease is partly due to risk factors such as smoking, diet, inactivity, obesity, excessive alcohol, and high cholesterol, which are associated with worse socioeconomic status. Haemostatic factors such as plasma fibrinogen levels are related to socioeconomic status so may be a further confounding factor of cardiovascular risk. Worse living conditions in childhood increase the risk of heart disease in later life. The relationship with socioeconomic status has varied with time. In the early to mid-twentieth century, heart disease was associated with the better-off but then became later associated with social deprivation. Access to medical care did not fully explain differences in socioeconomic status and cardiovascular outcomes. A systematic review identified other social risk factors for cardiovascular disease (Hemingway and Marmot, 1999). Job strain had a moderate association with coronary heart disease and people with low amounts of social support and smaller social networks had a moderate to strong association with heart disease.

Respiratory diseases such as asthma and chronic obstructive pulmonary disease (COPD) (Chapter 19 in Walker et al., 2014) are associated with exposure to environmental risk factors. These include atmospheric pollutants and occupational exposure to chemicals such as coal dust or silica and housing-related factors such as damp (which, as medical students, we were told was the biggest public health problem in Glasgow). Health-related behaviours such as smoking also increase risk and even diet. These types of factors tend to be associated with culture and worse socioeconomic status.

Globally there has been a large increase in the prevalence of type 2 diabetes, driven largely by socially influenced factors: changes in the diet, physically inactive lifestyle, obesity, urbanization, and other features of economic development. These factors have affected certain ethnic groups more than others, for example

African-Americans (Chapter 21 in Walker et al., 2014). Cancer risk (Chapter 11 in Walker et al., 2014) is also associated with social factors; even biological risk factors such as smoking, exposure to causative chemicals either in the living environment or through occupational exposure or diet are associated with social factors such as culture and social deprivation. Risks of sexually transmitted infections are influenced by sexual behaviour which is also strongly influenced by cultural factors (Chapter 14 in Walker et al., 2014) such as peer group pressure, parenting, oppression of women and sexual minorities.

The risk of infectious disease, for example, gastroenteritis (Chapter 13 in Walker et al., 2014)) and hepatitis A (Casadevall and Pirofski, 1999; Chapter 24 in Walker et al., 2014) is often strongly influenced by cultural, social, and economic factors such as poverty, access to clean drinking water, systems to treat and remove human sewage, crowded housing with increased proximity to other cases, and food preparation techniques (and avoidance of certain foods because of cultural taboos). The toll of gastroenteritis in developing countries is high: 3-4 million deaths annually, and 50% are elderly people or infants (Chapter 13 in Walker et al., 2014). In the United Kingdom, we should thank the poorly paid people who built our water and sanitation systems in the past as they have saved more lives than contemporary doctors.

TB has been described as a 'social disease' with strong links between it and social factors. Improvements in outcome and reduction in infection rates in the United Kingdom were due to improvements in social conditions, such as reduction in overcrowded housing and improved nutrition, even before the introduction of effective antibiotics (Ortblad et al., 2015). TB is both associated with poverty and social exclusion as well as being a cause of poverty through its debilitating effects on, for example, the ability to work and cost of treatment (Ortblad et al., 2015). Today, over two-thirds of cases in England and Wales occur in the most socially deprived areas (Lipman and White, 2015) and other at-risk populations include the homeless (Rangaka et al., 2015).

Poverty-related causal determinants of TB include poor living conditions (e.g. overcrowding), malnutrition, risk behaviours commoner in the less well-off (e.g. smoking or heavy alcohol use), and poor access to healthcare (Ortblad et al., 2015). Recent increases in TB prevalence in Eastern Europe post-communism's collapse have been caused by social upheaval, worsening social conditions, and lack of access to healthcare (Chapter 19 in Walker et al., 2014). To achieve the WHO target of 90% reduction of incidence of TB by 2035 we will need a 'biosocial' approach that addresses important social factors that increase risk of TB (Ortblad et al., 2015). An example is Chile's 14-point social reform plans from the 1930s to reduce TB which included measures such as increased wages, improved housing, improved working conditions, and compulsory unemployment insurance (Ortblad et al., 2015).

Research into adverse childhood events (ACEs) has identified several effects on physical health. The commonest method of measuring ACEs is a questionnaire for adult participants asking if they were exposed to a variety of stressors during childhood: psychological abuse, physical abuse, sexual abuse involving contact, witnessing substance abuse in the household, someone in the family had mental illness, witnessed violent treatment of mother or stepmother, and criminal behaviour in the household

(Felliti et al., 1998). Some caution applies about the reliability of detecting childhood adversity using questionnaires in adults.

A prospective study based on reports from parents and school from the UK National Childhood Development Study identified different effects on all-cause mortality in men compared to women. Both genders had moderate associations between mortality and adverse childhood events, but in men two or more recorded ACEs increased mortality, but for women there was a greater effect that increased the higher the number of recorded ACEs (Bellis et al., 2014). A 20-year prospective study from the United States (with ACEs recorded at baseline by questionnaire) found no association with mortality in women but moderate associations with physical or emotional abuse in women and an increased effect with multiple types of abuse. These effects could not be accounted for by childhood socioeconomic status, personality traits, or adult depression (Chen et al., 2016). Three mechanisms have been suggested for this increased mortality: increased rates of physical and mental health problems with increased mortality, increased high-risk behaviours for health (e.g. smoking or excessive drinking), or 'early-life programming of biological systems' with persistent adverse effects (Shalev et al., 2016).

Several studies using retrospective assessments of ACEs have shown associations with high-risk health behaviours. The retrospective nature of these studies introduces uncertainty as proof of causality. In a Welsh study, participants with four or more ACEs had very strong associations with heroin or crack cocaine use, strong associations with smoking and high-risk drinking, and a moderate association with poor diet (Bellis et al., 2015). An earlier study from the United States, also using a retrospective questionnaire to identify ACEs, found that participants with six or more ACEs had strong to very strong associations with heavy alcohol use or drug misuse and moderate to strong associations with smoking or multiple sexual partners and a moderate association with physical inactivity or obesity (Felliti et al., 1998).

A 30-year follow-up compared participants with documented child maltreatment with matched control participants. Different types of abuse had different health consequences which included higher haemoglobin levels, lower albumin levels, poor peak airflow, malnutrition, higher HbA1c, poorer oral health, and problems with vision. There was an intermediate interaction with childhood and adult socioeconomic status, high-risk health behaviours (e.g. smoking), and mental health (Widom et al., 2012). Childhood adversity is also associated with pro-inflammatory states which can increase risk of ill-health. See Table 12.2 for further discussion of the link between childhood adversity and increased inflammatory markers.

Several general medical conditions have been demonstrated to have associations with ACEs, usually at least partly caused by high-risk health behaviours. Liver disease risk increased with higher number of ACEs measured retrospectively, with a moderate association in participants with six or more ACEs with up to 50% of this increased risk due to high-risk health behaviours such as heavy alcohol use (Dong et al., 2003). Most types of ACEs have a moderate association with ischaemic heart disease and participants with seven or more ACEs had a strong relationship. The increased risk was due to both biological factors, for example, smoking, physical inactivity, diabetes, and high blood pressure, and psychological risk factors such as depression and anger (Dong et al., 2004). There was a strong relationship in participants with six or more ACEs assessed retrospectively and lung cancer and particularly associated with premature death. This relationship is partly explained by higher rates of smoking in this group but still persisted at a much weaker level of association once smoking was controlled for (Brown et al., 2010a).

Social factors including socioeconomic adversity and childhood trauma have a significant effect on risk for physical health problems, increased mortality, and some general medical conditions, and this relationship is similar in strength to mental health conditions. Adverse social factors such as social inequality and injustice or poverty lead to the clustering of multiple health conditions, both physical and mental (Singer et al., 2017). Social factors ae the biggest determinants of health status.

Adverse social consequences of diagnosis

This section will very briefly discuss some of the negative social consequences of a diagnosis both in mental health and general medicine. It will review the evidence for stigma and for loss of human rights such as loss of liberty and being given treatment without valid consent.

Stigma has been described as a 'mark' which discredits someone in interactive social processes (Goffman, 1963). Some stigmatizing medical conditions lead to people being discredit*able* as not always visible or can be hidden once recovered (e.g. intermittent episodes of bipolar disorder), or discredit*ed* as always visible (Gray, 2002). Stigma for mental health conditions is often greater than general medical conditions (Ben-Zeev et al., 2010). Self-stigma occurs where people internalize stereotypes which lowers self-esteem and reduces self-efficacy (Corrigan and Bink, 2016) and giving up on life goals (Ben-Zeev et al., 2010). Fear of stigma can lead to delay seeking treatment (Corrigan and Bink, 2016). Public stigma refers to how the public treat people with medical conditions; their stereotypes lead to prejudice then discriminatory behaviours (Corrigan and Bink, 2016).

Examples of stereotypes/prejudices about mental health conditions include dangerousness, lack of competence, and responsibility for their problems, leading to discrimination such as avoidance (with reduced employment/housing opportunities), coercion (forced admissions and treatment), and segregation in asylums (Corrigan and Bink, 2016). Structural stigma is exemplified by policies and laws of private- and public-sector entities restricting opportunities for people with stigmatized conditions—intentionally or unintentionally (Corrigan and Bink, 2016)—such as detaining people for treatment regardless of mental capacity, or having voting rights reduced (Sartorius, 2002), and also includes reduced access to general medical healthcare, contributing to increased mortality (Hert et al., 2011).

Stigma against mental health conditions is common in the United States (Corrigan and Bink, 2016) and the United Kingdom (Crisp et al., 2000), often despite reasonable knowledge about treatment, prognosis, and contact with people with mental health conditions. Stigma against mental health conditions varies in different non-Western cultures (Corrigan and Bink, 2016).

Diagnostic categories may increase stigma by groupness, homogeneity, and stability (Ben-Zeev et al., 2010) because they 'group' people together on the basis of a similarity of their problem, and this group can acquire harmful stereotypes in people's minds. People may overestimate degree of homogeneity amongst people who meet criteria for the same diagnosis; that is, they assume that all features are present in everyone and the diagnosis can be equated with the person. People may overestimate degree of stability of mental health conditions and think they will not recover. One study suggested thinking of mental health conditions as on a continuum with health may view people with these conditions as less 'different' and more likely to recover than categorical models (Corrigan et al., 2016).

A review of two meta-analyses of biogenetic explanations for mental health conditions effects on stigma found small to medium effects on blame reduction/lack of responsibility for developing the condition (the largest effect but lack of evidence that it reduced discrimination), increased desire for social distance/avoidance (but not in experimental studies), greater pessimism about outcomes, and association with dangerousness and/or unpredictability, and reduced empathy amongst clinicians—a 'mixed blessing' for stigma (Haslam and Kvaale, 2015). The authors accepted that we should not exclude biological factors including genetics from mental health. Ironically, the authors stereotyped medical approaches as biogenetic in mental health when, as emphasized in this book, it is usually biopsychosocial.

Schizophrenia is a highly stigmatized condition amongst the public; for example, people meeting schizophrenia criteria are viewed as dangerous (Crisp et al., 2000). Changing the name in Japan to one less associated with prognostic pessimism may have reduced media stories associating the condition with dangerousness or other negative aspects (Aoki et al., 2016). Personality disorder is a condition that is highly stigmatized by clinicians. Psychiatrists given case vignettes that differed in certain details such as whether the diagnosis was personality disorder tended to describe people with that diagnostic label as 'manipulative, attention-seeking, annoying, and in control of their suicidal urges and debts', suggesting personality disorder diagnosis facilitates pejorative judgements and discrimination (Lewis and Appleby, 1988). Careless use of diagnostic constructs increases stigma, but without diagnostic constructs, stigma against people with mental health conditions would not be eliminated (Sartorius, 2002). Reports from developing countries where access to psychiatry is limited and psychiatric diagnostic constructs are not used by the populace confirm that social exclusion and harmful stigma can exist without diagnostic terminology.

Many general medical conditions are also stigmatized and some of them are described in Table 13.3. Words such as 'leper' to describe leprosy sufferers indicate the associated stigma, and even conditions that exist on a spectrum with health or do not pose a risk to others such as acne vulgaris are also stigmatized.

People with mental health conditions may be subject to restriction of rights, such as being detained in hospital against their wishes or being given treatment without valid consent. Patients may be subject to pressure from mental health professionals known as 'informal coercion' (to distinguish from legally enforced coercion) such as persuasion, inducements, interpersonal leverage, and threats (Valenti et al., 2015).

Table 13.3 Stigmatised general medical conditions.

General Medical Condition	Notes	Reference
Food allergy	Teenagers may avoid carrying adrenaline injector because of stigma. Teenagers feel socially isolated by allergy,	Chapter 4
Acne vulgaris	Negative effects on self-esteem especially adolescence (suffer bullying, school avoidance, impaired ability to form relationships, achieve employment) despite acne being on a spectrum with health and near-universal amongst adolescents.	Chapter 28
Vitiligo	Stigma varies per population; can resemble leprosy so stigma tends to be greater in areas where leprosy is common.	Chapter 28
Alopecia areata	Psychological effects of alopecia can be significant.	Chapter 28
Excessive hirsutism in females	Associated with stigma and distress. Another condition that exists on spectrum with health.	Chapter 28
Epilepsy	Associated with stigma through history and across cultures. Effects of self-stigma, public stigma, and structural stigma may cause more problems to the person than clinical effects of illness.	Jacoby and Austin, 2007
Tuberculosis	Fear of infection seems to be main cause; can lead to delay in seeking treatment. TB treatment used to involve segregation into sanatoriums.	Courtwright and Turner, 2010
HIV	Self-stigma and public stigma are prominent including from health services, affects use of health services, seeking and concordance with treatment, and quality of life. HIV and AIDS related stigma can be said to be in four stages: at risk/pre-diagnosis, at diagnosis, latent—between illness and health, and social/physical death. Shame and stigma delays seeking treatment.	Chambers et al., 2015 Alonzo and Reynolds, 1995 Fortenberry et al., 2002
Gonorrhoea	Shame and stigma delays seeking treatment.	Fortenberry et al., 2002

Table 13.3 Continued

General Medical Condition	Notes	Reference
Genital herpes	Stigma consists of four elements: personalized stigma, disclosure concerns, negative self-image, and concern with public attitudes.	Wang et al., 2016a
Obesity	Individuals with obesity are highly stigmatized—common stereotypes are that they are 'lazy, unmotivated, lacking in self-discipline, less competent, non-compliant, and sloppy',	Puhl and Heuer, 2009
Lung cancer	Social stigma often based on public view of personal responsibility for illness by smoking even if non-smoker. Can feel blamed by health professionals.	Raleigh, 2010
Leprosy	Stigma affects leprosy sufferers' 'physical, psychological, social and economic well-being'.	Rafferty, 2005
Psoriasis	Stigma was the most powerful predictor of depressive symptoms for psoriasis patients.	Lakuta et al., 2017

Source: data from (Walker et al., 2014) and other sources listed

There is rightful concern over treatment and detention against someone's will and some people will always regard it as wrong (Lidz, 1998). To place these concerns in context, a US survey of 142 participants attending day hospital with at least one admission revealed high levels of distressing experiences in psychiatric settings including physical assault (31%), sexual assault (8%), witnessing traumatic events (63%), being forced to take medication against their will (27%), and 'takedowns' (i.e. physical restraint) (29%) (Frueh et al., 2005). This probably reflects experience over several admissions but it indicates the perils people face on admission to psychiatric wards. Service-user experiences of inpatient care from several countries including the United Kingdom were reviewed (Cutcliffe et al., 2015), and several common themes emerged: a lack of warm therapeutic interactions; lack of respect; limited information or choice on treatment; lack of access to any psychotherapy; coercive/custodial/controlling/inhumane practices, and over-reliance on medication.

A review of European mental health legislation showed differences in minor and major aspects; a major variation is whether presence of 'mental disorder' for treatment is sufficient or if some element of heightened risk is additionally necessary to justify detention (Salize et al., 2002). Use of detention for mental health problems from 1998–2000 varied significantly across Europe (Salize and Dressing, 2004) from 6/100,000 people in Portugal to 218/100,000 people in Finland (in England it was 93/100,000 people including individuals admitted informally who then later converted to formal detention). Service provision such as bed availability is likely to have a strong effect on these differences. There is an increasing use of compulsion. In England, for example (Care Quality Commission, 2016), 30,913 inpatients at a single time point at the end of 2008/9 were formally detained under the Mental Health Act (29.0% of all mental health inpatients) compared to the end of 2014/15 when 54,225 inpatients were formally detained (51.4% of all mental health inpatients).

Sometimes patients are admitted or treated regardless of their objection when they lack decision-making capacity to agree to admission or treatment. Conceptualizing capacity in mental health conditions is influenced by the MacArthur Treatment Competence study model which requires presence of four abilities: able to express a choice about treatment; able to understand information relevant to the treatment decision; able to appreciate significance of that treatment information for one's own situation; and able to reason with relevant information in logical processes of weighing treatment options (Applebaum and Grisso, 1995). A systematic review of mental capacity in psychiatric patients stated that clinicians tended to overestimate capacity, impairments in capacity were common even in patients who agreed to admission, a median figure of 29% of inpatients lacked decision-making capacity, capacity was more frequently impaired in schizophrenia than depression, and that a significant proportion of patients detained under the Mental Health Act had decision-making capacity (Okai et al., 2007).

A comparison of psychiatric and medical inpatients assessed using the MacArthur Competence Test in London (Owen et al., 2013) found impaired capacity in 29.6% of medical inpatients and 51.8% of psychiatric inpatients. Psychiatric inpatients were more likely to show impairments in appreciating that relevant information applied to them without this being distorted (in patients with psychosis or severe mood disorders), and medical inpatients were more likely to show impairments in reasoning (in patients with cognitive impairments, about 25% of the medical sample), but both types of impairment were common in medical and psychiatric inpatients with impaired capacity. Although the proportion of patients with impaired decision-making was lower in medical wards, the numbers of medical inpatients are higher than psychiatric inpatients, thus suggesting admission and/or treatment without capacitous consent may be close in absolute numbers for medical patients compared to psychiatric patients.

Some have suggested admission and/or treatment without capacitous consent for both physical and mental health problems should be combined under the same legislation to reduce stigma (Dawson and Szmukler, 2006). Detention in hospital against a person's will, even if they have capacity, can also occur for certain infectious diseases if the infected person is thought to be a risk to the public (Selinger, 2009). In the United Kingdom, examples include plague, smallpox, AIDS, anthrax, rabies, and TB (Enhorn v Sweden, 2006). This use of enforced detention for people with potentially hazardous infections such as TB as a last resort occurs across other legal jurisdictions such as Sweden (Enhorn v Sweden, 2006), Israel (Weiler-Ravell et al., 2004), and New York (Ball and Barnes, 1994), but is used much less frequently than detentions for mental health conditions. Medical treatments including injections and major surgery have been used in patients who refuse them or unable to consent but have been judged to lack capacity. However, these treatments are usually justified on the basis of risk of harm to the patient or others whereas, for comparison, in some jurisdictions, presence of a mental disorder without risk is sufficient to justify treatment (Salize et al., 2002).

Stigma is greater for mental health conditions but it also exists for general medical conditions. Use of compulsion such as admitting and/or treating without valid consent/opposition is commoner for mental health conditions than for general medical conditions but exists for both types of problems.

Conclusions

There is increased risk caused by social difficulties and/or childhood trauma for developing both general medical and mental health conditions with overlap in similarity of magnitude of some increased risks though intermediary mechanisms may differ. Social factors are the most important determinants of health status. Reducing social adversity and childhood trauma would improve the physical and mental health of the population. Life events and stresses/hassles are a common risk factor for mental health problems and more specific to mental health problems.

Social factors are often inadequate to solely explain the nature and severity of people's mental health problems without taking into account psychobiological factors. Given the greater effect of culture on how mental health conditions are expressed there is some overlap between psychiatric and general medical diagnostic constructs rather than near total overlap.

Mental health conditions do seem associated with greater stigma (some of this seems related to categorical nature of diagnostic constructs) and also with greater use of coercion than for general medical conditions but this also occurs for general medical conditions, hence the conclusion of some overlap (see Table 13.4).

Table 13.4 Social factors in psychiatric diagnostic constructs compared to general medical diagnostic constructs.

	No Overlap	**Some Overlap**	**Near Total Overlap**
Is the condition caused by social difficulties and/or traumatic events?		X	
Is the diagnosis associated with stigma?		X	
Is the diagnosis associated with a restriction of liberty?		X	

Chapter 14

Clinical utility of diagnosis

Box 14.1 Questions to compare diagnostic constructs of psychiatry with general medicine

- Does the condition have uniform prognosis (does the condition have a predictable unitary outcome)?
- Does the condition have different outcomes from other conditions?
- Does the condition predict differences in treatments given and their effectiveness?
- Is the use of the diagnosis justified due to some utilitarian reason such as relieving distress or risk?
- Is there a need for clinical information beyond the diagnosis in clinical decision making?

This chapter compares clinical utility of psychiatric diagnostic constructs to general medical diagnostic constructs often under stressful conditions such as time pressure or fatigue (see Box 14.1). Clinical utility is defined as communicating clinical information, choosing effective interventions to improve clinical outcomes, and predicting future clinical management need (First et al., 2004), including what treatments are most effective. Other information with clinical utility attached to diagnostic constructs are dealt with in other chapters such as associated clinical picture (Chapter 10), co-occurring conditions (Chapters 10 and 11), and treatment responses (Chapter 14).

Clinical utility of psychiatric diagnostic constructs

Allen Frances, the DSM-IV taskforce chair, concluded that the DSM system had mixed evidence of utility for clinical communication, education, research, epidemiological and forensic purposes, but it was still of great clinical use (Frances, 2016). Clinical utility in this chapter is compared to not using any classification at all, for example using a generic term such as 'mental health' or 'distress' for everyone seen by clinicians.

Before effective medical treatments existed, Kraepelin observed that mood disorder episodes (he combined unipolar depression and bipolar disorder into manic-depression) tended to last 6–8 months but were often recurrent, with good mental health and functioning in between episodes (Kraepelin, 1921). Evaluating evidence for unipolar depression's outcomes is complicated because of the use of differing definitions for depression, its remission, and relapse/recurrence (Belsher and Costello, 1988; Burcusa and Iacono, 2007), and the effects of treatment.

Average duration for depressive episodes varies depending on the population studied. Approximately 20% of untreated participants meeting depression criteria who were on a treatment waiting list met remission criteria after 4–8 weeks (Posternak and Miller, 2001). A Finnish primary care study reported median duration of 20 weeks (Riihimäki et al., 2014), and in an American epidemiological study the mean duration of depression was 16 weeks (Kessler et al., 2003). Some studies of clinical populations also found median duration of 20 weeks (Judd, 1997), but one UK study of mostly severe depression reported mean recovery time of 12 months and median 7 months, suggesting the mean was increased by some participants with very long durations of depression (Kennedy et al., 2003). Prolonged duration of depressive episodes in a minority has also been reported in other studies. In the Finnish study only 70% had achieved remission by 5 years (Riihimäki et al., 2014); in a Japanese study of depressed participants seeking psychiatric care (Kanai et al., 2003) 86% had achieved remission after 6 years; and a Danish prospective follow-up of participants receiving psychiatric care after their first episode of depression found 83.3% achieved remission after 5 years (Bukh et al., 2016).

A review of older studies summarized depressive episode recovery rates: 54% achieve remission by 6 months, 70% by 12 months and 88% by 5 years (Judd, 1997). Research indicates depressive episodes may last many months and over 10% of people may have an episode lasting more than 5 years, but is also shows that people who are depressed for 2 years have approximately 50% chance of recovering by 5 years. Increased duration of depression was associated with younger age of onset or suicidal ideation (Bukh et al., 2016), increased severity of depression (Kennedy et al., 2003; Riihimäki et al., 2014), co-occurring substance use disorder ((Riihimäki et al., 2014), or anxiety (Bukh et al., 2016), or a history of childhood trauma (Nanni et al., 2012).

Risk of depression recurrence after recovery from a depressive episode (either full relapse or partial relapse where some depressive symptoms return but the person does not meet all the criteria for depressive episode) is high. Earlier reviews of recurrence in depression summarized recurrence of depressive episodes as 22–27% by 6 months, 36–40% by 12 months, and 50–80% by 2 years or longer (Belsher and Costello, 1988), and a median lifetime number of 4 episodes of major depression with 80% chance of recurrence after the first episode (Judd, 1997). More recent studies have also confirmed high rates of recurrence with either full or partial relapses (Kennedy et al., 2003; Riihimäki et al., 2014; Bukh et al., 2016). One study, which followed up patients prospectively for 12 years after a depressive episode measured weekly level of symptoms, reported high levels of persistent depressive symptoms which were present in 59% of the weeks which were usually below the level of full relapse (Judd et al., 1998).

Multiple factors are associated with increased recurrence of depression in individual studies or reviews of the evidence and are summarized in Table 14.1. Recurrent episodes of melancholia/endogenous depression are less closely associated with triggering stressful life events than other types of depression (Brown et al., 1994).

Table 14.1 Prognostic factors associated with increased recurrence in depression.

Adverse Prognostic Factor	Reference
Severity of first depressive episode	Kessing, 2004; Burcusa and Iacono, 2007; Bukh et al., 2016
Social stressors including stressful life events and/or lack of social support	Belsher and Costello,1988
History of recurrence predicts increased future risk of recurrence and decreased time between episodes	Burcusa and Iacono, 2007; Kessing et al., 2004
Persistent neuroendocrine dysregulation after clinical recovery	Belsher and Costello, 1988
Residual depressive symptoms at time of recovery from depressive episode, indicating partial response to treatment	Kania et al., 2003; Bukh et al., 2016
Family history of mental health problems particularly mood disorders suggesting genetic contribution to risk of recurrence and/or effect on childhood	Burcusa and Iacono, 2007
Psychological factors, e.g. negative cognitions and 'neurotic' personality traits	Burcusa and Iacono, 2007
History of childhood trauma	Nanni et al., 2012; Nelson et al., 2017b
Co-occurring anxiety disorders	Burcusa and Iacono, 2007; Riihimäki et al., 2014
Co-occurring personality disorder	Riihimäki et al., 2014
'Double depression' with co-occurring dysthymia or depressive episode in bipolar disorder	Burcusa and Iacono, 2007
Co-occurring substance misuse disorders	Burcusa and Iacono, 2007
Younger age of onset of first depressive episode	Burcusa and Iacono, 2007

Gender, marital status, and socioeconomic status have not been convincingly shown to increase recurrence rates (Burcusa and Iacono, 2007).

There is some evidence of diagnostic stability for depression in future episodes of mental health problems, that is an episode of depression predicting the next episode of mental health problems will also have a similar clinical picture. Diagnostic stability for depression measured as a percentage retaining the same diagnosis after a period of time (usually years) varies across studies; for example, 75.2% by the end of the second clinical contact but dropping to 43.8% by the tenth clinical contact as a main diagnosis (Kessing, 2005), 40.3–66.7% across a variety of care settings such as outpatient or inpatient (Baca-Garcia et al., 2007), 56.4–72.8% across admissions (Kessing, 2004), and 79% in admissions who were then followed up (Kim et al., 2011). Stability varies with setting of care, for example, a depression diagnosis made in inpatient care is more stable than one made in outpatients (Baca-Garcia et al., 2007), and severe depression is more stable than moderate depression, which is in turn more stable than mild depression (Kessing, 2004). Stability of diagnosis over multiple time points is lower, about 37.5% for at least 75% of clinical evaluations for mild to moderate depression (Baca-Garcia, 2007). The diagnosis of depression may change in individuals because depressive symptoms exist as part of a spectrum of internalizing/emotional disorders (see Chapter 11), and the diagnosis may change on subsequent contacts to another diagnosis in this spectrum, or change to depression from another diagnosis in this spectrum (Lahey et al., 2014).

The rate of conversion of diagnosis from unipolar disorder to bipolar disorder after a first episode of depression in Denmark has been observed to be 6.3% after 2 years and 8.3% by 5 years (Bukh et al., 2016). An 11-year follow-up of white Americans (Akiskal et al., 1995) noted switching to bipolar disorder occurred in the first 5 years: 3.9% converted to bipolar 1 disorder and 8.6% to bipolar 2 disorder. Other important predictive information attached to the depression diagnostic construct such as mortality and appropriate treatment will be discussed later in this chapter.

Kraepelin regarded course and outcomes of mental health problem and treatment response as a valid basis of grouping them into diagnostic categories (Hoenig, 1983). His other major grouping distinct from manic depression was dementia praecox, which he viewed as having invariably chronic deteriorating course, resulting in major social and clinical impairments ((Hoenig, 1983; Kazanetz, 1989) despite 12.5% of his sample recovering (Hoenig, 1983). Kraepelin recognized there may be periods of remission during this decline (Kazanetz, 1989). It was quickly realized that some patients presented with intermediate states between manic depression and dementia praecox (Kendell and Gourlay, 1970), now usually called schizoaffective disorder, and that other types of psychotic illness could be seen that were neither dementia praecox nor manic depression (Kazanetz, 1989), with other psychiatrists describing diagnostic categories for these, for example, cycloid psychosis (Kendell and Gourlay, 1970). Kraepelin could not identify any 'pathognomic' symptoms confirming the diagnosis but described instead greatly heterogeneous clinical pictures (Hoenig, 1983). Eugen Bleuler coined the term schizophrenia to replace dementia praecox and changed the diagnostic concept to a broader construct including a greater range of people (Hoenig, 1983), and regarded it as a heterogeneous diagnostic construct that included many different conditions. Kurt Schneider described 'first-rank' symptoms that helped identify schizophrenia in the absence of organic disease (Hoenig, 1983).

Does modern research agree with Kraepelin? Comparing results of different studies is complicated by methodological issues such as different assessment methods, different diagnostic criteria, differing definitions of outcomes or the effects of treatments, or use of mixed samples of participants with first-episode psychosis or chronic psychosis (Jobe and Harrow, 2005; Jääskeläinen et al., 2013; Morgan et al., 2014). Samples including broad diagnostic criteria of all non-organic psychosis may give better outcomes than samples composed of participants who only meet schizophrenia criteria (Menezes et al., 2006). Studies using narrow diagnostic criteria using schizophrenia criteria influenced by Schneider or Kraepelin with long duration of symptoms and/or premorbid poor functioning tend to show worse outcomes than studies using broad diagnostic criteria based on Bleuler and/or only requiring shorter periods of symptoms (Hegarty et al., 1994). Untreated psychosis episodes (not just schizophrenia) may last on average 61 weeks (but with a large diversity in range of 10 to 213 weeks) before contact with services (Penttilä et al., 2014).

Earlier reviews of outcome from long-term follow-up of participants meeting criteria for schizophrenia—some studies followed up for several decades—recognized that outcomes were variable and good outcomes were present in far higher proportions of people than Kraepelin believed (Angst, 1988; Hegarty et al., 1994; McGlashan, 1998; Jobe and Harrow, 2005) disproving the 'myth' of inevitable decline for all people who meet schizophrenia criteria (Harding and Zahniser, 1994; Zipursky et al., 2013; Zipursky and Agid, 2015).

A recent meta-analysis of recovery in schizophrenia (Jääskeläinen et al., 2013)—with recovery defined as improvements in both clinical and social domains and evidence that improvements in at least one of these two domains had persisted for at least 2 years—estimated that a median 13.5% of participants met criteria for recovery (with an annual 1.4% of participants meeting recovery criteria) but results were skewed so median was felt to be more reliable than the mean of 16.4%. When factors such as first-episode or recurrent psychosis, gender, or diagnostic criteria were taken into account there were no significant differences between studies. This study concluded recovery rates, defined in this way, have not changed, despite the introduction of antipsychotics. An earlier meta-analysis, which defined recovery as substantial improvement in functioning and no psychotic symptoms (Hegarty et al., 1994), found that recovery rates improved with use of antipsychotics and/or broad diagnostic criteria and deteriorated more recently as studies tended to use narrower diagnostic criteria; that is, the apparent worsening of outcomes was due to use of diagnostic criteria associated with worse outcomes.

A systematic review looked at the average frequency of types of outcome in studies following up participants after a first episode of schizophrenia spectrum psychosis (Menezes et al., 2006). Outcomes were divided into good, intermediate, or poor but these were defined differently between studies. For studies with longer than 2 years' follow-up 24.6% of participants had good outcomes (including recovery but also other outcomes regarded as good), 54.5% had intermediate outcomes, and 30.8% bad outcomes. For follow-up over 2 years, 58.9% participants experienced relapse, 30.1% were employed, and 39.3% in functional recovery. Studies using narrowly defined schizophrenia criteria had worse outcomes than studies using broadly defined criteria.

Three studies with long follow-up will be discussed to give a more vivid picture of outcomes. A Dutch study (Wiersma et al., 1998) with 15-year follow-up of 82 first contact, broad, non-affective psychosis criteria for schizophrenia (including acute reactive psychosis) found 11% of the sample having a continuous episode of psychosis during the 15 years, another 10% improved but still had persistent symptoms after partial remission, 12.2% had a full remission after one episode, 14.6% experienced multiple episodes followed by remission, 40% experienced multiple episodes and partial remission with persistent symptoms between episodes, and 12.2% unknown outcomes.

A Canadian study followed up 128 participants after first admission for schizophrenia (Newman et al., 2012) until death or up to 34 years. On average participants spent 24.2% of person-years with no or mild symptoms, 28.7% of person-years with moderate symptoms and 47.1% of person years with severe symptoms. At the end of the study or at time of death for social functioning, about one-quarter were in each category of high functioning, mild to moderate dysfunction, severe dysfunction, and inability to function as defined by SOFAS (scale measuring social functioning).

In the UK AESOP study (Morgan et al., 2014) following first episode psychosis for up to 10 years, participants in the broad non-affective psychosis category (including schizophrenia, schizoaffective disorder, delusional disorder, and other psychotic illnesses, but excluding depressive psychosis and bipolar disorder) 39.7% were symptom-free for at least 2 years by end of follow-up, demonstrating that late recovery from symptoms is possible and the symptoms may plateau or even improve after about 5–10 years (McGlashan, 1988).

Various factors outlined in Table 14.2 are associated with worse outcomes (such as more relapses, worse social functioning, or increased self-harm) in participants who meet schizophrenia criteria, as well as improved outcomes.

For developing countries, improved employment outcomes may be due to jobs being easier to find for people with psychosis in agrarian economies, and difficulties in accessing healthcare may explain reduced service use (Kulhura et al., 2009). There is a danger that romanticized Western views of developing countries underplay the severe problems people meeting criteria for psychosis diagnostic constructs face in these countries (Burns, 2009), and whilst outcomes may be better in some parts of the developing world, it may well be worse in other parts, particularly for mortality and suicide (Cohen et al., 2008).

A meta-analysis of diagnostic stability of first-episode psychosis found high rates of stability for schizophrenia: 85–95% at follow-up (Fusar-Poli et al., 2016a). This figure seems high compared to other research studies where diagnostic stability is in the range 72.9–83% after 3–10 years (Amin et al., 1999; Heslin et al., 2015). In clinical practice, diagnostic stability may be less than in research studies; one study measured prospective diagnostic reliability of 68.3–92.2%, depending on setting, and diagnostic stability of schizophrenia diagnosis of 49% as measured by being recorded in at least 75% of clinical evaluations in multiple settings (Baca-Garcia et al., 2007). This lower figure over multiple clinical assessments could be because a substantial minority of participants with an initial diagnosis of other psychotic conditions (e.g. up to one-third of those with initial diagnosis of delusional disorder) at follow-up meet schizophrenia criteria instead (Heslin et al., 2015; Fusar-Poli et al., 2016a). Diagnostic stability for bipolar disorder is also high: 76.4–78% for bipolar disorder with psychosis in research studies (Amin et al., 1999; Heslin et al., 2015) and for clinical practice 49.4–91.5% depending on setting, but only 23.1% across at least 75% of clinical evaluations (Baca-Garcia et al., 2007). In clinical settings, diagnostic stability for bipolar disorder and schizophrenia was higher for inpatient and emergency settings than for outpatient settings, suggesting the more severe cases have higher diagnostic stability (Baca-Garcia et al., 2007).

Table 14.2 Prognostic factors for schizophrenia/psychosis.

Prognostic Factors for Worse Outcomes	**Reference**
Poor premorbid social functioning	McGlashan, 1986; Ram et al., 1992; Alvarez-Jimenez et al., 2012; Marchesi et al., 2015 by the inverse: good premorbid functioning associated with better outcome
Mood-incongruent psychotic symptoms	Angst, 1986; Harrow et al., 2000
Negative symptoms	Jobe and Harrow, 2005; Dikeos et al., 2006; Marchesi et al., 2015
Insidious onset	Wiersma et al., 1998
Cognitive impairment	Jobe and Harrow, 2005; Keefe and Fenton, 2007
Male gender	Lewis, 1992; Haro et al., 2011; Morgan et al., 2014. Female gender is associated with good prognostic factors and male gender with poor prognostic factors (Abel et al., 2010)
Medication non-adherence	Alvarez-Jimenez et al., 2012
Persistent substance misuse	Alvarez-Jimenez et al., 2012
Long duration of untreated psychosis	Marshal et al., 2005; Penttilä et al., 2014
Critical comments from carers	Alvarez-Jimenez et al., 2012
History of childhood trauma	Lysaker et al., 2001; Conus et al., 2010

Prognostic Factors for Better Outcomes	Reference
Mood symptoms early in course of the condition especially depressive symptoms	McGlashan, 1986; Jobe and Harrow 2005; Haro et al., 2011
Early remission within three months of treatment with improvements in symptoms, functioning, and subjective well-being	Lambert et al., 2008
Social factors such as being in paid employment or living independently or being socially active/not isolated	Ram et al., 1992; Haro et al., 2011
Less/no family history of schizophrenia	McGlashan, 1986
Treatment involving combination of psychotherapy and medication	Menezes et al., 2006
Living in developing country	Menezes et al., 2006; Kulhura et al., 2009

Are there any differences in outcome between schizophrenia, schizoaffective disorder, unipolar depression—or simply depression—and bipolar disorder including mania? Results from several studies with long follow-up are summarized in Table 14.3. Direct comparisons are made more complex by different diagnostic criteria being employed (including whether they necessitated chronic symptoms and poor premorbid functioning for schizophrenia), differing methodologies, and differences in definitions of outcomes. Social outcomes tend to include employment, independent living, and/or relationship status. Clinical outcomes include severity of symptoms, long hospitalizations, or repeated relapses. Combined outcomes incorporate both clinical and social outcomes.

Table 14.3 Comparison of outcomes between schizophrenia and mood disorders.

Comparison	Outcomes from Studies
Schizophrenia v Depression	Schizophrenia has *worse* **social** (Tsuang et al., 1979; McGlashan, 1984; Harrow et al., 2000), **clinical** (Tsuang et al., 1979; Harrow et al., 2000), and **combined** outcomes (Tsuang et al., 1979; McGlashan, 1984; Harrow et al., 2000). *Mixed evidence* on worse **clinical** outcomes (McGlashan, 1984).
Schizophrenia v affective psychosis (bipolar disorder or depressive psychosis combined in one category)	Schizophrenia: *worse* **social** (Hohe-Schram et al., 1989; Harrow et al., 2000), **clinical** (Hohe-Schram et al., 1989; Harrow et al., 2000), and **combined** outcomes (Hohe-Schram et al., 1989; Harrow et al., 2000). *No differences* in **combined** outcomes but small numbers in affective psychosis group made it hard to achieve statistical significance (Strauss and Carpenter, 1972).
Schizophrenia v bipolar disorder (including mania)	Schizophrenia: *worse* **social** (Tsuang et al., 1979; Pope et al., 1980), **clinical** (Tsuang et al., 1979; Pope et al., 1980), and **combined** outcomes (Tsuang et al., 1979 ; Pope et al., 1980). *No differences* in **social**, **clinical,** or **combined** outcomes but small number of bipolar subjects made it hard to demonstrate significant differences (McGlashan, 1984).
Schizophrenia v schizoaffective disorder	Schizophrenia has *worse* **social** (Tsuang and Dempsey, 1979; Pope et al., 1980; Hohe-Schram et al., 1989; Marneros et al., 1990, , Harrow et al., 2000; Jäger et al., 2004), **clinical** (Pope et al., 1980; Hohe-Schram et al., 1989; Marneros et al., 1990; Harrow et al., 2000; Jäger et al., 2004), and **combined** outcomes (Tsuang and Dempsey, 1979; Pope et al., 1980; Harrow et al., 1989; Hohe-Schram et al., 1989; Jäger et al., 2004). Schizophrenia: *worse* disability of functioning (Marneros et al., 1990). *No differences* on **social** ((Williams and McGlashan, 1987), **clinical** (Williams and McGlashan, 1987), or **combined** outcomes (Williams and McGlashan, 1987).

(*continued*)

Table 14.3 Continued

Comparison	Outcomes from Studies
Bipolar disorder v depression	*No differences* in **social**, **clinical,** and **combined** outcomes (Tsuang et al., 1979). Bipolar disorder has *worse* **clinical** outcomes (Angst, 1986; Angst et al., 2003), **social** and **combined** outcomes *not measured*.
Affective psychosis v depression	Affective psychosis: *worse* **social** (Harrow et al., 2000), **clinical** (Harrow et al., 2000), and **combined** outcomes (Harrow et al., 2000).
Schizoaffective disorder v bipolar disorder	Schizoaffective disorders: *worse* **clinical** (Tsuang and Dempsey, 1979) and **combined** outcomes (Tsuang and Dempsey, 1979). Schizoaffective disorders: *no difference* in **social**, **clinical,** and **combined** outcomes (Pope et al., 1980; Williams and McGlashan, 1987) but low numbers of manic patients (Williams and McGlashan,1987) make it hard to demonstrate significant differences.
Schizoaffective disorder v depression	Schizoaffective disorders: *worse* **clinical** (Tsuang and Dempsey, 1979; Harrow et al., 2000), **social** (Harrow et al., 2000), and **combined** outcomes (Tsuang and Dempsey, 1979; Williams and McGlashan, 1987; Harrow et al., 2000). Schizoaffective disorder: *mixed evidence* of worse **clinical** outcomes (Williams and McGlashan, 1987)
Schizoaffective disorder v affective psychosis	Similar **social** (Harrow et al., 2000 Hohe-Schram et al., 1989 ; Jäger et al., 2004), **clinical** (Hohe-Schram et al., 1989; Harrow et al.,2000 ; Jäger et al., 2004) and **combined** (Hohe-Schram et al., 1989 ; Jäger et al., 2004) outcomes for schizoaffective disorder compared to affective psychosis. *Worse* **combined** outcomes for schizoaffective disorder (Harrow et al., 2000)

Summarizing these results, there is a 'rank order' of diagnostic constructs with increasing chances of better outcomes: schizophrenia, schizoaffective disorder, bipolar disorder/affective psychosis, then depression (Harrow et al., 2000). Schizoaffective disorder is closer for chances of good outcomes to affective disorders than schizophrenia (Marneros et al., 1990). The AESOP study found a combined 'non-affective psychosis' category, including schizophrenia and schizoaffective disorder, had worse clinical, social, and combined outcomes than manic psychosis/bipolar (Morgan et al., 2014). These results are averaged over groups of participants meeting specific diagnostic criteria but there is overlap in outcomes between these diagnostic constructs for individuals—some people who meet the criteria for schizophrenia will have worse outcomes than those who meet criteria for depression—but they do have predictive utility for relative risk of good or poor outcomes.

Mood-incongruent psychotic symptoms are associated with worse outcomes across diagnostic categories (Angst, 1986; Harrow et al., 2000). Psychotic symptoms without mood symptoms for periods of at least 10 days was associated with worse long-term combined outcomes and episodic mania had better long-term combined outcomes than no or chronic mania (Kotov et al., 2013). Another study found that in bipolar disorder, that those without psychotic symptoms had worse outcomes (Burton et al., 2019), which may indicate some difference in prognostic factors compared to schizophrenia.

These diagnostic constructs may represent areas of symptom dimensions (Reininghaus et al., 2013) that have prognostic implications (Harrow et al., 2000) rather than truly separate entities, but as summaries of prognostic information they have utility compared to not using any classification at all.

Mortality is obviously an important outcome. Evidence from systematic reviews and meta-analyses confirms that psychiatric diagnostic constructs are associated with differing rates of mortality and also different likelihood of deaths caused by suicide or accident (Harris and Barraclough, 1988; Joukamaa et al., 2001; Chesney et al., 2014; Walker et al., 2015a). Mortality rates are usually compared by calculating the standardized mortality ratio (SMR) or using the relative risk compared to a reference population. The increased mortality of mental health conditions has multifactorial causes: higher rates of smoking causes increased deaths from smoking-related disease (Joukamaa et al., 2001); other lifestyle factors such as inactivity or substance use also increases physical health mortality (Correll et al., 2015); associated social factors linked to increased mortality (see Chapter 13), reduced access to healthcare (Correll et al., 2015), suicide (Harris and Barraclough, 1998), or other 'unnatural deaths' such as accidents (Joukamaa et al., 2001); and sometimes mental health conditions are associated with physical health risk factors such as schizophrenia's association with abnormal glucose metabolism (Pillinger et al., 2017). Psychiatric medication is also linked with adverse effects on physical health (Correll et al., 2015), but there is mixed evidence on overall beneficial or adverse effect on mortality (see Chapter 15).

For comparison with mental health conditions, the SMR for moderate smoking is 2.0, that is, twice the rate of the reference population, and for heavy smoking was 2.4–2.7 (Chesney et al., 2014). Substance misuse disorders are associated with increased mortality, particularly opioid misuse (Chesney et al., 2014) having a SMR 14.7, with other substance misuse disorders including alcohol misuse registering a SMR 4–8 (Chesney et al., 2014). Anorexia nervosa is also associated with high mortality with an SMR of approximately 6 (Chesney et al., 2014), partly due to relatively large increases in mortality due to direct effects of starvation or its physical health consequences, suicide, substance misuse, and other 'unnatural deaths' such as victim of homicide or undefined cause (Papadopoulos et al., 2009). Personality disorder is also associated with similar high mortality with an SMR of 5 in men, 6 in women, with higher figures for women with borderline personality disorder diagnosis; causes of mortality in this latter group are due to large increases in deaths due to substance misuse or suicide and other 'unnatural deaths' (Björkenstam et al., 2015). Personality disorder and anorexia mortality figures are taken from the most severe cases that were admitted to hospital. Nevertheless, anorexia-related mortality seems higher than bulimia nervosa which has an SMR of 1.9 (Chesney et al., 2014), indicating utility in differentiating between the two diagnostic constructs.

SMRs for other diagnostic constructs include schizophrenia at an SMR of 2.5, depression with an SMR of 1.6 (both from Chesney et al., 2014), and bipolar disorder with an SMR of 2.05 (Hayes et al., 2015). It may be that mortality for depression has been overestimated by low-quality studies and that once the effects of other mental health conditions and behaviours that impact on health such as smoking are accounted for there is no significant effect of depression on mortality (Miloyan and Fried, 2017), but there is increased risk of suicide (Harris and Barraclough, 1997).

The causes of excess mortality in schizophrenia are probably multifactorial including environmental and lifestyle factors such as diet and smoking, poverty and poor healthcare (Brown et al., 2010b). The effects of medication will be discussed in Chapter 15. Suicide was much commoner in a British community sample of people with a schizophrenia diagnosis followed up for 25 years than in the general population and mostly occurred in the first 5 years of follow-up (Brown et al., 2000; Brown et al., 2010b) and mortality related directly to diabetes was also elevated but 70% of the excess mortality was due to smoking-related diseases such as cardiovascular disease which reflected over double the prevalence of smoking compared to the reference population (Brown et al., 2000, 2010). Similar results were obtained from a large cohort in the United States, which also noted additional contributions to mortality from alcohol or substance misuse related diseases (Olfson et al., 2015).

Direct comparisons between studies are difficult due to heterogeneity of results and methods. In one meta-analysis using relative risks, psychoses (including schizophrenia) had significantly higher mortality rates than bipolar disorder, which had non-significantly higher mortality than depression, which had significantly higher mortality than anxiety conditions (Walker et al., 2015a). Different diagnostic constructs are associated with predictive utility for differing mortality rates and causes of mortality.

For people who present with psychotic symptoms, six important categories have been suggested that influence treatment decisions and outcome predictions (Frances, 2016). For depression, Goldberg suggested six important additional subdivisions/important co-occurrences with important clinical implications, also summarized in Table 14.4, which emphasized the importance of other important information, such as co-occurring conditions or atypical presentations, that influences clinical management. The psychosis section focused on separating psychosis into different diagnostic constructs based on the context in which psychotic symptoms occur.

Several treatments benefit the same type of symptoms across different diagnostic constructs and even different types of symptoms that define different diagnostic constructs. As an example of the latter, antipsychotics are effective at reducing manic symptoms in mania (Cipriani et al., 2006; Scherk et al., 2007; Smith et al., 2007), as well as reducing psychotic symptoms in both schizophrenia (Leucht et al., 2013a; Turner et al., 2012, which included unpublished trial data) and mania (Johnstone et al., 1988). On the other hand, some treatments are effective for the same types of

Table 14.4 Depression and psychosis classification.

Classification	Clinical Implication
Depression	
Major depression	Heterogeneous construct, milder stress-reaction forms may improve without treatment; identify if caused by remediable biological or medical cause (see Chapter 12); other variants, e.g. bipolar depression, melancholia, atypical or psychotic depression may differ for treatment and outcomes (see this chapter)
Depression presenting with somatic symptoms	Patients often need explanation of links between emotional states and somatic symptoms, understandably patients may focus on their somatic symptoms. I would add need to be careful of diagnostic overshadowing and missing a medical illness causing both somatic symptoms and depression.
Depression with panic attacks	Treating depression is a priority but patient needs education around panic attacks and CBT for panic.
Depression in people with obsessional personality traits	May display both depressive symptoms, prominent ruminations, and compulsive behaviours. Will need CBT for obsessional features in addition to treating depression.
Depression in people with physical illness	Often missed but can be recognized by enquiring about depressive cognitions. Treatment can improve mortality and concordance with medical care. Beware interactions between psychiatric and medical medications.
Depression presenting with 'pseudo-dementia'	Depression in present with marked cognitive impairment in the elderly and be confused for dementia (age-related brain changes may also increase chances of misdiagnosis). Important to differentiate from dementia. If depression is treated, then marked improvement in cognitive impairment results.
Psychosis	
Psychotic like experiences commonly found in the community (see Chapter 9)	If not associated with marked distress and/or impaired functioning, then medical intervention not required.
Psychosis caused by intoxication or withdrawal from substances including alcohol or cannabis (see Chapter 12)	Need to focus on reducing consequences of substances and reducing further use of them in the future; in the short term may need appropriate medical treatment depending on the substance.
Psychosis caused by medical disease (see Chapter 12)	Clinical focus should be primarily on the causative disease.

(continued)

Table 14.4 Continued

Brief/acute/reactive psychosis	Associated with better prognosis (Fusar-Poli et al., 2016b) if does not develop into schizophrenia or affective psychosis and may benefit from use of antipsychotics in the short term but unclear for how long to continue (Castagnini and Galeazzi, 2016).
Psychosis as part of depression or bipolar disorder (I would also add psychosis associated with another mental health condition or in specific situations, e.g. post-partum psychosis Bergink et al., 2016)	May benefit from antipsychotics for psychosis but focus needs to be on the primary condition. Usually different prognostic and treatment implications than schizophrenia (see this chapter).
Psychosis as primary feature causing distress, functional impairment and/or risk	Worth differentiating schizophrenia from delusional disorder as the latter often has important differences in the clinical picture and reduced responsiveness to antipsychotics, (Peralta and Cuesta, 2016), both conditions may benefit from antipsychotics for a long period.

Source: data from Goldberg, 2011 and Frances, 2016

symptoms but not always in every diagnostic construct. Lithium and valproate (in various formulations) is effective in reducing acute manic symptoms (Smith et al., 2007), but lithium is ineffective for the treatment of psychotic symptoms of schizophrenia (Leucht et al., 2015a), and there is no convincing evidence of valproate's effectiveness for psychotic symptoms in schizophrenia (Wang et al., 2016). Lithium is, however, effective in reducing psychotic symptoms in mania (Bowden et al., 2005). The Northwick Park study, often quoted as an example of lack of specificity of psychiatric medications that examined effectiveness of different treatments across dimensions of symptoms, had too few people in each group to demonstrate significant differences for all but large effects such as antipsychotics in elated mood (Johnstone et al., 1988). Examining the graphs, lithium seems to have an effect in reducing psychotic symptoms only in participants with elated mood, but the sample sizes were too small for the difference to be significant.

Antidepressants have some effectiveness for depressive symptoms in unipolar depression (Turner et al., 2008, which included unpublished trial data). Use of antidepressants in bipolar depression is problematic due to antidepressant-induced mania (Goldberg and Truman, 2003)—far commoner in bipolar depression than unipolar depression (Angst, 1985)—and there is only mixed evidence that prescribing mood stabilizers (e.g. valproate or lithium) at the same time may be beneficial in preventing this with strongest evidence for lithium (Goldberg and Truman, 2003). Antidepressants combined with mood stabilizers or antipsychotics had a smaller effect size for reducing depressive symptoms in bipolar depression than unipolar depression and should only be used for short periods due to risk of inducing mania (McGirr et al., 2016).

Combination of antipsychotics with antidepressants is superior to either antipsychotic or antidepressant alone for psychotic depression (Wijkstrata et al., 2017), although this conclusion was based on a small number of studies (Smith, 2017). Lamotrigine has modest benefit in reducing depressive symptoms in bipolar depression but benefits may be greater in more severely depressed patients (Geddes et al., 2009), and has little benefit in unipolar depression (Amann et al., 2011), although this may be due to methodological problems such as short duration of trials in unipolar depression combined with lengthy titration time to reach effective doses leading to insufficient time for benefit to show (Zavodnick and Ali, 2012). Antidepressants may be ineffective for the treatment of depression in people with Alzheimer's disease (Banerjee et al., 2013; Orgeta et al., 2017).

Melancholia is said to be associated with different responses to treatment than other depression diagnostic constructs such as reduced placebo response in antidepressant trials, and possibly is more likely to require tricyclic antidepressants instead of selective serotonin reuptake inhibitor (SSRI) antidepressants, greater response to electroconvulsive therapy (ECT), and is less likely to respond to psychotherapy (Brown, 2007; Fink and Taylor, 2007; Parker et al., 2010; Carroll, 2012). From a medication point of view, there is often little difference between depression and many anxiety diagnostic constructs, with antidepressants being effective for both. Antidepressants have similar effectiveness for anxiety symptoms and depression symptoms (Roest et al., 2015, which included unpublished trials). There are some minor differences such as starting with low doses in panic disorder due to anxiety side effects or higher doses being used in obsessive–compulsive disorder (Chapter 15 in Cookson et al., 2002).

Diagnostic categories may offer clinical utility to psychotherapists for 'conceptualizing diagnostic entities' (First et al., 2004) and differences in treatment. There are, for instance, differing cognitive behavioural models for panic disorder (Clark, 1986), obsessive–compulsive disorder (Salkovkis, 1999), and depression (Beck, 1964, 2008). These diagnostic construct-specific models can form the basis of models altered for individuals in therapy. These separate models have led to variations in cognitive behavioural therapy for these diagnostic constructs such as different behavioural experiments (Beck et al., 1987; Wells, 1997). There are developments in 'transdiagnostic' psychotherapeutic approaches focusing on common approaches across different diagnostic constructs (Mansell et al., 2009; Gros et al., 2016). Diagnostic constructs can give information about how effective psychotherapy may be. There is evidence for individual psychotherapy being ineffective for mania (Oud et al., 2016). Cognitive behavioural therapy is far superior at reducing the symptoms of depression than psychotic symptoms of schizophrenia and at preventing relapse in depression compared to schizophrenia and bipolar disorder (Lynch et al., 2010).

Psychiatric diagnostic constructs are not associated with unitary outcomes but they do have predictive utility with useful information on the range of likely outcomes that may overlap but differ in terms of probabilities from other diagnostic constructs. These outcomes include recurrence of problems and impaired functioning. They also have clinical utility in giving information on the likelihood of effectiveness of different treatments. This information attached to the diagnostic construct helps guide clinical management. Diagnosis often needs supplemented by additional useful information in a broader 'diagnostic formulation'.

Clinical utility of general medical diagnostic constructs

This section will summarize evidence on general medical conditions with variable outcomes before discussing how some general medical diagnostic constructs are used for clinical utility reasons. Several general medical conditions are specifically noted to have markedly variable outcomes influenced by other factors than diagnosis.

Mortality associated with angina can vary greatly from 1–20% over a 4-year period associated with factors such as degrees of positive response to an exercise stress test. Conversely, development of collateral vessels with improved blood supply can cause improvement of angina symptoms (Chapter 18 in Walker et al., 2014). Coronary arterial disease 5-year survival ranges vary from greater than 90% to less than 30% influenced by number of vessels affected and left ventricular function (Chapter 18 in Walker et al., 2014).

Prognosis following myocardial infarction (MI) is variable; 12% mortality for those who survive the initial effects of the MI by 1 month and 20% by 6–12 months, 25% by 5 years, and 50% at 10 years. This is affected by multiple factors such as recurrent ischaemia or amount of damaged heart muscle, promoting the use of risk stratification to help estimate prognosis (Chapter 18 in Walker et al., 2014). A GRACE score can be calculated in acute coronary syndromes, particularly unstable angina and non-ST elevation MI, to guide clinical management (Timmis, 2015). GRACE score is based on multiple prognostic indicators such as degree of heart failure, age, or elevated cardiac enzymes, and can be used to predict risk of in-hospital and mortality up to six months after an acute coronary syndrome (Fox et al., 2006). This can vary greatly, for example from < 0.2% to < 52% for in-hospital mortality, a 250-fold degree difference in risk for acute coronary syndrome as a whole but an approximately 20-fold variation for in-hospital mortality for many cases of MI (Chapter 18 in Walker et al., 2014).

Asthma outcomes vary from controlled, partially controlled, or uncontrolled, depending on the number of clinical features present such as need for rescue inhalers/ treatments, limitation of activities, or lung function (Chapter 19 in Walker et al., 2014). Diffuse parenchymal lung disease has highly variable prognosis; some individuals may live for many years barely affected by symptoms whilst others may die within months (Chapter 19 in Walker et al., 2014). TB is well-known to have a great variety of outcomes; some eradicate the bacillus entirely, about 10% progress from primary infection to recurrent pulmonary infection (although relapse may occur after several years) to disseminated infection in multiple sites with many possible complications (Chapter 19 in Walker et al., 2014), with social factors important for differences in outcomes (Ortblad et al., 2015).

Thyrotoxicosis caused by Graves' disease has four broad types of outcome; 60% have either prolonged hyperthyroidism or alternating hyperthyroidism and normal thyroid functioning and the rest have a short period of hyperthyroidism followed by normal thyroid functioning or later onset of hypothyroidism (Chapter 20 in Walker et al., 2014). In thyrotoxicosis as a whole, relapse after stopping treatment is common but not invariable; at least 50% do relapse, usually within two years (Chapter 20 in Walker et al., 2014).

Liver cirrhosis has poor but variable prognosis. Child–Pugh classification or MELD scores can be used to improve prognostic accuracy based on factors such as serum bilirubin or presence of ascites (Chapter 23 in Walker et al., 201). The most severe Child–Pugh classification ('C') has 42% 1-year survival and 0% 10-year survival rate, whilst the least severe ('A') has 42% 1-year and 25% 10-year survival rate (Chapter 23 in Walker et al., 2014). Alcoholic hepatitis also has poor but variable prognosis, with use of either the Maddrey or the Glasgow alcoholic hepatitis score to guide clinical management based on prognosis. The Glasgow alcoholic hepatitis score is based on factors such as age and serum bilirubin and 28-day mortality and can vary from 40% for score > = 9 to 80% for score < 9 (Chapter 23 in Walker et al., 2014).

Hepatitis B infection has variable outcomes: 90–95% recover from initial infection, 5–10% develop chronic infection (but some recover later) and less than 1% progress to liver failure (Chapter 23 in Walker et al., 2014). Primary biliary cirrhosis also has variable outcomes: median survival until death or liver transplant is 12 years if symptomatic, but if asymptomatic then 75% live 15 years or greater (Chapter 23 in Walker et al., 2014). The consequences of gallstone disease vary greatly: 80% are asymptomatic, jaundice occurs in less than 10% of cases, and gallbladder perforation is seen in 10–15% (Chapter 23 in Walker et al., 2014). Hepatocellular cancer is staged to guide treatment and inform prognosis: in the very early stages 5-year survival rates are 40–70% but by the advanced stage it is 6–14% (Chapter 23 in Walker et al., 2014).

Prognosis in haematological neoplasms (from benign to malignant), indeed, for many neoplasms, can be highly variable. Five-year survival rates for acute myeloid leukaemia can vary from 21–76%, depending on prognostic factors such as presence of identified genetic abnormalities (Chapter 24 in Walker et al., 2014). Myelofibrosis patients' survival varies from 1 year to more than 20 years (Chapter 24 in Walker et al., 2014). Median survival in low-risk myelodysplastic syndrome is 5.7 years but only 0.4 years in high-risk patients (Chapter 24 in Walker et al., 2014). Non-Hodgkin's lymphoma prognosis varies as measured by the international prognostic index (IPI), based on factors such as age, clinical stage of illness, and performance status, with 5-year survival rates of 25% in patients with high-risk scores to 75% 5-year survival in low-risk score patients (Chapter 24 in Walker et al., 2014).

Gout sufferers may have only one episode, others may experience a relapsing course but may be gout-free for years, whilst some have a rapid relapse within 12 months and develop chronic gout after multiple attacks with joint damage and deformity (Chapter 25 in Walker et al., 2014). Epilepsy has variable long-term outcomes even with effective treatments: half are free of seizures for at least five years untreated, one-fifth have been seizure-free for at least five years whilst on medication, and the rest experience seizures despite being on medication (Chapter 26 in Walker et al., 2014). Multiple sclerosis (MS) prognosis is highly variable and hard to predict, especially early in the illness, with 15% of patients having only one episode (Chapter 26 in

Walker et al., 2014), 15% have progressive deteriorating course from the onset (primary progressive MS) and the rest having a variable remitting–relapsing course with progressive deterioration setting in after 10–15 years in 50% of cases (secondary progressive MS) with overlapping pathological mechanisms between these types (Galea et al., 2015; Ontaneda et al., 2017).

Cervical myelopathy can also show great variety in outcome, from spontaneous improvement to stabilization to progression with sphincter dysfunction or pyramidal signs (Chapter 26 in Walker et al., 2014). Poliomyelitis infection results in heterogeneous outcomes from asymptomatic seroconversion to recovery from infection to paralysis with variable recovery—that is, from complete recovery to varying degrees of disability—or death (Chapter 26 in Walker et al., 2014). Cerebrovascular accidents (strokes) are associated with variable outcomes: 20% mortality within 1 month and at least 50% have impaired functioning that varies per area of the brain affected (Chapter 27 in Walker et al., 2014). The risk of recurrence is 5–15% by 1 week, up to 15% in the following year, then 5% annually (Chapter 27 in Walker et al., 2014).

Basal cell carcinoma has variable outcome, depending on thickness of tumour and other factors, with 10-year survival rates ranging from < 10% for advanced disease including metastases to 95% if thickness is < 1mm (Chapter 27 in Walker et al., 2014). Psoriasis tends to have two broad types of course: an early-onset form with worse outcomes and a later-onset form with more benign prognosis (Chapter 27 in Walker et al., 2014). Vitiligo is also associated with variable outcomes; some may regain pigment in the lesions but for others, their lesions remain the same or become unpredictably larger (Chapter 27 in Walker et al., 2014).

Multiple factors can affect prognosis which are often combined into a prognostic index to aid management of many medical conditions which often include demographic variables such as age, measures of disease severity or metastatic spread, and other risk factors for poor outcome such as smoking. Examples include the famous Glasgow Coma Scale used to measure consciousness as well as give prognostic information (Teasdale and Jennett, 1974, 1976). Modified Blatchford score, incorporating factors such as haemoglobin and systolic blood pressure, can be used to predict need for intervention in acute gastrointestinal bleeding (Blatchford et al., 2000; Chapter 22 in Walker et al., 2014). CURB-65 (confusion, urea, respiratory rate, blood pressure, and age greater than 65) scores are used to guide management of pneumonia such as whether inpatient admission is needed (Chapter 19 in Walker et al., 2014).

The DAS28 score measuring disease activity in rheumatoid arthritis (calculated using a formula with data such as number of involved joints) is used to measure response to treatment and inform clinical decision-making such as use of biological treatments (Chapter 25 in Walker et al., 2014). The Bath Ankylosing Spondylitis Index is also used to measure disease activity and guide clinical decisions such as the use of anti-tumour necrosis factor therapy (Chapter 25 in Walker et al., 2014).

Several medical diagnostic constructs are used to identify situations where medical intervention is justified at least partly on the basis of reducing distress or risk. Hirsutism not caused by obvious pathology is designated as a medical condition if it causes distress; further investigation of hirsutism may reveal a causative condition such as polycystic ovarian syndrome in women (Chapter 20 in Walker et al., 2014).

Acne vulgaris is another condition that, like hirsutism, exists on a spectrum with health but is recognized as a medical condition where treatment is justified to reduce the extent of the illness and to improve emotional health (Chapter 28 in Walker et al., 2014). In some cases, conditions have benign outcomes but it is important to diagnose them accurately as confusing them for other conditions may lead to harm from treating the wrongly diagnosed condition. For example, familial hypocalciuric hypercalcaemia, if confused for primary hyperparathyroidism, may lead to an unnecessary parathyroidectomy (Chapter 20 in Walker et al., 2014). Benign conditions may not cause problems and only be discovered incidentally but they may need to be monitored or treated in case they become dangerous, such as pre-cancerous or potentially cancerous lesions (see also Table 12.7).

Some medical conditions are identified and treated because they are associated with increased risk of developing further medical conditions with or without increased mortality. Examples include obesity, often defined using body mass index, fasting plasma glucose, total serum cholesterol, and blood pressure where higher values are associated with increasing risk of vascular diseases such as ischaemic heart disease, strokes, or aortic aneurysm, but these effects may lessen with age (Singh et al., 2013). For body mass index, there is also increased risk of mortality at lower ends of values in the population (Prospective Studies Collaboration, 2009).

Most vascular events (e.g. heart attacks or strokes) occur at the middle of the normal range for these risk factors (e.g. blood pressure) so it may be better to try to modify these risk factors in everyone rather than just identify and treat people in high-risk categories (Viera, 2017). Nevertheless, usual practice is to identify thresholds for these risk factors that identify people for whom the risks of treatment are outweighed by the benefits (e.g. reducing risks of complications) (Chapter 18 in Walker et al., 2014). These thresholds are established by committees of experts, some of whom have links to pharmaceutical companies even if this is in the form of research grants (Chapter 3 in Taylor, 2013), to define diagnostic constructs such as hypertension, type 2 diabetes, or hypercholesterolaemia/hyperlipidaemia. People who meet criteria for these diagnostic constructs are then offered interventions at least partly on the basis of preventing complications associated with these diagnostic constructs such as retinopathy (which differs between diabetes and hypertension), vascular events, and chronic kidney disease (Chapters 16, 18, and 21 in Walker et al., 2014).

Hypertension is often asymptomatic (Chapter 18 in Walker et al., 2014), hypercholesterolaemia is usually asymptomatic apart from cholesterol deposits over the body (Chapter 16 in Walker et al., 2014), and type 2 diabetes lacks the dramatic symptoms of type 1 diabetes, often presenting instead with non-specific symptoms like fatigue or with infections (Chapter 21 in Walker et al., 2014).

For the prevention of cardiovascular disease events clinicians commonly use risk indexes that calculate probability of vascular events over a time period to identify individuals at high risk and offer appropriate interventions (Viera, 2017). These risk indexes include the Framingham Risk score (Kannel et al., 1976), QRISK (Hippisley-Cox et al., 2007), and QRISK2 (Hippisley-Cox et al., 2008), and calculate risk using demographic data such as age and clinical factors such as blood pressure, serum cholesterol, and smoking status. Statins were recommended if the risk index predicted 20% or greater chance of a cardiovascular event in 10 years (Chapter 16 in Walker et al., 2014), but this threshold for prescribing statins was dropped to 10% or greater chance in 10 years by NICE (NICE, 2014a).

As inflammatory, coagulation, and immune system processes contribute to many medical conditions, medications, such as steroids, that have an effect on any of these systems are used across several conditions rather than being specific to one condition (see Chapters 20, 26, and 41 in Harvey et al., 2011).

Many medical conditions have variable rather than unitary outcomes and other information apart from diagnosis is commonly used in clinical decision-making. Some medical diagnostic constructs, including common conditions, are used at least in part for utilitarian reasons such as identifying people at high risk of medical problems or the use of a diagnostic construct for a condition that is not a disease is justified because of distress caused by the condition. Some medications, such as steroids, are used for many medical conditions.

Clinical utility of alternative classifications

Psychological formulations achieve clinical utility in part by being used during psychotherapy (e.g. Beck et al., 1987; Wells, 1997) as well as including predictive information from psychological science (Flinn et al., 2014), including diagnosis if part of the formulation. The clinical utility of formulation depends on the information it contains. Psychological formulation should be a joint enterprise between clinician and client (Division of Clinical Psychology, 2011), but it is not always possible to collect enough information in certain situations due, for example, to limited consultation time or if the client is unable to communicate effectively. It is inappropriate as sole classification for certain situations, especially organic conditions such as dementia.

Shortcomings of diagnosis in mental health (see Chapter 11) have led to calls for use of dimensional systems (Widiger and Samuel, 2005) or a symptom/complaint-based classification (Bentall, 2006). Whether based on symptoms or dimensions of symptoms, several categorical choices are made as part of this classification, making them akin to 'diagnosis by proxy'. Some of these categorical decision processes are listed below for classifying depressive or psychosis symptoms/decisions including interactions *between* symptoms/dimensions.

The amount of data required to record and process—administratively and cognitively—for symptom/dimensional classification is enormous. If a classification system uses 10 symptoms/dimensions coded as present/absent, it would have 10 examples of only 1 symptom/dimension present, 45 examples of two symptoms/dimensions present, 360 examples of three symptoms/dimensions present, and 2520 examples of 4 symptoms/dimensions present, and so forth exponentially (Phillips, 2016), compared to just under 300 disorders listed in DSM-5 (APA, 2013).

Imagine the numbers if symptoms or dimensions were coded as absent, mild, moderate, or severe, or more than ten symptoms/dimensions were to be used? Trying to remember and use clinical utility information such as prognosis and treatment responses for each of these symptom/dimensional states will be very difficult in brief appointments or under pressure such as in emergencies or the very early hours of the morning. More than one diagnosis is frequently used for a patient but rarely more than a handful per individual, and diagnosis is easier to use in these circumstances.

Given the high number of different mental health symptoms, which symptoms/dimensions should we choose to use (Williams, 2016)? There are high degrees of correlation between mental health symptoms with some community studies suggesting a single '*p*' psychopathology factor underlying other factors such as internalizing/externalizing/psychosis (Lahey et al., 2012; Caspi et al., 2014). Any symptom/dimensional classification will lose information if it excludes any symptoms as multiple symptoms are likely to be present.

Accepting this loss of information, one can choose between three broad groups: internalizing, psychosis, and externalizing (for the latter, substance misuse will be omitted for reasons of brevity). For internalizing problems, 11 dimensions have been suggested to describe anxiety/depression symptoms and associated personality temperament (Brown and Barlow, 2009). The complexity of this system precludes use except in long appointments in non-urgent settings. Using an appropriate diagnostic category for a problem is a better solution for short appointments and urgent care settings even if multiple diagnoses are often used.

A single psychosis category with five dimensions has been recommended to replace current diagnostic categories (Van Os and Reininghaus, 2016). The problem is that there are multiple versions of these factors that are often created by post-hoc factor analysis of symptom-rating scores in research studies and often do not fit the data from other studies (van der Gaag et al., 2006a). DSM-5 uses eight dimensions alongside the diagnosis of schizophrenia though even more dimensions could have been used (Barch et al., 2013). Follow-up studies comparing standard diagnostic categories with dimensions created by post-hoc factor analysis of participants who meet psychosis diagnostic criteria tend to show that diagnostic categories have significant predictive utility but that dimensional models were superior overall (e.g. van Os et al., 1996, 1999; Rosenman et al., 2003; Dikeos et al., 2006). This is unsurprising as these studies are comparing one information unit type (diagnostic categories created before the study) versus multiple information units (psychosis category with multiple dimensions optimized post-hoc to describe the sample) for predicting outcomes. Given the complexity of dimensional systems, making them difficult for use in short appointments or urgent situations, and the need to incorporate additional information, such as lifetime course (van Os et al., 1999 and Table 14.5) and complementary predictive information from diagnosis and dimensions (Demjaha et al., 2009), the best compromise for clinical practice and research is to start with a diagnosis then add as much dimensional information as possible (Allardyce et al., 2007; Demjaha et al., 2009; Russo et al., 2014).

A disputed view is that diagnostic criteria of personality disorder constructs do not correspond well to general population personality traits (Shedler et al., 2010), therefore making little sense to describe them as 'personality' disorders. There are high degrees of stigma attached to personality disorder diagnostic constructs (Lewis and Appleby, 1988). DSM-5 has offered an alternative ('hybrid') model where people who have personality traits related to general population personality models that

Table 14.5 Some categorical decisions for symptoms/dimensions of depressive and psychotic symptoms.

Decision	Clinical Implication
Both Depression and Psychosis	
Duration, severity, and frequency	Are the symptoms of sufficient duration and severity occurring frequently enough to indicate a mental health problem that requires help? Symptoms or experiences that last for brief periods of time and/or of mild (or less) severity and/or are highly infrequent may not require intervention or be regarded as a problem.
Impairment of functioning and/or distress and/or risk	Is there sufficient evidence of reductions in functioning or failure to reach potential in functioning or associated distress or increased risk to justify intervention or describe someone as having a mental health problem?
Appropriate experiences/ responses taking into account cultural factors such as religion, within the expected range of responses to stressors	Is the person describing what others from a similar cultural background would regard as appropriate and not indicating a mental health problem? For example, low mood in response to bereavement is expected and hallucinations of the deceased can occur as part of grieving. How people experience and display grief can vary between cultures. On the other hand, if reaction to difficulties is within a culturally appropriate range then may still meet criteria for mental health problem; as an example, flashbacks and nightmares and other features meeting criteria for PTSD after sexual assault would still be regarded as a culturally appropriate response but the diagnostic construct is used in part to help choose the best treatments to reduce distressing symptoms. Even if within cultural normal range then help can be given trying to support with cause of the distress. Reactions outside the culturally normal range are more likely to meet criteria for a mental health problem.
Presence of medical disease/ illness directly causing the symptoms through disease processes (not as a psychological reaction to the medical illness)	Identified organic causes of mental health problems means treating the causative mechanisms is usually the priority. Absence of organic cause, i.e. functional mental health problems often require focus on different causes (e.g. social) and different treatments.
Direct effects of substances or withdrawal from substances (including alcohol)	If the symptoms experiences are caused by substances (through intoxication or withdrawal) then treatment and management will focus on substance misuse. Treatments of resultant symptoms may either not be needed, for only a short period of time, or be different from symptoms not related to substances.
Effects of medication	Several medications cause mood or psychotic symptoms either as a side effect or during withdrawal. It is important to recognize this and take steps to reduce the adverse effect.
Physiological extremes	Hallucinations can occur as someone is going to sleep or waking up and do not require treatment. Other physiological extremes such as prolonged lack of sleep can cause mood or psychotic symptoms.

Table 14.5 Continued

Decision	Clinical Implication
Currently no symptoms but has had episodes of ill-health in the past/general course information	People with mental health problems often have relapsing/remitting courses. For periods of time they can have few/no symptoms. A cross-sectional measure assessing symptoms at this time may find little difference from people without a history of mental health problems, therefore a classification system will need additional information to record this past history of mental health problems and their nature. Details of course of illness, e.g. insidious onset will also be useful
Depression	
History of manic symptoms in the past or manic symptoms currently	Care needs to be taken with antidepressants. May benefit from mood stabilizer or antipsychotic. Mixed state of depression and manic symptoms may not respond as well to lithium. Lamotrigine may benefit depression if history of manic symptoms in the past but not presently.
Psychotic symptoms also present	More likely to benefit from addition of antipsychotic to treatment for depression. Mood incongruent psychotic symptoms associated with worse outcome.
Co-occurring anxiety problems	If using antidepressants some adjustments to dosing may be needed. Will often require psychoeducation at minimum or psychotherapy
Co-occurring cognitive impairment	Important to identify if cognitive impairment is caused by depression (pseudo-dementia) in which case it is likely to improve dramatically if depression is treated. Treatment responses for depressive symptoms may vary if cognitive impairment caused by brain disease, e.g. for newer antidepressants in Alzheimer's disease less effective
Psychosis	
Cultural and religious norms	Different cultures and religions may have different beliefs about how the world functions, the influence of the supernatural or deities and so forth that can be wrongly labelled as psychotic symptoms.
Presence of manic symptoms	If manic symptoms co-occurring with psychotic symptoms may respond to lithium. Manic symptoms also associated with better outcomes.
Presence of cognitive impairment	If cognitive impairment is due to a dementia or delirium, then the management and outcomes of psychotic symptoms is different. Cognitive impairment in a functional psychosis is associated with worse outcomes.
Course of the mental health problems	Insidious onset is associated with worse outcomes. Depressive symptoms present during first episode psychosis is associated with better outcomes.
Presence of mood incongruent symptoms	Associated with worse outcomes

lead to distress/impaired functioning and/or meet criteria for prototypical personality disorder categories will meet personality disorder diagnostic construct criteria (Hopwood et al., 2012; Skodol et al., 2015). A better alternative is to split these two types of constructs.

Classification of personality should involve validated tools for assessment of general population personality traits using dimensional measures. The prototypical personality disorder categories could drop the 'personality disorder' and just keep the title, for example schizotypal and psychopathy. Borderline personality disorder should instead be called 'complex trauma' for the up to 90% of cases with a history of childhood trauma (Zanarini. 2000), naming both an important aetiological factor as well as indicating the additional complex interaction of psychobiological factors (see Chapters 12 and 13). Remaining cases without history of childhood trauma could be described as 'affective instability' present in over 90% of people who meet borderline personality disorder criteria (Zimmerman et al., 2017). Complex PTSD (or cPTSD) has been suggested as an alternative for borderline personality disorder (Hernan, 1992; Kulkarni, 2017) but not everybody who meets criteria for borderline personality disorder meets criteria for cPTSD (Resick et al., 2012; Ford and Courtois, 2014; Kulkarni, 2017).

Despite greater accuracy of depicting present symptoms, symptom/dimensional models have worse clinical utility than diagnostic systems (First, 2005b; Williams, 2016); they still need thresholds for decision-making, are incompatible with other healthcare specialties, struggle with symptom fluctuation (someone who recovered or in-between episodes may have a similar symptom profile to someone with no history of problems), lack of established standards (like DSM and ICD for diagnosis), lack of information on course, and presence/absence of aetiological factors (Table 14.6), without adding further dimensions and hugely increased complexity in assessment and treatment planning (especially for symptoms as would need to assess and remember prognostic and treatment information about many symptoms and relationship with other symptoms). Symptom/dimensional and formulation classifications are unsuitable for administrative/statistical and other functions of diagnosis such as access to benefits (see Chapter 2).

Clinicians whose regular contacts with patients have durations close to an hour can use complicated and lengthy classification systems and so may find the greater detail afforded by symptom/dimension classifications more useful. Researchers who often have the time to collect large amounts of data may not have to make clinical decisions during their assessments and can use computerized databases to store and manipulate data may also find symptom/dimension classifications useful.

Conclusion

There is evidence of overlap between psychiatric and general medical constructs for clinical utility, particularly for variability of outcomes, use of diagnostic criteria decided by committees of experts, and use of clinical information apart from the diagnosis. For psychiatric diagnostic constructs, there is evidence of some differences in outcomes and responses to treatments. However, it is easier to measure variables relevant for clinical purposes in general medicine directly. Therefore, for all these questions, the conclusion of some (not near total overlap) seems fairest (see Table 14.6).

Psychological formulation has utility but is unlikely to be helpful in all clinical scenarios. Dimension- or symptom-based classification may have greater validity, still involves categorical choices, and has limitations in clinical utility. Alternative classifications have compatibility problems with the healthcare system for collecting date for administration or statistics or for access to benefits.

Table 14.6 Utility of psychiatric diagnostic constructs compared to general medical diagnostic constructs.

	No Overlap	Some Overlap	Near Total Overlap
Does the condition have uniform prognosis?		X	
Does the condition have different outcomes from other conditions?		X	
Does the condition predict differences in treatments given and their effectiveness?		X	
Is the use of the condition justified due to some utilitarian reason such as relieving distress or risk?		X	
Are clinical management decisions based on recognizing the condition?		X	
Is there a need for clinical information beyond the diagnosis in clinical decision-making?		X	

Chapter 15

Treatments in psychiatry compared to general medicine

Box 15.1 Questions to compare psychiatric treatments with treatments in general medicine and psychotherapy

- How effective are the treatments used?
- How harmful are the treatments used?
- Does the treatment used have a disease-reversing mechanism of action that produces the clinical benefit?

This chapter will examine the evidence for medication in psychiatry and general medicine and for psychotherapy (see Box 15.1). Treatment effectiveness is measured by its ability to achieve treatment objectives (see Chapter 5). The difference between two treatments (sometimes 'control' treatments like placebo) may be *statistically significant* but this is not the same as *clinically significant* (Chapter 7 in Sackett et al., 1991) as outlined in Table 15.1. Some treatments, for example, insulin for type 1 diabetes, show sufficient clinical benefit to not require randomized controlled trials (RCTs) (Glasziou et al., 2007). Ideally, information is taken from good quality RCTs or meta-analysis combining the results of several RCTs (Laupacis et al., 1988).

The important point about NNT (number needed to treat) is that the doctor does not know in advance which patient would benefit versus comparator. If NNT = 10, the doctor could not identify which of his 10 patients would be the one to benefit before starting treatment. It also does not mean that the other nine patients are only harmed; they may benefit from the placebo effect. NNH (number needed to harm) gives us the estimate of who was harmed versus the comparator. Effect sizes can be converted to NNT and vice versa in an approximate fashion if the comparator event rates are known (Furukawa, 1999; Furukawa and Leucht, 2011).

Psychiatric treatments

This section will summarize information on clinical effectiveness, adverse effects, and mechanisms of actions for antidepressants and antipsychotics. It will then briefly discuss lithium and electroconvulsive treatment (ECT). The lack of knowledge of biological aetiology (see Chapter 12) means cure is unlikely so treatment objectives are

Table 15.1 Estimating clinical significance.

Type of outcome	Clinical significance measures	Reference
Continuous Sequentially ordered numeric values, e.g. serum cholesterol or blood pressure or number of illness events, e.g. relapses. Psychiatric symptom rating scale scores often analysed as if they were continuous variable.	Effect size is difference in means between two groups (standardized mean difference) expressed as proportion of standard deviation (Cohen uses pooled standard deviation but other methods exist) 0.2 = small 0.5 = medium 0.8+ = large (based on Cohen's judgement) For correlations measured as '*r*' 0.1 = small 0.3 = medium 0.5 = large	Cohen, 1992
Categorical Outcomes different from each other and not sequentially ordered, e.g. death, recovered from illness, whether relapsed during follow-up. Continuous outcomes can be *simplified* to create categorical outcomes, e.g. response to antidepressant defined as 50% reduction of HAMD scores. This simplification leads to loss of information. Often needs combined with effect size as threshold effects may confuse interpretation (e.g. 49% reduction HAMD not response but 50% reduction is).	Relative risk reduction (RRR) is reduction in rate of unwanted events expressed as difference in event rates between a treatment versus comparator (e.g. placebo) event rate and divided by comparator event rate. 50% RRR almost always and 25% RRR often clinically significant. Relative benefit increase (RBI) is increase of desired events, e.g. clinical response expressed as differences in event rate in a treatment versus comparator and divided by comparator event rate.	Laupacis et al., 1988; Chapter 7 in Sackett et al., 1991; Furukawa, 1999
	Absolute risk reduction (ARR) is difference in rates of unwanted events between a treatment and comparator. Absolute benefit increase (ABI) is difference between rates of desired event between a treatment and comparator. Useful additional info to RRR/RBI, e.g. reduction in relapse from 30–15% has same RRR (50%) as from 0.5– 0.25% but ARR greatly different (15% vs 0.25%)	
	Number Needed to Treat (Benefit) (NNT/NNB) for one patient to experience stated benefit (or reduced unwanted event) from a treatment compared to comparator is reciprocal of ARR/ABI (1/ARR or 1/ABI). So ARR of 5% is NNT = 20. Can also be used for adverse events (where it is NNH, Number Needed to Harm).	

to relieve current distress/reduce symptoms, limit functional deterioration, and then to prevent recurrence after the episode has improved. Evidence is mostly from adults (18–65 years old) although some studies include older participants. Most RCTs use placebos and blinded assessments. Confidence intervals are not stated but are taken into account if they indicate non-significant results. Measures of effectiveness are in relation to placebo unless stated otherwise.

Antidepressant efficacy studies often use rating scales measuring depressive symptoms, for example the Hamilton Depression Rating Scale (Hamilton, 1960) which was intended as a diagnostic tool, not an outcome rating scale, and is flawed as an outcome measure (Bagby et al., 2004). Categorical outcomes are usually based on rating scale scores. Table 15.2 summarizes evidence for effectiveness of antidepressants for depression and anxiety. The evidence of antidepressants effectiveness and adverse effects presented below groups together different medications and conceals the differences between them.

The small effect sizes in Table 15.2 may be partly because of the depression rating scales used measure many symptoms (Bagby et al., 2004), whereas antidepressants have greater effects on core depressed mood/psychic anxiety (Hieronymus et al., 2016) and core emotional symptoms (Chekroud et al., 2017), although using only these symptoms will slightly increase the effect size, at best to medium. Tricyclic antidepressants have similar effectiveness to selective serotonin reuptake inhibitors (SSRIs) but amitriptyline has a very small superiority (effect size 0.14) over SSRIs (Anderson, 2000), and dual-action tricyclics (acting on noradrenaline and serotonin) have small superiority (effect size 0.3) over SSRIs in depressed inpatients (Anderson, 1998), but these conclusions may be affected by publication bias of SSRI trials with the best results (Anderson, 2000; Turner et al., 2008).

Placebo response in antidepressant RCTs may increase with time reducing the gap between antidepressants and placebo (Walsh et al., 2002), but more recent analysis suggested that antidepressant response rates also increased with time and the antidepressant–placebo gap has remained constant (Khan et al., 2017). Placebo response may differ from antidepressant response in some respects with increased expectation of pill effectiveness particularly associated with placebo response (Leuchter et al., 2014). Other potential common factors between antidepressant and placebo responses include increased therapeutic contact and therapeutic alliance (Rutherford and Roose, 2013; Leuchter et al., 2014). Placebo response viewed a spontaneous remission should be further researched to identify active components which can then be encouraged in clinical practice (Cuijpers and Cristea, 2015).

Earlier meta-analysis suggested placebo had less benefit in more severely depressed participants (Kirsch et al., 2008; Fournier et al., 2010), but meta-analysis including patient-level data from RCTs showed severity had no effect on placebo effectiveness in depression (Rabinowitz et al., 2016, but this meta-analysis included a small number of quetiapine studies) or anxiety (De Vries et al., 2016b). Some contend antidepressant benefits in RCTs are due to participants and/or researchers realizing which participants are taking active antidepressants (becoming 'unblinded'), which leads to depression scores being rated as improved or are caused by psychoactive effects such as sedation (Moncrieff, 2015b) or cognitive slowing (Yeomans et al., 2015).

In a meta-analysis of antidepressants compared to anticholinergics ('active placebos'), to maintain blinding by mimicking tricyclic antidepressant side effects (Moncrieff et al., 1998) effect size for antidepressants was 0.21 (after excluding one trial with an atypically large effect size), indicating that after controlling for potential 'unblinding', antidepressants are still significantly more effective than 'active placebo'. The effect size is slightly smaller but anticholinergics reduced Hamilton depression rating scores by over 50% in an open trial, probably due to psychoactive intoxicating effects (Kasper et al., 1981). Anticholinergics did not show significant benefit over placebo in a double-blind RCT but there is a visible difference in the graph of results favouring anticholinergics and the study was underpowered to show statistical significance except for large effects (Gillin et al., 1995). Antidepressants showed significant small benefit over anticholinergics that might in themselves also reduce depression rating scores. A meta-regression found no significant relationship between experiencing adverse events (potentially causing 'unblinding') and antidepressant efficacy (Barth et al., 2016). The evidence suggests 'unblinding' is not an explanation for antidepressant superiority compared to placebo.

That core emotional symptoms show greater response rather than insomnia or cognitive speed items (Hieronymus et al., 2016; Chekroud et al., 2017) suggests that the benefit of antidepressants is not due to psychoactive effects but more direct effects on emotion.

Antidepressant RCTs are designed to demonstrate 'efficacy' (i.e. are more effective than placebo) which they have done but the results are hard to translate into 'effectiveness' in patients seen in clinical practice (Parker et al., 2003), with the possibility that antidepressants may be more effective compared to placebo in clinical practice (Kasper and Dold, 2015). RCT participants are not typical of patients in clinical practice making results less generalizable (Zimmerman et al., 2015), including being more likely to experience placebo response (Montgomery, 2015). Problems with how antidepressant RCTs are designed and conducted contribute to the problem of proving efficacy including pressure to recruit causing inflation of participants' depression rating scores initially to get them into a study that rapidly drop on assessment after randomization to a treatment group by researchers without this incentive to recruit. This can lead to high apparent response rates in placebo groups and masks any effectiveness of antidepressants (Khan and Brown, 2015).

Use of arbitrary average minimum differences in rating scores in groups rather than individuals to decide if antidepressants are clinically effective has been criticized (Parker et al., 2003; Chapter 7). More worrying is the fact that many antidepressant RCTs are rated as having high risk of bias (Jakobsen et al., 2017), often through sloppy practices, for example, not reporting if 'blinding' is maintained (Parker et al., 2003). Knowing the magnitude of effect of this bias is important. One of the most important is if the pharmaceutical industry funded the RCT, and this has been shown to be significant but of small impact in studies comparing antidepressants with psychotherapy and even controlling for this antidepressants have similar efficacy to psychotherapy (Cristea et al., 2017b).

Table 15.2 shows a significant but small advantage for antidepressants compared to placebo on depression rating scores but a reasonable NNT for response to treatment

Table 15.2 Effectiveness of antidepressants in depression and anxiety.

Outcome	Study Type	Results	Reference
Continuous Depression rating scale scores	Meta-analysis of RCTs including unpublished trials	Effect size 0.31 (mixed SSRIs, SNRIs, other)	Turner et al., 2008
		Effect size 0.30 including studies after Turner (mixed SSRIs, SNRIs, other)	Gibertini et al., 2012
	Meta-analysis of TCAs in published primary care studies, often low-quality studies	Effect size 0.42 (also 0.34 by 4 weeks and 0.5 if only high-quality intent to treat studies included)	Arroll et al., 2005
Average reduction of depression rating scale scores	Average from multiple types of studies in depression	40% reduction of symptoms in blinded trials for antidepressants 40% reduction of symptoms in blinded trials for psychotherapy 30% reduction of symptoms in blinded trials for placebo	Khan and Brown, 2015
Categorical Response of Depression to Treatment (usually defined as 50%+ reduction depression rating scale scores), equivalent to CGI-I 2 'much improved'. Leucht et al., 2013B	Meta-analysis of antidepressant RCTs submitted to Swedish regulatory authorities	48% antidepressant vs 32% placebo NNT 6–7	Melander et al., 2008
	Meta-analysis of SSRI RCTs including unpublished trials	48.9–49.7% antidepressant vs 38.4–40.0% placebo. NNT approximately 10	Jakobsen et al., 2017 (S2 data)
	Meta-analysis of SSRI RCTs including from registered drug company RCTs	50.7% antidepressant vs 38.7% placebo. NNT 8–9	Barth et al., 2016

Categorical Remission from Depression defined as < 8 points on Hamilton or < 10 points on Becks or MADRS scales Equivalent to CGI-S 'borderline ill'. Leucht et al., 2013B	Meta-analysis of SSRI RCTs including unpublished trials	34.3% antidepressant vs 25.5% placebo NNT approximately 11	Jakobsen et al., 2017
Categorical Combined Depression Remission and/or Response	Meta-analysis of studies of depression set in primary care	NNT for TCAs 8.5 and 6.5 in SSRIs	Arroll et al., 2016
Categorical Relapse rates in participants that responded to antidepressants in acute phase and randomized to maintenance antidepressants or placebo	Meta-analysis of RCT depression relapse rates; most studies up to 12 months but a few up to 36 months	6 months 15% antidepressants vs 34% placebo relapsed RRR=55.9%, NNT approximately 5 12 months 16% antidepressant vs 40% placebo relapsed RRR = 60%, NNT approximately 4 18–36 months 24% antidepressant vs 63% in placebo relapsed RRR=61.9%, NNT approximately 2.5	Geddes et al., 2003
		< 12 months, average 8.35 months 23.3% antidepressants vs 49.4% placebo relapsed RRR = 52.8%, NNT 4.4 > 12 months antidepressants vs placebo RRR = 50.7% NNT 3.8	Sim et al., 2016
		Withdrawal reactions after randomization to placebo may account for some relapses but persistent benefit and some in antidepressant group also stopped meds suggest at least some benefit is due to antidepressants.	

(*continued*)

Table 15.2 Continued

Outcome	Study Type	Results	Reference
Continuous Anxiety rating scale scores	Meta-analysis of RCTs including unpublished trials in anxiety using SSRIs and SNRIs	Anxiety disorders (social anxiety disorder, PTSD, OCD, panic disorder, and generalized anxiety disorders) effect sizes ranging from 0.27–0.39 depending on diagnosis with average effect size 0.33 for SSRIs/SNRIs.	Roest et al., 2015
		For social anxiety disorder, PTSD, OCD, and generalized anxiety disorders effect size 0.20–0.43	De Vries et al., 2016b
Quality of Life (QOL)/Functioning in Depression	Meta-analysis of SSRI RCTs including unpublished trials	SSRIs superior to placebo on QOL measures.	Jakobsen et al., 2017
	Meta-analysis searching databases for RCTs on depression spectrum conditions	Antidepressant vs placebo had effect size 0.31 on QoL and effect size 0.27 for functioning measures.	Kamenov et al., 2017
Qualitative Antidepressant users' views	Anonymous online questionnaire open-ended question 1747 New Zealand participants	Positive (54 %), negative (16 %), and mixed (28 %) experiences Positive themes: necessary for disease treatment (like taking medication for e.g. diabetes), life-saver, meeting social obligations, getting through difficult times, a stepping stone to further help (such as being able to engage in therapy). Mixed themes: benefits vs side effects, calmer but not myself, fear of dependence versus stopping meds, finding one that works. Negative themes: ineffective, unbearable side effects, loss of authenticity/emotional numbing, masks real problems, loss of control.	Gibson et al., 2016b

CGI-S = Clinical Global Impression Severity CGI-I = Clinical Global Impression Improvement

SSRI = Selective Serotonin Reuptake Inhibitors. SNRI = Serotonin and Noradrenaline Reuptake Inhibitors. TCA = tricyclic antidepressants

PTSD = Post traumatic stress disorder OCD = obsessive-compulsive disorder

but less so for remission, and very clinically significant benefit in preventing recurrence in those with an acute phase response as well as benefits in limiting functional deterioration. The small average reduction in symptom scores compared to placebo is often seen in general medicine medications regarded as effective (Khan and Brown, 2015).

Table 15.3 discusses nature and frequency of antidepressant adverse effects. Inert substances used as placebos can also be associated with participants experiencing adverse effects (the 'nocebo' effect).

There are high rates of adverse events even in the placebo group due to combination of nocebo effects and possibly physical symptoms associated with depression being attributed to medication even if it is a placebo. SSRIs increase fear and anxiety in the short-term, probably through serotoninergic effects on the bed nuclei striae terminalis (Ravinder et al., 2013; Marcinkiewcz et al., 2016). Antidepressants can also cause mania, especially if there is a pre-existing diagnosis of or family history of bipolar disorder (Goldberg and Truman, 2003). There is some evidence of increased mortality but also of reduced mortality, depending on what criteria are used to select studies.

Data from 527,907 insured US patients showed adherence with an antidepressant regime is not good;41% by 3 months, 31% by 6 months, and 21% by 12 months, with tricyclics having half the adherence rates of SSRIs (Keyloun et al., 2017). Rates of adherence to antidepressants are similar to long-term general medicine drugs such as antihypertensives (Chapter 1 in Pendleton et al., 1984).

For individuals, clinical utility of antidepressants will depend on the balance of effectiveness in themselves, desirability of treatment objectives (e.g. reduced symptoms/ preventing relapse) compared to their burden of side effects. Withdrawal effects are common and the patient should be warned of these. Appropriate tapering off from antidepressants should be used when they are discontinued and contingency planning if withdrawal syndromes occur should be put into place. Many people find these medications helpful. If effective in the acute phase, maintenance antidepressants have clinically significant benefit in preventing relapse.

There is little evidence that antidepressants cure deficiencies of monoamines that are causing the depression (Healy, 2015). Their named pharmacological action—most inhibit reuptake of monoamines from synapses—happens quickly but clinical benefits appear later, sometimes after weeks (Harmer et al., 2017). Antidepressants may cause compensatory mechanisms over several weeks that improve mood, perhaps by ultimately reducing brain serotonin levels (Andrews et al., 2015). There are often complex synaptic changes including desensitization of the 5HT1A autoreceptor with long-term antidepressant use, and hippocampal neurogenesis may occur (Mnie-Filali et al., 2013). Antidepressants may cause clinical benefit by improving neuronal plasticity and resilience by effects on neurotrophic chemicals such as Cyclic adenosine monophosphate (cAMP) and brain-derived neurotropic factor (BDNF) (Manji et al., 2003; Castrén and Rantamäki, 2010). Biological effects may complement psychological effects described below, or may be the biological substrate of them; that is, the psychological effects listed below are embodied by these biological changes (Harmer et al,, 2017).

Antidepressants very quickly reduce processing of negative emotional stimuli and increase recognition of positive emotional stimuli which ultimately leads to

Table 15.3 Antidepressant adverse effects.

Outcome	Study Type	Results	Reference
Proportion of Participants Experiencing Adverse Events	Meta-analysis of SSRI RCTs including registered drug company RCTs	77.6% antidepressants vs 65% placebo NNH 8–9.	Barth et al., 2016
Serious Adverse Events	Meta-analysis of SSRI RCTs including unpublished trials Meta-analysis of clinical study reports of antidepressant RCTs as harms under-reported in main RCT data	2.7% antidepressants vs 2.1% placebo (also includes some unlikely related to intervention, e.g. viral gastroenteritis) NNH 167. All-cause mortality NNH 598.	Jakobsen et al., 2017
		Suicide NNT 9115 (i.e. antidepressants very slight benefit in reducing suicide) Suicides, acts, preparations, and threats of self-harm and suicidal ideation NNH 1432. Aggressive acts NNH 535. Akathisia (including inner restlessness) NNH 880.	Sharma et al., 2016
		The <https://rxisk.org/antidepressants/> website says FDA data show more suicides in antidepressant group than placebo but does not give specific figures.	
Adverse Events (10 commonest for SSRIs); many adverse effects commoner in antidepressants than placebo, e.g. 84 in Jakobsen et al., 2017	Meta-analysis of SSRI RCTs including unpublished trials	Nausea NNH 9. Sexual dysfunction NNH 11. Somnolence NNNH 13. Drowsiness NNH 14 Anorexia (loss of appetite) NNH 15. Tremor NNH 16. Asthenia (weakness) NNH 18. Diarrhoea NNH19. Insomnia NNH 19. Abnormal ejaculation NNH 19 (in males).	Jakobsen et al., 2017 S2 data

Withdrawal/discontinuation syndromes on stopping antidepressants	Expert and systematic reviews of evidence	Seen with all types of antidepressants, can vary from mild to severe and lead to difficulties stopping antidepressants, can be misdiagnosed, e.g. as depression relapse, commoner in short half-life drugs, can vary greatly in clinical features. Incidence variable, e.g. 46–78% (placebo 22%), commoner in paroxetine, least common fluoxetine for SSRIs.	Haddad and Anderson, 2007
		Highly variable rates of withdrawal/discontinuation syndromes from SSRIs depending on how measured from 0% to over 80% of varying severity compared to 0–13.5% in placebo. Significantly commoner in SSRI than placebo. Commonest in paroxetine.	Fava et al., 2015
Tricyclic adverse effects	Pharmacology textbooks and research on toxicity and adherence	Tricyclics associated with greater adverse effects than SSRIs including more likely to have anticholinergic side effects such as blurred vision, dry mouth, constipation.	Chapter 12 in Harvey et al., 2012
		Tricyclics more toxic in overdose than SSRIs, over 20 times higher fatality rates per prescription numbers.	Hawton et al., 2010
		Participants stopping treatment due to adverse effects more common for tricyclics compared to SSRIs in RCTs. This advantage in tolerability for SSRIs may not exist when compared to newer tricyclics or heterocyclics.	Anderson and Tomenson, 1995; Hotopf et al., 1997; Arroll et al., 2005
Mortality	Meta-analysis of observational studies comparing mortality between those taking and not taking antidepressant then controlling for comorbidities	Increased mortality risk of 33% overall in 'general population' participants but no significant increased mortality in those with cardiovascular disease or a combined 'general population' and cardiovascular sample. Observational studies may not control for hidden confounding factors, e.g. through use of randomization so confidence in results is reduced. Excluded at least one study with reduced mortality in those prescribed antidepressants in a large cohort study of 93,653 (Scherrer et al., 2011); this study was identified by a systematic review of interventions for mortality in mental health as the only study of antidepressants and mortality with good enough quality to be included in the review (Baxter et al., 2016). The meta-analysis of Maslej et al., 2017 may be effected by selection bias of studies.	Maslej et al., 2017

SSRI = Selective Serotonin Reuptake Inhibitors

improvement in mood consistent with cognitive theories of depression (Harmer et al., 2009). A systematic review of fMRI studies concluded that this pattern was reflected in normalized patterns of brain activity with increasing activity to positive stimuli and reduced activity with negative stimuli. However, in depressed, not healthy, participants, an increase in dorsolateral prefrontal cortex activity with this 'bottom-up' change in emotional reactivity lead to improvements in mood (Ma, 2015). This suggests antidepressants work by compensating for effects of depression by indirect compensation acting on an opposing mechanism (see Chapter 5).

Symptoms associated with psychosis are highly diverse and the choice of how and which symptoms are assessed can impact antipsychotic trials results summarized in Table 15.4. The commonest scale, PANSS (Kay et al., 1987), gives a combined score and three subscale scores (which contribute equally to the combined score): positive (e.g. hallucinations or grandiosity), negative (e.g. blunted affect), or general (e.g. depression or anxiety). The older Brief Psychiatric Rating Scale (Overall and Gorham, 1962) is slightly more weighted towards positive symptoms which antipsychotics are more effective at reducing (Leucht et al., 2017). Many RCTs for antipsychotics include comparison groups with reference antipsychotics (with previously demonstrated efficacy, e.g. haloperidol). 'First-generation antipsychotics' refers to older antipsychotics, sometimes called 'typicals', and 'second generation' refers to newer antipsychotics, sometimes called 'atypicals'. The evidence presented in Table 15.4 again groups together different medications and conceals differences between them.

Placebo response is smaller compared to antidepressant trials (Lepping et al., 2011), but this has increased recently and also increases the longer the duration of study (Rutherford et al., 2014). Antipsychotics have small to medium benefit, particularly on positive and manic symptoms, and small benefit on quality of life and functioning. They have greater benefit compared to placebo on participants with more severe symptoms at baseline (Furukuwa et al., 2015). Antipsychotics have clinically significant benefit in preventing recurrence.

Antipsychotic studies are often of short duration. A meta-analysis of studies where participants meeting schizophrenia criteria were randomized to placebo or remained on antipsychotic demonstrated persistent clinical benefit over one year (Takeuchi et al., 2017). In a naturalistic 20-year follow-up study, several participants, who tended to have good prognostic factors at onset, were not taking antipsychotics and did not have psychotic symptoms (Harrow et al., 2014). The study is not very informative as participants were not randomized to antipsychotics or no antipsychotics, and it seems likely that people with an intrinsic good prognosis are more likely to recover and stop treatment without experiencing relapse and needing to restart medication.

A Dutch study randomized first-episode psychosis participants in sustained remission on antipsychotics for six months to either gradual discontinuation (65 participants) of their antipsychotics or continued antipsychotic (63 participants) (Wunderink et al., 2007). The treatment was then adjusted depending on clinical need, and in the first 18 months, relapses were twice as common in the discontinuation group, of whom only 20% were able to have stopped medication completely (Wunderink et al., 2007). At seven years' follow-up, data were available on 52 discontinuation participants and 51 maintenance participants (Wunderink et al., 2013).

Table 15.4 Effectiveness of antipsychotics in psychosis/schizophrenia and mania.

Outcome	Study Type	Results	Reference
Continuous Psychosis rating-scale scores	Meta-analysis of RCTs of eight SGAs including unpublished trials	Effect size 0.44.	Turner et al., 2012
	Meta-analysis of RCTS including from FDA and pharmaceutical industry databases using direct and indirect comparisons, mostly SGAs	Effect size of clozapine 0.88 (large), other effect sizes depending on drug vary from 0.33–0.66.	Leucht et al., 2013a
	Meta-analysis of 60 years of RCTs from trial registries, FDA databases and other sources. RCT results controlled for small trials and publication bias. Oral FGAs and SGAs except clozapine as it is more effective than the rest.	Effect size 0.38 for psychosis rating symptoms overall. Effect size 0.45 for positive symptoms. Effect size 0.35 for negative symptoms. Effect size 0.27 for depression. Pharmaceutical industry sponsorship associated with *smaller* effect sizes (by 0.16); publication bias for more effective studies noted (also seen in Turner et al., 2012).	Leucht et al., 2017
Average reduction of psychosis rating scale scores	Meta-analysis based on previous meta-analysis and literature search.	PANNS FGAs 21% reduction, SGAs 28% reduction, placebo 5.5% reduction. BPRS FGA 39.9% reduction, SGAs 49.6% reduction, placebo 7.3% reduction. PANNS changes compared to placebo equivalent to 'minimal improvement' on CGI-I (i.e. noticeable improvement but less than 'much improved'). BPRS changes compared to placebo halfway between CGI-I 'minimal improvement' and 'much improved' (Leucht et al., 2006).	Lepping et al., 2011

(*continued*)

Table 15.4 Continued

Outcome	Study Type	Results	Reference
Categorical Response of Psychosis to Treatment			
Minimal Response 20%+ reduction PANSS or BPRS score or CGI-I 'minimally improved' or better	Meta-analysis of 60 years of RCTs from trial registries, FDA databases, and other sources. RCT results controlled for small trials and publication bias. Oral FGAs and SGAs except clozapine.	51% antipsychotics vs 30% placebo NNT 5.	Leucht et al., 2017
Good response 50%+ reduction PANSS or BPRS score or CGI-I 'much improved' or better		23% antipsychotics vs 14% placebo NNT 11-12. (stated as 8 in paper but by my calculation closer to 11-12).	
'Dramatic response' trajectory with 70%+ PANNS reduction	Data from two RCTs analysed for trajectory of responses.	43/251 antipsychotics vs 0/117 combined placebo and very low dose antipsychotic NNT 6.	Marques et al., 2011
Categorical Relapse rates in participants that responded to antipsychotics in acute phase and randomized to antipsychotics or placebo	Meta-analysis of RCTs identified from trial registries and contacting pharmaceutical companies.	In blinded studies, 28% relapse rate antipsychotics vs 64% antipsychotics by 7–12 months. Relative risk reduction 56% NNT 3.	Leucht et al., 2012a
Continuous Quality of Life and Functioning in psychosis	Meta-analysis of 60 years of RCTs from trial registries, FDA databases, and other sources. RCT results controlled for small trials and publication bias. Oral FGAs and SGAs except clozapine.	Quality of life effect size 0.35. Functioning effect size 0.34.	Leucht et al., 2017

Continuous Mania symptoms-rating scale scores	Meta-analysis of published/unpublished SGA RCTs in acute mania from trial registries/databases.	Effect size 0.45.	Scherk et al., 2007
	Meta-analysis and network analysis of published/unpublished RCTs from trial registries/databases.	Effect size Haloperidol 0.54. Effect size SGAs 0.44.	Yildiz et al., 2015
Categorical response of mania to treatment Response 50%+ reduction of mania rating scores Remission (Young Mania Rating Scale Score < 12)	Meta-analysis of RCTs identified from searching Cochrane and EMBASE databases.	RCTs < 6 weeks NNT 5.1, RCTs 6–12 weeks NNT 4. RCTs < 6 weeks NNT 5.4, RCTs 6–12 weeks NNT 4.	Derry and Moore, 2007
		Harder to interpret studies on prevention of relapse due to problems with methodology of studies.	Goodwin et al., 2016
Discontinuation due to lack of efficacy in long-term follow-up of 12 months plus	Double-blind or open label RCTs in first episode, chronic, or older patients.	Approximately 25% of participants discontinue antipsychotics because of lack of efficacy; second or third commonest reason for discontinuation.	Lieberman et al., 2005; Kahn et al., 2008; Jin et al., 2013
Qualitative Antipsychotic Users' views	Qualitative research on small samples.	Mixed experiences of medication. In acute phase helps with reducing mental chaos, reducing psychotic symptoms or they become less distressing or compelling and can help with mood. Side effects regarded as potentially hindering recovery, e.g. by sedative effects or reduction of participation in activities.	Gray and Keane, 2016
		Some people found medication helpful but many expressed a desire for treatment to include additional forms of help such as therapy.	Bjornestad et al., 2017

CGI-S = Clinical Global Impression Severity CGI-I = Clinical Global Impression Improvement; FGA = First generation antipsychotic, SGA = Second generation antipsychotic

Medication status varied greatly within both groups and there were no large differences between the groups. Average dosage difference in the previous two years in participants taking antipsychotics was not objectively large between the two groups (2.2 mg haloperidol dose equivalent in discontinuation group versus 3.6 mg in the maintenance group). There were participants not taking antipsychotics over the past two years in both groups (14 in discontinuation group, 8–12 in maintenance group, with 11–12 towards end of follow-up); 6–7 in discontinuation group and 2–5 in maintenance group were taking a very low dose of antipsychotic (1 mg or less haloperidol dose equivalent).

Symptomatic remission was common in both groups (about two-thirds of participants) but functional remission was significantly higher in the discontinuation group compared to the maintenance group (46.2% versus 19.6%) as was recovery—combined symptomatic and functional remission—(40.4% versus 17.6%). Differences in relapse rates were no longer significant between both groups.

It is unclear if assessments were blinded. Given the relatively small difference between both groups for medication use, it may be that the important lesson is to try to stop medication in first-episode psychosis patients who are asymptomatic for a period (six months is possibly too short). Some patients will only have a single episode so do not need medication for years, whilst others may recover after several years so can trial stopping medication then (see Chapter 14). Even if patients need to restart antipsychotics, the break from medication may improve long-term functional outcomes, but this study needs replicated. Intermittent antipsychotic dosage, using only during psychotic episodes then tapering off afterwards but restarting if symptoms recur, is associated with far higher relapse rates than continuous medication (De Hert et al., 2015).

It is important to avoid overmedication. Meta-analysis of older antipsychotic RCTs found that doses of approximately 16–40% of maximum dose was the optimum dose range. Higher doses had non-significant clinical benefits but significantly increased side effects (Bollini et al., 1994).

An expert review concluded that most patients who meet schizophrenia criteria probably have improved outcomes with long-term use of antipsychotics, but some patients may benefit from either short-term antipsychotic use or non-medication alternatives (Goff et al., 2017).

There are a wide range of adverse effects associated with antipsychotics and the risk of developing these side effects varies greatly between different antipsychotics (Haddad and Sharma, 2007). Information for adverse effects in Table 15.5 will therefore often be presented as a range rather than combined figures.

In double-blind or open-label RCTs lasting 12 months or in first episode, chronic or older patients median time to antipsychotic discontinuation for any reason is about 6 months, but this varies between different medications (Lieberman et al., 2005; Kahn et al., 2008; Jin et al., 2013). About 16–50% of discontinuations are because of side effects (with tolerability varying greatly between different medications), one of the commonest reasons for stopping antipsychotics along with lack of efficacy and patient choice (Lieberman et al, 2005; Kahn et al., 2008; Jin et al., 2013).

Table 15.5 Antipsychotic adverse effects.

Type of Outcome	Type of Study	Results	Reference
Selected Adverse Events	Meta-analysis of RCTS including from FDA and pharmaceutical industry databases using direct and indirect comparisons, mostly SGAs.	Weight gain 0.09–0.74 effect size EPSEs (indicated by using medication treating it) by central parameter of credible interval (1 = equal frequency of placebo); clozapine = 0.31, others 0.81–4.76 with almost all above 1. Prolactin increase –0.22 (i.e. reduces prolactin) to 1.3 (large effect size to increase), most increase prolactin QTc prolongation using 'odds ratio' to placebo but 0 (not 1) equals placebo rate (may actually be effect size). –0.1 to 0.90 (most increase odds of QTc prolongation) Sedation odds ratio with 1 equals placebo rate. Odds ratio varies from 1.42–8.82.	Leucht et al., 2013a
Selected Adverse Events	Meta-analysis of 60 years of RCTs from trial registries, FDA databases and other sources. RCT results controlled for small trials and publication bias. Oral FGAs and SGAs except clozapine.	EPSEs (indicated by use of medication to treat) 19% drug vs 10% placebo, NNH 11–12. Sedation 14% drug vs 6% placebo, NNH 12–13. Weight gain: Effect size 0.40. Prolactin increase: Effect size 0.43. QTc prolongation: Effect size 0.19.	Leucht et al., 2017

(*continued*)

Table 15.5 Continued

Type of Outcome	Type of Study	Results	Reference
Selected Adverse Events in bipolar disorder trials (NNH from my own calculations)	Meta-analysis of RCTs identified from searching Cochrane and EMBASE databases.	< 6 weeks Weight 8% drugs vs 2% placebo NNH 16–17. Akathisia 10% drugs vs 4% placebo NNH 16–17. EPSE 20% drugs vs 6% placebo NNH 7–8. Tremor 7% drugs vs 3% placebo NNH 25. Somnolence 26% drugs vs 8% placebo NNH 5–6. 6–12 weeks Weight gain 23% drugs v. 4% placebo NNH 5–6. EPSEs 10% drugs vs 7% placebo NNH 33. Somnolence 30% drugs vs 11% placebo NNH 5–6. Depression 11% drugs vs 8% placebo NNH 33. > 12 weeks Weight gain > 7% 17% drugs vs 2% placebo NNH 6–7. Somnolence 6% drugs vs 4% placebo NNH 50.	Derry and Moore, 2007
Type 2 diabetes	Systematic reviews and expert reviews.	Prevalence of type 2 diabetes varies from 3.9–13.2% for different antipsychotics vs 2.9% in antipsychotic naïve participants.	Vancampfort et al., 2016
		Risk is higher for certain antipsychotics such as olanzapine, risperidone, and clozapine.	Vancampfort et al., 2016; Ho et al., 2014
Metabolic Syndrome	RCT of 99 first episode drug-naïve schizophrenia measuring BP, lipids, fasting blood glucose, waist circumference (increased by weight gain); prescribed olanzapine, haloperidol, or risperidone.	Males more affected than females but antipsychotics depending on type increase risk of different metabolic syndrome aspects.	Saddichha et al., 2008

	Compared to MH outpatient controls.	Prevalence of metabolic syndrome varies per definition and drug type from 0–25% in antipsychotic group compared to 0–2% in MH outpatient controls.	Correll et al., 2017
Cardiovascular disease	Meta-analysis	Increased prevalence of metabolic syndrome thought to explain association with higher rates of cardiovascular disease in people prescribed antipsychotics	Corell et al., 2017
Mortality	Population databases identifying cohorts of people with diagnosis of schizophrenia and medication status often with duration of follow-up over several years up to 11 years	Highest mortality in those not taking antipsychotics followed by those on high dose of antipsychotics. This suggests not taking antipsychotics increases mortality. As these are cohort studies potential hidden confounders reduce confidence in conclusions (e.g. see De Hert et al., 2010). Higher dose association with mortality may reflect more severe schizophrenia condition causing increased mortality not the higher dose antipsychotic used to treat it.	Tiihonen et al., 2009; Cullen et al., 2012; Torniainen et al., 2014; Tiihonen et al., 2016
Tardive dyskinesia- TD- (Stigmatizing and distressing abnormal movements often in mouth region)	Up to 4-year follow-up of 352 participants free of TD at baseline.	Annual incidence of tardive dyskinesia 5.6% per year; non-significantly lower for SGAs compared to FGAs. Higher if combined FGAs and SGAs prescribed for participant.	Woods et al., 2010
	SOHO study of SGAs followed over 2 years; 9,104 no TD at baseline.	0.78% annual incidence with 80% persistence (this seems closer to clinical experience with lower rates of TD seen than in past with FGAs).	Tenback et al., 2010
	50 years or older participants who met DSM-IV schizophrenia criteria in urban, suburban and rural India.	Tardive dyskinesia found in both medicated and non-medicated participants; follow-up over 18 months showed tardive dyskinesia, and parkinsonism symptoms fluctuated in both medicated and never medicated participants suggesting extra-pyramidal symptoms are part of the condition but also associated with anti-psychotics.	McCreadie et al., 1997; McCreadie et al., 2002b

(continued)

Table 15.5 Continued

Type of Outcome	Type of Study	Results	Reference
Subjective Reports of Unpleasant Experiences	Commentary paper	Antipsychotic-induced apathy, emotional indifference, mental 'fogginess', 'blankness', and 'clouding'; 'neuroleptic dysphoria'.	Jones, 2012
	Content analysis of database of online comments about medication	Sedation, cognitive impairment, emotional flattening/ indifference, parkinsonism, akathisia, sexual/metabolic syndrome side-effects.	Moncrieff et al., 2009c
Loss of Brain Volume Schizophrenia also has effect on brain volumes (see Table 12.3)	Meta-analysis	Total cortical grey matter effect size: –0.1 (controls) vs –0.24 (antipsychotics) only significant difference; small in size.	Vita et al., 2015
	Systematic review	Some evidence for brain volume loss especially in frontal lobe and increased ventricle size in antipsychotic users.	Moncrieff and Leo, 2010
	Follow-up of over 200 first episode schizophrenia participants with MRI scans over 7 years	Duration of episodes associated with loss of brain volume particularly frontal lobe; antipsychotics at higher doses and for longer periods associated with brain tissue loss; severity of illness less associated with brain volume loss, and number of relapses little effect. Average amount of brain volume loss due to antipsychotics is small but will be greater in some individuals and are cumulative over time and at high doses.	Ho et al., 2011; Andreassen et al., 2013
	Meta-analysis with meta-regression	FGAs associated with more brain volume loss than SGAs.	Vita et al., 2015
	Comparison of brain volume and functioning in unmedicated vs medicated first episode psychosis participants	Thinner dorsolateral prefrontal and temporal cortex in medicated vs unmedicated participants but higher dorso-lateral prefrontal cortex activation and behavioural perfor-mance in medicated vs unmedicated participants..	Lesh et al., 2015

Examples of other adverse events associated with antipsychotics	Systematic review of adverse events	Many other adverse events listed including anticholinergic effects (constipation, dry mouth, blurred vision), raised prolactin, sexual dysfunction, postural hypotension, seizures, discontinuation syndromes, cardiac arrhythmias, cerebrovascular accidents in elderly.	Haddad and Sharma, 2007

FGA = First generation antipsychotic, SGA = Second generation antipsychotic EPSEs = extrapyramidal side-effects (e.g. parkinsonism, akathisia, dystonia, tardive dyskinesia). MH= mental health

The clinical utility of antipsychotics for an individual again depends on the balance of effectiveness in achieving treatment objectives (and how valued they are) with the adverse effects they experience.

Antipsychotics have actions on many receptors but it is thought that reducing the activity of dopamine type 2 receptors is key to their effect on psychotic symptoms (Kapur, 2003; Kapur et al., 2006). Clinical effectiveness is linked to occupation of this receptor but this may be briefer for second-generation antipsychotics and clozapine (Seeman and Tallerico, 1998; Kapur and Seeman, 2001). Even at high occupancy levels, significant numbers of patients do not respond to antipsychotics, reflecting the diversity of factors involved in psychosis and the fact that dopaminergic system abnormalities are often absent in people who meet criteria for schizophrenia (see Table 12.4; Howes and Kapur, 2014).

'Avoidance response' is avoiding an aversive stimulus. In rats, reduction of conditioned avoidance response by test compounds is a good predictor of antipsychotic activity in humans, and for antipsychotics with established antipsychotic efficacy is significantly superior to benzodiazepines for this effect (Li et al., 2007). Early trials of antipsychotics reported that they did not eliminate hallucinations or delusions but participants were 'less disturbed by them' (Elkes and Elkes, 1954) and that antipsychotics were more effective than sedating drugs like barbiturates (Casey, 1960). Factor analysis of 99 participants (including 8 antipsychotic-naïve) meeting schizophrenia spectrum criteria reported two main factors of therapeutic response to antipsychotics: detachment towards symptoms (by far the commonest factor), and eradication/elimination of symptoms (Mizrahi et al., 2005). In 17 participants meeting schizophrenia spectrum criteria (60% antipsychotic-naïve), antipsychotics had greatest effect on behavioural impact of psychotic symptoms but also significant effects on cognitive preoccupation and emotional improvement with later effect on conviction, that is, degree of belief in the reality of the symptoms (Mizrahi et al., 2006). Preoccupation and distress, which are reduced by antipsychotics, are some of the characteristics that differentiate clinical psychotic symptoms from non-clinical psychotic-like experiences in non-clinical populations (David, 2010).

Antipsychotics may act by reducing salience (degree of importance and relevance that the patient places on the psychotic symptoms) and motivational effects of psychotic symptoms thus leading to indifference/reduction of distress initially and sometimes reduction of psychotic symptoms by 'extinction and unlearning' (Kapur, 2003; Kapur et al., 2006). For example, reducing strong emotional arousal by delusional beliefs may allow patients to notice and incorporate disconfirmatory information, thus reducing delusional conviction. Mechanism of antipsychotic action could be indirect compensation by acting on an opposing mechanism and/or inducing a compensatory state (indifference) that mitigates the unpleasant/distressing effects of psychotic symptoms.

Lithium's effectiveness in bipolar disorder will now be briefly discussed. There is little good-quality evidence of lithium's effectiveness in the acute treatment of depression (Bhagwagar and Goodwin, 2002). For acute mania, a network meta-analysis concluded lithium had effect size of 0.45 on continuous manic symptom rating scores compared to placebo (Yildiz et al., 2015). Response in acute mania, defined by 50%

or greater reduction in mania rating symptom scores, was present in 44% of lithium participants versus 31% placebo participants' NNT 8 (Bowden et al., 1994).

Systematic reviews and meta-analysis of lithium's effectiveness in relapse prevention is complicated by even slow withdrawals of lithium increasing lithium's apparent benefit by inducing mania in those switched to placebo but also higher rates of dropouts in placebo group boosting apparent effectiveness of placebo (Burgess et al., 2001). A meta-analysis (Severus et al., 2014) concluded 34% of lithium participants versus 56% placebo participants experienced relapse—clinically significant relative risk reduction of 39% and NNT 5—and that lithium was more effective in preventing manic than depressive episodes. Data on patients with bipolar disorder diagnosis from Swedish national registries were analysed and researchers concluded that lithium had clinically significant relative risk reduction of 33% of hospital admissions for bipolar disorder (Joas et al., 2017). Meta-analysis of RCTs demonstrated lithium's significant benefit in reducing suicides versus placebo (relative risk reduction up to 100%) and overall mortality (Baldessarini et al., 2006; Cipriani et al., 2013), but other meta-analyses found non-significant reduction of suicide risk but their conclusions may have been due to lack of power (Burgess et al., 2001) or including a poor-quality study with markedly different results than the other studies (Hawton and Pirkis, 2017; Riblet et al., 2017).

Lithium is used to relieve current distress (particularly mania), prevent recurrence, and prevent later complication (suicide).

In a meta-analysis, side effects were common in lithium-treated participants (odds ratio of 2.35 times more likely in lithium participants than placebo participants) including tremor, somnolence, diarrhoea, hypercalcaemia, and hypothyroidism (Burgess et al., 2001). A meta-analysis of adverse effects associated with lithium concluded that there were higher risks of reduced urinary concentrating ability, hypothyroidism, and weight gain (McKnight et al., 2012). Long-term lithium treatment is associated with declining kidney function and risk of chronic kidney disease (Shine et al., 2015). Increased risk of renal impairment may at least in part be due to effects of bipolar disorder or co-occurring conditions such as smoking (Kessing et al., 2015).

Responsiveness to lithium as a maintenance treatment may be inherited (Grof et al., 2002) and this may be partly related to a single nucleotide peptide associated with phospholipid regulation (Song et al., 2016). Stem cell research suggests hyperexcitable nerve cells found in bipolar disorder participants may become less excitable in lithium-responders perhaps by acting on mitochondria and calcium signalling (Mertens et al., 2015). These findings are not confirmed and lithium's mechanism of action is unknown.

Electroconvulsive therapy—where an electric current is passed through either both cerebral hemispheres (bilateral ECT) or only the non-dominant (usually the right) hemisphere (unilateral ECT)—to induce the seizure that is the actual therapeutic agent, is one of the most controversial treatments in psychiatry (Kolar, 2017). ECT is associated with many side effects, more commonly headaches, confusion, pain/muscle soreness, and less commonly fractures/soft tissue trauma (reduced by anaesthetics and muscle relaxants), burns, and cardiovascular and respiratory problems, amongst others (FDA, 2011). Although some confusion and cognitive impairment is temporary and improves quickly after treatment completion (Semkovska and McLoughlin, 2010), there is evidence of persistent cognitive impairment in some patients, for example, retrograde amnesia for autobiographical memories, lasting at least six months especially if bilateral ECT or sinewave stimulation is used (Sackeim et al., 2007). This cognitive impairment can vary in severity, and for some patients outweighs any clinical benefit (Robertson and Pryor, 2006).

Evidence for depression and ECT will be discussed below as this is the commonest clinical indication, but ECT is also used to treat mania, catatonia, and schizophrenia. ECT is regarded as particularly effective in older adults (Kerner and Prudic, 2014). Meta-analysis often combines studies using different ECT techniques and it is hard to completely 'blind' assessors to treatment group. The patients who seem to most benefit from ECT—the most severely depressed or those with depression and dementia—are also hard to get capacitous consent to include in studies. Often, simulated ECT (where the ECT procedure is copied including anaesthetic apart from ECT) is the control treatment. Methodological concerns include trials where simulated ECT is only used for a few sessions then switching to ECT due to ethical concerns of withholding treatment from severely depressed patients (who are extremely distressed, may be suicidal, and/or not eating or drinking) and problems with blinding raters to treatment group because of obvious ECT side effects (Read and Bentall, 2010).

Meta-analysis concluded ECT was superior to simulated ECT with effect size 0.908, superior to antidepressants with effect size -0.802, and bilateral ECT superior to unilateral ECT, and higher electrical dose superior to lower dose (UK ECT Review Group, 2003). A later meta-analysis results showed high-dose right unilateral ECT was as effective as bilateral ECT but had less cognitive side effects (Kolshus et al., 2017). A meta-analysis of good treatment response, defined as 50% reduction of Hamilton Depression Rating Scale score or a score of 10 or less or clinical judgement of 'recovered' or 'markedly improved', had a higher odds ratio 2.83 times more likely in ECT versus sham ECT and odds ratio 11 times more likely versus pill placebo (Pagnin et al., 2004).

Significant clinical response in RCTs are estimated to have been shown in 70–90% of participants meeting depression criteria for given ECT, and whilst response rates may be lower in community samples, it still has superior effectiveness compared to other depression treatments (Prudic et al., 2004). ECT is more effective for severe forms of depression, for example with delusions or psychomotor agitation/retardation, but control groups often improve to the same level as ECT group by one month after treatment is completed (Read and Bentall, 2010), although this may in part be due to ECT participants worsening after ECT treatment finishes (Prudic et al., 2004). After ECT treatment is completed a systematic review found 37.7% relapse by 6 months and 51.1% by 12 months and that antidepressants halve risk of relapse compared to placebo (Jelovac et al., 2013). One RCT demonstrated maintenance ECT (i.e. repeated treatments after acute treatment is finished at reduced frequency) reduces relapse rates in older adults (Kellner et al., 2016), but there is little evidence that maintenance ECT reduces relapse rates (Jelovac et al., 2013).

This large advantage of ECT compared to simulated ECT is strong evidence for effectiveness, even taking into account methodological concerns, and this is reinforced by evidence of large superiority over antidepressants. ECT relieves current distress/

reduces symptoms in the short term, particularly for severe forms of depression, but it does not prevent further recurrence after the treatment is ended and there is little evidence for maintenance treatment.

It has been suggested that ECT has a therapeutic benefit by causing a traumatic brain injury (TBI), giving the appearance of improving depression (Chapter 3 in Moncrieff, 2009a). TBI is associated with increased depression (Perry et al., 2016) so is unlikely to cause states resembling apparent improvement of depression. ECT is associated with increase in BDNF levels and subsequent increased neuroplasticity and evidence of hippocampal neurogenesis (Castrén and Rantamäki, 2010). Despite these findings, mechanism of action of ECT is largely unknown.

Psychiatric treatments have demonstrated efficacy to varying degrees but are not cures and often have partially to totally unknown mechanisms. They can be associated with serious side effects. There are often important mental health problems that lack medications recommended to treat them such as impaired cognition in schizophrenia (Keefe et al., 2015) or the core features of borderline personality disorder (NICE, 2009). Many psychiatric medications are variations of drugs that had their clinical efficacy established over 50 years ago (Anderson and McAllister-Williams, 2016). Antiepileptics are often tried in mental health conditions and some have established efficacy (see Chapter 14).

Lack of knowledge of biological systems that either cause or compensate for mental health symptoms (see Chapter 12) means current prospects for new medications with improved efficacy are not high. Improving effectiveness of medications currently depends on discovering better ways of utilizing them in clinical practice. Innovative treatments have been developed, such as transcranial magnetic stimulation (TMS) most commonly used in depression that has not responded to treatment (Hardy et al., 2016). NNT for response of depression (50% reduction of depression rating scale scores) is 6 and for remission is 8 (Berlim et al., 2014) and it is less effective than ECT (Berlim et al., 2013). The optimum TMS techniques are still be determined but some methods are superior to others (Brunoni et al., 2017).

There are also concerns about potential bias in the evidence base for effectiveness of medication and psychotherapy effectiveness, for example, researcher allegiance to a treatment including pharmaceutical industry sponsorship, over-emphasizing small differences, changing trial protocols and/or statistical analysis to increase the chances of positive results, and publication bias for positive results (Leichsenring et al., 2017), including preferentially submitting positive results over negative studies (Lenzer and Brownlee, 2008).

General medical treatments

This section briefly overviews effectiveness and adverse effects of selected general medical treatments and notes mechanisms of action that do not reverse disease or are unknown.

Comparing effectiveness of psychiatric medications directly with those of general medical treatments has been performed using meta-analytic estimates of effectiveness of treatments chosen on the basis of either being the 20 most common treatments from a US health informatics source (Leucht et al., 2015b), or treatments for the commonest conditions identified from medical and psychiatric textbooks (Leucht et al., 2012b). NNTs for some of the drugs with highest gross sales in the United States in terms of dollar value are also listed (Schork, 2015). Effectiveness is in comparison with placebo unless otherwise stated.

Data on the effectiveness of medical and psychiatric treatments to allow comparison will be presented in Tables 15.6 and 15.7; Table 15.6 will present effectiveness data using effect size whilst Table 15.7 will use NNT. Only some of the treatments are listed.

Psychiatric treatment effectiveness tends to lie in the middle of the range of general medical treatments effectiveness but with some medical treatments being far more as well as far less effective (Leucht et al., 2012b). Sometimes there are differences in the nature of outcomes. Some general medicine medication outcomes may be more objective or valuable, such as preventing death or achieving cure, but reducing distress is still a worthwhile outcome. Most mental health conditions have lower mortality than many general medical conditions with events such as suicide being relatively rare even over many years compared to death following myocardial infarction. This makes it harder for psychiatric medications—even if they had an anti-suicide effect—to achieve low NNTs for mortality.

Antibiotics targeting micro-organisms sensitive to their effects can have high cure rates but not everybody is cured due to the pharmacological action of the antibiotic as demonstrated by an NNT = 3 for cystitis. There is more knowledge about causative pathways for general medical conditions (see Chapter 12), hence more medications are available to achieve cure or affect disease processes.

Some medications target risk factors for medical conditions (a surrogate outcome) in order to prevent these conditions or improve outcomes for these conditions if already present. For cardiovascular disease risk factors, antihypertensives lower blood pressure, statins lower cholesterol, metformin reduces plasma glucose, and aspirin inhibits platelet aggregation.

Whilst metformin is effective for reducing plasma glucose and is relatively safe, there is little good evidence that it reduces rates of cardiovascular events, mortality, or other micro/macrovascular complications (Boussageon et al., 2016). Even when effective in reducing mortality or cardiovascular events, the benefits these drugs offer are greater in those at higher risk (contrast NNTs for statins in primary or secondary prevention). Whether statins in primary prevention have sufficient benefit is a controversy that has featured in print media (Mathews et al., 2016). In people over 60 years old, lowering low-density lipoprotein (LDL) cholesterol may not reduce mortality (Ravnskov et al., 2016), suggesting that statins may be less useful in this age group and possibly harmful in the over 75s (Han et al., 2017).

For people over 75 years old, aspirin causes much higher risks of gastrointestinal haemorrhage without the addition of proton pump inhibitors (Li et al., 2017), thus reducing aspirin's benefit/risk balance. Even when medication is shown to affect a biological risk factor or other surrogate outcome, there is no guarantee of clinically significant benefit.

A systematic review of surgical procedures compared with placebo controls (e.g. simulated surgery where everything is identical, such as use of anaesthesia, but

Table 15.6 Effectiveness of treatments using effect size.

Condition and Medication	Outcome	Effectiveness Effect Size	Reference
General Medical Treatments			
Chronic Hepatitis C Interferon	Viral Load Reduction	2.27	Leucht et al., 2012b
Reflux Oesophagitis Proton Pump Inhibitor	Remission	1.39	Leucht et al., 2012b
Pain Oxycodone and Paracetamol	50% pain reduction	1.04	Leucht et al., 2015b
Chronic Obstructive Pulmonary Disease Tiotropium	Forced expiratory volume	0.99	Leucht et al., 2015b
Parkinson's disease Levodopa	Reduction of Symptoms	0.93	Leucht et al., 2015b
Type 2 Diabetes Metformin	Reducing fasting glucose Mortality	0.87 0.03	Leucht et al., 2012b Leucht et al., 2015b
Rheumatoid arthritis Methotrexate	Reducing tender joints	0.86	Leucht et al., 2012b
Cystitis Antibiotics	Cure	0.85	Leucht et al., 2012b
Migraine Sumatriptan	Pain-free after two hours	0.83	Leucht et al., 2015b
Hypertension Antihypertensives	Reduction in systolic/diastolic blood pressure	0.56/–0.54	Leucht et al., 2012b
Asthma Corticosteroids	Forced expiratory volume	0.56	Leucht et al., 2012b
Ulcerative Colitis 5-acetyl salicylic acid	Remission	0.44	Leucht et al., 2012b
Chronic Obstructive Pulmonary Disease Corticosteroids	Forced expiratory volume Exacerbations	0.36 0.20	Leucht et al., 2012b
Multiple Sclerosis Interferon	Exacerbation	0.34	Leucht et al., 2012b
Overactive Bladder Anticholinergics	24-hour micturition	0.23	Leucht et al., 2015b
Antibiotics Otitis media	With pain after treatment	0.22	Leucht et al., 2012b

(continued)

Table 15.6 Continued

Condition and Medication	Outcome	Effectiveness Effect Size	Reference
Psychiatric Treatments			
Schizophrenia Antipsychotics	Relapse prevention	0.92	Leucht et al., 2012b
Depression Electroconvulsive therapy	Reduction depressive symptoms	0.908 (vs simulated ECT and some methodolog-ical concerns)	UK ECT Review Group, 2003
Attention Deficit Hyperactivity Disorder Methylphenidate	Reduction of teacher-rated symptom scores	0.78	Leucht et al., 2012b
Depression Antidepressants	Prevention of relapse	0.64	Leucht et al., 2012b
Bipolar disorder Lithium	Prevention of relapse	0.47	Leucht et al., 2012b
Mania Lithium	Reduction of manic symptoms	0.45	Yildiz et al., 2015
Psychosis Antipsychotics	Reduction of psychotic symptoms	0.38–0.44	Table 15.4
Depression Antidepressants	Reduction of depressive symptoms	0.30–0.42	Table 15.2
Anxiety Antidepressants	Reduction of anxiety symptoms	0.2–0.43	Table 15.2
Dementia Anticholinesterase inhibitors	Cognitive assessment rating scales Not worse	0.41 0.26	Leucht et al., 2012b

without surgical procedure itself) found only 49% of such RCTs demonstrated significant superiority for surgery and benefits over placebo were usually in the small range (Wartolowska et al., 2014). Many of these RCTs were for minor procedures such as endoscopy and not for life-threatening conditions, and they used more subjective outcomes such as symptoms, for example, pain or functioning.

Research evidence in all medicine is affected by similar concerns in psychiatry: publication bias, pharmaceutical industry influence on result, over-extrapolating evidence of significant clinical benefit from study results (such as surrogate outcomes), and unclear conflicts of interests in researchers (Goldacre and Heneghan, 2015). Financial ties of principal investigators are associated with higher chances of studies reporting significant benefit (Ahn et al., 2017). The marketing by the pharmaceutical industry is often out of proportion to the clinical benefit of the marketed medication (Greenway

Table 15.7 Effectiveness of treatments using NNT.

Condition and Medication	**Outcome**	**Effectiveness NNT**	**Reference**
General Medical Treatments			
Reflux oesophagitis Proton pump inhibitor	Remission	2	Leucht et al., 2012b
Autoimmune Hepatitis Prednisolone +/– azathioprine	Prevent 1 death	2.7	Chapter 23 in Walker et al., 2014
Cystitis Antibiotics	Cure	3	Leucht et al., 2012b
Rheumatoid arthritis Adulimab	ACR50–50% disease reduction	4	Schork, 2015
Symptomatic heart failure Angiotensin receptor blocker	Prevent 1 admission for heart failure or death	8	Chapter 18 in Walker et al., 2014
Acute ischaemic stroke Thrombolysis with rTPA	Prevent 1 death or disability in those treated	9	Chapter 27 in Walker et al., 2014
Ulcerative Colitis 5-acetyl salicylic acid	Remission	12.5	Leucht et al., 2012b
Variceal bleeding and cirrhosis Propranolol	Reduced variceal bleeding Prevent 1 death	10 16	Chapter 23 in Walker et al., 2014
Secondary prevention of cardiovascular disease in patients with pre-existing cardiovascular disease Statins	Prevent 1 major vascular event	10	Collins et al., 2016
Multiple Sclerosis Interferon	Prevent Exacerbation	14	Leucht et al., 2012b
Otitis Media Antibiotics	Free of pain	16	Leucht et al., 2012b
Multiple Sclerosis Glatiramer acetate	Relapse-free	16	Schork, 2015
Chronic obstructive airways disease Fluticasone/salmeterol	Prevention of 1 exacerbation	20	Schork, 2015
Acute coronary syndrome Aspirin	Prevent death, myocardial infarction, or stroke	20-25	Chapter 18 in Walker et al., 2014

(*continued*)

Table 15.7 Continued

Condition and Medication	Outcome	Effectiveness NNT	Reference
Hypertension ACE inhibitors	Prevent 1 cardiovascular event	25	Leucht et al., 2012b Leucht et al., 2015b
Osteoporosis Bisphosphonates	Prevention of fracture	33	Leucht et al., 2015b
Secondary prevention after myocardial infarction Beta-blocker	Prevention of 1 death Prevention of non-fatal myocardial re-infarction	48 56	Chapter 18 in Walker et al., 2014
Secondary prevention of serious vascular events Aspirin	Prevent 1 serious vascular event	66	Leucht et al., 2015b
Primary prevention cardiovascular disease (no prior events) Statins	Prevent 1 composite cardiovascular outcome (e.g. stroke or MI) Prevent 1 death	68 250	Chou et al., 2016b
Psychiatric Treatments			
Schizophrenia Antipsychotics	Relapse prevention	3	Leucht et al., 2012b
Depression Antidepressants	Relapse prevention	2.5–5	Table 15.2
Bipolar disorder Lithium	Relapse prevention	5	Severus et al., 2014
Mania Antipsychotics	Response to treatment	5.4	Table 15.4
Depression Antidepressants	Response to treatment	6–10	Table 15.2
Depression Antidepressants	Remission	11	Table 15.2
Schizophrenia Antipsychotics	Good response	11	Table 15.4
Dementia Anticholinesterase inhibitors	Not worse	14	Leucht et al., 2012b

and Ross, 2017). Introduction of trial methodology pre-registration and transparent reporting may be responsible for reducing frequency of trials reporting significant results (Kaplan and Irvin, 2015).

There is overlap in effectiveness of psychiatric and general medicine treatments. Some general medicine treatments are more effective (but others less effective) than psychiatric treatments and may achieve more desirable outcomes such as preventing death or cure, but reduction of mental health symptoms or preventing them returning is still a worthwhile objective. Research evidence in general medicine has similar concerns to that in psychiatry. Better knowledge of the biological factors involved in general medicine does not always lead to greater clinical benefit but general medicine has a superior record in developing new medications and improving the efficacy of their treatments.

Adverse drug reactions (ADRs) are common and are responsible for 3% of primary care consults and 7% of hospital admissions in the United Kingdom (Chapter 2 in Walker et al., 2014). Commonest medication classes that caused ADRs leading to admission in one study in descending order of frequency were: anti-infective agents, hormones including steroids, chemotherapy for cancer, anticoagulants, analgaesics and psychotropic drugs, for example, antidepressants (Weiss et al., 2013). One or more ADRs occurred in approximately 15% of inpatients during their admission, most commonly caused by diuretics, opioid analgesics, and anticoagulants (Davies et al., 2009). Deaths due to ADRs were estimated at 106,000/year in the United States (Starfield, 2000), which would be sixth most common cause of death in that country (CDC, 2016). A Swedish study estimated ADRs were responsible for 3% of all deaths and were the seventh commonest cause of death (Wester et al., 2008), and it further analysed a small sample of 49 deaths, finding that about 20% were on psychiatric drugs (usually antidepressants), but about 80% of fatal ADRs were due to general medicine medications, apart from one anaesthetic-related death. The two predominant causes of death were gastrointestinal haemorrhage and haemorrhagic stroke. The four commonest types of drugs involved in descending order of frequency were: anticoagulants, platelet inhibitors, nonsteroidal anti-inflammatories (NSAIDS), and antidepressants. Psychiatric medications in this study had a lower rate of fatal ADRs amongst people taking medications in the whole cohort of deaths, compared to anticoagulants, platelet inhibitors, and NSAIDs. The commonest fatal ADR for psychiatric medications was haemorrhage, especially gastrointestinal haemorrhage. Medication can cause fatal ADRs and psychiatric medications contribute towards this but to a lesser degree than general medicine medications.

A selection of drugs noted as commonly causing ADRs (Chapter 2 in Walker et al., 2014) are listed in Table 15.8. Other drugs and side effects are mentioned because they are common and/or significant as well as cognitive side effects for coronary artery bypass graft (CABG), a common cardiac surgery procedure. Chemotherapy for cancer

Table 15.8 General medical medication adverse effects.

Medication	Adverse effect	Reference
ACE inhibitors, e.g. lisinopril	Renal impairment, hyperkalaemia; less commonly neutropoenia.	Chapter 2 in Walker et al., 2014
Alpha-interferon	Common side-effects include fatigue, depression, irritability, bone marrow suppression; autoimmune thyroid disease.	Chapter 23 in Walker et al., 2014
Aminoglycoside antibiotics, e.g. gentamicin Amphotericin antifungal	Acute tubular necrosis in renal nephrons or loss of renal nephron tubular function.	Chapter 17 in Walker et al., 2014
Antibiotics, e.g. amoxicillin	Nausea, diarrhoea.	Chapter 2 in Walker et al., 2014
Antibiotics for TB—rifampicin, isoniazid	Acute hepatitis. Isoniazid only—drug-induced lupus syndrome, arthritis/arthralgia.	Chapters 23 and 25 in Walker et al., 2014
Anticoagulants, e.g. warfarin	Bleeding, e.g. gastrointestinal, intracranial.	Chapter 2 in Walker et al., 2014
Aspirin and other NSAIDs	Renal impairment, gastric side effects, e.g. dyspepsia, gastrointestinal bleeding. In the United Kingdom, responsible for 65,000 emergency admissions; 7,000 gastrointestinal bleeding episodes, and 2,000 deaths. Risks higher in over 75s of major and fatal bleeds for aspirin including gastrointestinal and intracranial bleeds if not given proton pump inhibitor. Celecoxib, rofecoxib, diclofenac, ibuprofen, and naproxen may increase the risk of myocardial infarction.	Chapter 2 in Walker et al., 2014; Bally et al., 2017; Li et al., 2017
Beta-blockers, e.g. atenolol	Cold peripheries, bradycardia.	Chapter 2 in Walker et al., 2014
Calcineurin inhibitors used topically, e.g. tacrolimus	Initial stinging and burning limits tolerability; immunosuppressive effects and can cause photosensitivity.	Chapter 28 in Walker et al., 2014
Digoxin	Nausea and anorexia, bradycardia.	Chapter 2 in Walker et al., 2014
Dithranol	Highly irritant; skin stained brown; light hair acquires purple discolouration.	Chapter 28 in Walker et al., 2014

Table 15.8 Continued

Medication	Adverse effect	Reference
Diuretics, e.g. furosemide	Dehydration, electrolyte imbalance (e.g. hypokalaemia), hypotension, renal impairment; cramp and secondary gout.	Chapters 2 and 25 in Walker et al., 2014
Fumaric acid ester therapy	Common side effects are diarrhoea, flushing, and lymphopenia.	Chapter 28 in Walker et al., 2014
Insulin	Hypoglycaemia.	Chapter 2 in Walker et al., 2014
Levodopa	Postural hypotension, nausea and vomiting; dyskinesias; hallucinations.	Chapter 26 in Walker et al., 2014
Opioid analgaesics	Nausea and vomiting, confusion, constipation.	Chapter 2 in Walker et al., 2014
Penicillamine	Glomerulonephritis; neutropaenia If Wilson's disease and long-term treatment, one-third suffer rashes, protein-losing nephropathy, lupus-like syndrome, and bone marrow depression; myositis/myasthenia.	Chapters 17, 23, 24, and 25 in Walker et al., 2014
Adrenal steroids, e.g. prednisolone	Raised blood glucose, increased body fat, hirsutism, peptic ulcers, high blood pressure, osteoporosis, peripheral oedema, depression, euphoria, impaired wound healing, immunosuppression/increased infection, glaucoma, decreased growth in children, hypokalaemia. Major problem is discontinuation/withdrawal that can cause unpleasant and dangerous effects due to switching off endogenous steroid production.	Chapter 26 in Harvey et al., 2011
Sulphasalazine	Side effects in 20–45%: headache, nausea; blood dyscrasias.	Chapter 22 in Walker et al., 2014
Thiopurines, e.g. azathioprine	20% have to stop due to complications, e.g. flu-like syndrome with myalgia, nausea, and vomiting; hepatoxicity; pancreatitis; leukopenia in 3%.	Chapter 22 in Walker et al., 2014
Vitamin E	High doses associated with increased prostatic cancer risk and all-cause mortality.	Chapter 23 in Walker et al., 2014
Coronary artery bypass graft (CABG)	Stroke: 1–5%. Short-term cognitive impairments, resolving within 6 months: 30–80%. Long-term cognitive decline over 5 years: 30% or more.	Chapter 18 in Walker et al., 2014

has been omitted but is well-known to have severe side effects (thiopurines are also used in treatment of auto-immune disorders). The side effects listed are an incomplete list of ADRs associated with each medication.

Medication (both general medical and psychiatric) is an important cause of renal, gastrointestinal liver, haematological, musculoskeletal, and dermatological problems (Chapters 17, 22–25, and 28 in Walker et al., 2014). The commonest cause of Cushing's syndrome is steroid medication (Chapter 20 in Walker et al., 2014). General medicine's treatments are associated with side effects and are more dangerous in terms of severe harm or mortality than psychiatric treatments, but they are used for conditions with higher mortality rates.

Chapter 5 included examples of mechanisms of actions for treatments. This section will review the evidence for general medicine treatments that do not act in disease-centred ways (e.g. treatment objective is not cure or mechanism of action is not remove cause of condition or reverse causal mechanism of condition) or have unknown mechanism of action that produces benefit. Some examples of these medications are listed in Table 15.9.

Omitted from Table 15.9 include numerous examples of medical interventions for conditions where cures are unavailable. Cystic fibrosis treatments, including physiotherapy and antibiotics, are often aimed at preventing structural/functional deterioration and later complication of chronic inflammation and airway infection (Chapter 19 in Walker et al., 2014. Sjogren's syndrome sufferers are prescribed various liquids to reduce dryness of bodily fluids (Chapter 25 in Walker et al., 2014). Many topical treatments in dermatology cannot cure or reverse disease processes but act by indirect compensation; for example, dithranol reduces cellular proliferation and increases cellular differentiation, underpinning its effectiveness in psoriasis (Chapter 28 in Walker et al., 2014).

Even when medications act on disease-causing mechanisms to achieve clinical benefit, the reverse of a therapeutic effect can occur. 5-aminosalicyclic acid can cause colitis and anti-TNF can cause psoriasis, even though these medications are used to treat these conditions (Cohen and Sachar, 2017).

General medicine treatments do not always have cure as an objective nor always act in a disease-centred way. Sometimes mechanism of action is unknown.

There is clear overlap between psychiatric and general medicine treatments for all three questions in Box 15.1. A systematic review suggested psychiatric treatments were in the middle of the range of effectiveness of medical treatments (Leucht et al., 2012). General medical treatments seem more dangerous but arguably they are often used in more dangerous conditions. General medical treatments do not always aim for cure or act in a disease-centred way but this is still commoner in general medicine than in psychiatry.

Psychotherapeutic treatments

I am not an expert in psychotherapy and some psychotherapy experts have disagreed with my conclusions in this section. I have had some training and experience in providing psychotherapy, particularly cognitive behavioural therapy, which may bias me towards favouring cognitive behavioural therapy.

Table 15.9 General medical treatments not acting in disease-centred ways.

Condition/ Medication	**Objective of Treatment (O)/ Mechanism of Action (M)**	**Reference**
Antihypertensives, e.g. beta blockers, calcium channel blockers	O—Limit structural or functional deterioration and prevent later complication. M—Compensate for effects of condition by indirect compensation by acting on opposing mechanism or by inducing a state that mitigates effect of condition.	Chapter 19 in Harvey et al., 2011; Chapter 18 in Walker et al., 2014
Antihypertensive Thiazide diuretic	O—Limit structural or functional deterioration or prevent later complication. M—Unknown/unclear.	Chapter 18 in Walker et al., 2014. Suggested mechanisms limited evidence in humans, Mussini et al., 2014
Antiarrhythmics e.g. calcium channel blockers, beta blockers	O—Limit structural or functional deterioration and prevent later complication. M—Compensate for effects of condition by indirect compensation by acting on opposing mechanism and/or compensate for effects of condition by inducing a state that mitigates effect of condition.	Chapter 17 in Harvey et al., 2011; Chapter 18 in Walker et al., 2014
Prevention of recurrence of thromboembolic events Anticoagulants, platelet inhibitors (Hypercoagulable states are present in some people who developed thromboembolic events)	O—Limit structural or functional deterioration and prevent later complication. M—Compensate for effects of condition by indirect compensation by acting on opposing mechanism.	Chapter 20 in Harvey et al., 2011; Chapter 18 in Walker et al., 2014
Primary/Secondary prevention of cardiovascular events (Primary hypercholesterolaemia rare, some even have normal or near normal cholesterol levels) Statins	O—Limit structural or functional deterioration and prevent later complication. M—Compensate for effects of condition by indirect compensation by acting on opposing mechanism, or by inducing a state that mitigates effect of condition.	Chapter 21 in Harvey et al., 2011; Chapter 18 in Walker et al., 2014
Type 2 diabetes Antidiabetics (not insulin), e.g. metformin, sulfonylureas	O—Limit structural or functional deterioration and prevent later complication, reduce symptoms (often few symptoms). M—Compensate for effects of condition by indirect compensation by acting on opposing mechanism, or by inducing a state that mitigates effect of condition.	Chapter 24 in Harvey et al., 2011; Chapter 21 in Walker et al., 2014

(continued)

Table 15.9 Continued

Condition/ Medication	Objective of Treatment (O)/ Mechanism of Action (M)	Reference
Haemochromatosis Venesection	O—Limit structural or functional deterioration and prevent later complication. M—Compensate for effects of condition by indirect compensation by acting on opposing mechanism.	Chapter 23 in Walker et al., 2014
Rheumatoid arthritis Sulfasalazine, Hydroxychloroquine, D-penicillamine, gold	O—Limit structural or functional deterioration, prevent later complication, relieve current distress/reduce symptoms. M—Unknown.	Chapter 25 in Walker et al., 2014
Anti-epileptics, e.g. carbamazepine, benzodiazepines, sodium valproate	O—Limit structural or functional deterioration, relieve current distress/symptoms, and prevent later complication. M—Compensate for effects of condition by inducing a state that mitigates effect of condition.	Chapter 15 in Harvey et al., 2011; Chapter 26 in Walker et al., 2014
Cluster headaches Lithium	O—Relieve current distress/reduce symptoms. M—Unclear/unknown.	Chapter 26 in Walker et al., 2014
Parkinson's disease Dopaminergic enhancing medications	O—Limit structural or functional deterioration, relieve current distress/symptoms. M—Compensate for effects of condition by direct compensation/replacement.	Chapter 26 in Walker et al., 2014
Parkinson's disease Antimuscarinics	O—Limit structural or functional deterioration, relieve current distress/symptoms. M—Compensate for effects of condition by indirect compensation by acting on opposing mechanism.	Chapter 26 in Walker et al., 2014
Malaria—plasmodium species Artemisinin (quinghaosu) derivatives as part of combination with other antimalarials	O—Cure. M—Unknown.	Chapter 7 in Walker et al., 2014
Tuberculosis Pyrazinamide	O—Cure. M—Unknown.	Chapter 19 in Walker et al., 2014
Mild Graves' ophthalmology Selenium	O—Limit structural or functional deterioration, relieve current distress/symptoms, and prevent later complication. M—unknown but may be antioxidant.	Chapter 20 in Walker et al., 2014

A suggested definition of psychotherapy is an intervention with focus on verbal communication (or using books supported by a therapist), structured, and purposeful therapist–client encounters, and the establishment of therapeutic relationships (Barth et al., 2013; Cristea et al., 2017a). Psychotherapy can be provided by one therapist to a single client (individual therapy) or to many clients (group therapy) and can also be provided to carers/significant people in the support network of the client, sometimes with the client present (family intervention/therapy). Psychotherapy requires cooperation between client and therapist so is ineffective if the client is unwilling or unable to participate if their condition is too severe at the time of psychotherapy; for example, they may not be able to concentrate on what the therapist says if in an extreme mood state.

There are problems with applying RCT paradigms to psychotherapy (Margison et al., 2000). The problems that make psychotherapy research hard to replicate and thus reduces confidence in scientific validity of research results include: researcher allegiance (to type of psychotherapy, e.g. for ideological or career advancement reasons); therapist/therapist supervisor allegiance (to type of psychotherapy); reviewer/editor/policy allegiance (may affect which psychotherapy studies are published); treatment integrity (whether interventions compared in a study are carried out according to their therapeutic model which can impact on their effectiveness and make it harder to replicate in research or clinical practice); therapist effects (the therapist may be better at one intervention than another thus skewing comparisons); overemphasizing small differences (statistical versus clinical significance); flexibility in design allowing researchers to cherry-pick outcomes to demonstrate desired results; underpowered studies; publishing bias and in meta-analysis selection bias to include studies of poor-quality and exclude studies of good-quality in order to achieve desired summative outcomes (Leichsenring et al., 2017). Some of these also affect medication studies but some are more of an issue in therapy issues; it is harder to standardize psychotherapy (due to therapist effects, for example) than medication preparation and dosage.

Pre-registration of trials and adhering to registered methodology may help prevent cherry-picking of outcomes, and providing access to the data allows others to check results (Coyne and Kok, 2014; Leichsenring et al., 2017). Adequate control interventions to compare with the psychotherapy under investigation is also problematic (Coyne and Kok, 2014). Kirsch argues that psychotherapy can be regarded as a placebo (it has treatment effects but no pharmacological action) and that valid control interventions display similar beneficial characteristics so no difference between control and psychotherapy intervention does not mean psychotherapy is ineffective (Kirsch, 2005). This argument is untenable as control groups are used in RCTs to measure more than non-specific treatment effects, such as natural fluctuations of severity in conditions (see Chapter 5).

The type of control intervention used may have dramatic effects on results of psychotherapy trials (Mohr et al., 2009). 'Treatment as usuals' (TAUs) value as control intervention depends on the consistency of TAU provided to different participants and its effectiveness in itself. However, it may provide information on benefits of adding psychotherapy to TAU (Mohr et al., 2009) but it does not elucidate whether the treatment model used is effective or whether it is the spending more time with empathic clinicians that is providing the benefit. Waiting list controls (those on waiting lists for treatment) are compromised as control intervention as waiting may have nocebo effects, worsening clinical states of participants, and giving exaggerated impressions of the comparison psychotherapy's benefits (Furukuwa et al., 2014). Pill placebo control is used in some RCTs; this also presents some issues but does allow easier comparison with medication placebo-controlled RCTs results. It also reduces a small bias in favour of pharmacotherapy if a pill placebo arm is also included in medication versus psychotherapy RCTs and if the raters are 'blinded' to treatment group (Cuijpers et al., 2015).

Another problem in both therapy and medication research is maintaining 'blindness' of researchers to treatment group when rating participants' response to treatments. In a meta-analysis of CBT for psychosis (CBTP), the benefits of CBTP on positive and general symptoms became dramatically reduced when only studies where raters were blinded to treatment group were included (Jauhar et al., 2014).

Undeclared researcher allegiances in psychotherapy systematic reviews and RCTs are common (Dragioti et al., 2015), as are undeclared conflicts of interest (which may affect interpretation of results) in reviews of psychotherapy (Lieb et al., 2016). These problems with psychotherapy research may inflate its apparent effectiveness (Coyne and Kok, 2014) and contribute to low rate of replication for highly quoted psychotherapy studies (Tajika et al., 2015). There is evidence of publishing bias in favour of trials showing psychotherapy is effective in depression and generalized anxiety disorder (Driessen et al., 2015; Flint et al., 2015; Cuijpers et al., 2016).

No research is perfect and rarely gives certainty. Instead, it gives varying degrees of confidence in the result and steps can be taken to improve psychotherapy research quality (Coyne and Kok, 2014; Leichsenring et al., 2017).

Psychotherapy is a complex intervention; treatment objectives may also be broader in nature and complementary to medical-type objectives. Suggested treatment objectives (Grosse and Grawe, 2002) include: coping with specific symptoms and problems (e.g. life difficulties); resolving interpersonal issues (e.g. intimacy); improving well-being/functioning (e.g. increased activity); addressing existential issues (e.g. processing of personal issues); personal growth (e.g. self-acceptance or emotional regulation); or residual categories not covered above. Understanding the client's predicament is also a psychotherapeutic goal, usually through co-constructed formulations (Division of Clinical Psychology, 2011). Treatment objectives vary between different psychotherapy types (Phillips, 2009) as well as between different conditions (Holtforth et al., 2009).

Table 15.10 offers a non-comprehensive summary of evidence of psychotherapy effectiveness. Some psychotherapy types or conditions are omitted.

Evidence-based 'bona fide' psychotherapies use therapists trained in viable treatment models described in professional books or manuals and based on theories of change (Leichsenring et al., 2017). Psychotherapy is an effective treatment for many conditions and can have similar degree of effectiveness as medication in psychiatry and general medicine. Psychotherapy has different degrees and nature of benefits depending on the condition it is treating. Psychiatric medication and psychotherapy often have complementary benefits and sometimes synergistic benefits. People may derive sufficient benefit from psychotherapy that they do not need psychiatric medication.

Table 15.10 Psychotherapy effectiveness.

Condition and Type of Therapy	Type of Therapy and Study	Results	Reference
Depression Reduction of Symptoms (Continuous)			
CBT	Meta-analysis RCTs from databases	High-quality studies vs WL 0.93; vs TAU 0.43. All quality studies vs PP 0.55.	Cuijpers et al., 2016
PDT	Expert review	PDT medium effect sizes vs inactive controls or PP.	Fonagy, 2015
Multiple psychotherapy types, e.g. CBT, IPT	Meta-analysis of RCTs from databases	Psychotherapy vs PP combined effect size 0.25 (calculated NNT = 7).	Cuijpers et al., 2014b
IPT	Meta-analysis of RCTs from databases and textbooks/papers 'depressive spectrum'	Expressed as weighted mean difference, i.e. average difference in depression rating scale scores between different groups; appear to be in small to medium effect size range; IPT superior to PP and CBT.	De Mello, 2005
Multiple psychotherapy types, e.g. IPT, CBT, PDT, ST	Network meta-analysis of RCTs from databases	Effect sizes vs WL 0.62–0.92, PP 0.29– 0.59, TAU 0.29–0.58 (social skills training no significant benefit vs PP and TAU).	Barth et al., 2013
CBT vs antidepressants	Meta-analysis of RCTs from databases	After controlling for studies with financial conflict of interest such as pharmaceutical industry sponsorship, no significant differences in effectiveness in reducing symptoms between CBT and antidepressants.	Cristea et al., 2016
	Meta-analysis of RCTs from databases and trial registries including unpub-lished of CBT vs second-generation antidepressants	Meta-analysis of RCTs showed no significant differences in symptoms, response, remission and discontinuations due to lack or tolerability or lack of efficacy between CBT and 2nd generation antidepressants	Amick et al, 2015
Multiple psycho-therapy types combined with antidepressants vs antidepressants alone	Meta-analysis of RCTs from databases and earlier meta-analyse for relevant RCTs	Effect size 0.43 (NNT = 4.2) favouring different types combined psychotherapy (e.g. CBT and IPT) and antidepressants vs antidepressants alone.	Cuijpers et al., 2014a

(continued)

Table 15.10 Continued

Condition and Type of Therapy	Type of Therapy and Study	Results	Reference
Depression—recurrence prevention			
Multiple psychotherapy types, e.g. MBCT, CT, IPT	Meta-analysis of RCTs from databases then meta-regression to identify factors predicting effectiveness	Combined different types of psychotherapy group (NNT = 5) and IPT, CT, and MBCT (NNT4–6) all reduced relapse rates vs TAU Combined different types of psychotherapy group had a reduction in relapse rates vs maintenance antidepressants (NNT = 13), individual psychotherapy types no significant difference vs maintenance antidepressants. Psychotherapy more effective if begun in acute phase then sessions dedicated to relapse prevention. In practice, some clients get booster sessions after acute phase therapy.	Biesheuvel-Leliefeld et al., 2015
Depression—Quality of Life (QOL) and functioning			
Multiple psychotherapy types, e.g. CBT, IPT	Meta-analysis of RCTs from databases 'depressive spectrum'	Effect size 0.35 on QOL for psychotherapy; effect size 0.35 on functioning. Compared to antidepressants, psychotherapy has benefit effect size 0.21 for QOL but no significant difference in functioning, Combined antidepressant/psychotherapy treatment was superior to either treatment alone both for functioning (effect size 0.32–0.34) and QOL (effect size 0.36–0.39)	Kamenov et al., 2017
Anxiety Reduction of Symptoms			
CBT for anxiety disorders	Meta-analysis of RCTs from databases	For GAD, PD, SAD Effect sizes (high quality results used when available) vs WL 0.61–1.0; vs TAU 0.27–0.45; vs PP 0.28–0.57	Cuijpers et al., 2016

Table 15.10 Continued

Condition and Type of Therapy	Type of Therapy and Study	Results	Reference
Psychotherapy (multiple types but mostly CBT or similar therapies) compared to medication (almost always antidepressants) for anxiety disorders	Meta-analysis of RCTs from databases and earlier meta-analyses	Non-significant differences between psychotherapy and medication for anxiety disorders as whole and SAD or PAD. Psychotherapy more effective for OCD effect size 0.64.	Cuijpers et al., 2013b
Behavioural therapy compared to serotonergic antidepressants for OCD	Meta-analysis of RCTs from databases	Behavioural therapy more effective (effect size 0.37) than antidepressants as a whole but no significant advantage over SSRIs.	Romanelli et al., 2014
Multiple psychotherapy types combined with antidepressants vs antidepressants alone for anxiety disorders	Meta-analysis of RCTs from databases and earlier meta-analyses	For anxiety disorders as a whole combined psychotherapy and antidepressant treatment advantage over antidepressants alone effect size 0.47 (NNT = 3.85). Combined psychotherapy and antidepressant treatment more beneficial for OCD (effect size 0.7 NNT = 2.63) and PD (effect size 0.54 NNT = 3.36). No significant differences for PTSD, SAD, and GAD.	Cuijpers et al., 2014a
Psychosis/Schizophrenia Reduction of Symptoms/Improvement of Functioning/ Reduction of Relapse			
CBT to reduce psychosis symptoms	Meta-analysis of RCTs from databases and papers and earlier meta-analyses	Variety of controls but only 'masking', i.e. blinding of raters to treatment group had significant effect on outcomes; random effects model to control for heterogeneity of study populations; most/all participants on antipsychotics. Overall symptoms (positive, negative, and other psychiatric symptoms) effect size 0.15 (i.e. below small). Positive symptoms: no significant benefit for CBT. Negative symptoms: effect size 0.13 (below small).	Jauhar et al., 2014

(continued)

Table 15.10 Continued

Condition and Type of Therapy	Type of Therapy and Study	Results	Reference
CBT for psychosis	Synthesis of qualitative studies on CBT clients' experiences for psychosis	Themes of changed attitude towards psychotic symptoms (no longer needed eliminated, acceptance of psychotic symptoms and improved coping); clients felt more empowered to disagree with their voices and experiences; changes in self-concept away from identifying themselves solely in terms of illness.	Berry and Hayward, 2011
Family Intervention for psychosis	Meta-analysis of RCTs from databases and papers and earlier reviews	Compared to TAU; reduced risk of relapse (NNT = 7); admission to hospital (NNT = 8), and improve concordance with medication (NNT = 6). Non-significant effects on social functioning or reduction of family burden.	Pharoah et al., 2010
Cognitive Remediation Behavioural training to improve cognitive processes	Meta-analysis of RCTs from databases and papers and contacting researchers in field	Beneficial to global cognition (effect size 0.448); differing benefits in cognitive subdomains particularly social cognition and reasoning/problem solving (effect sizes 0.651 and 0.572 respectively); and functioning (effect size 0.418). Benefits durable for global cognition and functioning. Combining cognitive remediation with psychiatric rehabilitation improved benefit for functioning.	Wykes et al., 2011
CBT to reduce relapse	Meta-analysis of RCTs from databases and papers and meta-analyses. No RCTs with < 10 participants/ treatment group included	Two trials excluded as five years between therapy and assessment and judged unlikely to attribute differences in relapse rate to therapy. Relapse had to meet predefined criteria not just, e.g., hospitalization Controls either TAU or ST. No significant difference in relapse rates between CBT and controls	Lynch et al., 2010

Table 15.10 Continued

Condition and Type of Therapy	**Type of Therapy and Study**	**Results**	**Reference**
Borderline Personality Disorder/Emotionally Unstable Personality Disorder			
Psychotherapy multiple types e.g. CBT, DBT and transference-focussed therapy based on PDT	Meta-analysis of RCTs from databases and papers and meta-analyses Standalone–borderline specific therapy vs TAU or control therapy Add-on: Both groups TAU and one group Borderline specific therapy in addition	Results from end of treatment and after more than two years follow-up if available. End of treatment combined therapy outcomes in standalone (effect size 0.32, NNT = 5.56) and add-on therapies (effect size 0.40, NNT = 4.50) for variety of outcomes combined (and similar size for individual outcomes) such as borderline symptoms; self-harm; anxiety/depression symptoms. Follow-up: no significant differences except for standalone combined outcome (effect size 0.56, NNT = 3.25) and self-harming behaviour (effect size 0.58, NNT = 3.14). Only DBT (effect size 0.34 NNT = 5.26) and PDT-based approaches (effect size 0.41, NNT = 4.39) more effective than controls.	Cristea et al., 2017a
Mania/Bipolar			
Multiple psychotherapy types, e.g. individual/group CBT	Meta-analysis of RCTs from databases and papers and meta-analyses	Discussion of NICE Guidelines on bipolar disorder (NICE, 2014B) meta-analyses. Individual CBT beneficial on bipolar depression end of treatment vs TAU effect size 0.31 but no benefit after 12 months. No benefits for individual CBT vs active control treatments in bipolar depression or for group CBT in bipolar depression. No benefits for individual CBT in relapse prevention if largest RCT included (was excluded by NICE). No psychotherapy recommended for mania.	Jauhar et al., 2016

(continued)

Table 15.10 Continued

Condition and Type of Therapy	Type of Therapy and Study	Results	Reference
	Meta-analysis searching databases and earlier meta-analyses and papers for relevant RCTs	Many analyses: often of low or very low-quality studies or involving few studies sometimes as few as one study. Individual psychotherapy vs TAU benefit end of treatment in depression effect size 0.23. Active control treatments superior to individual psychotherapy for bipolar depression. No benefits for mania at end of treatment. May be benefit for psychotherapy in relapse vs TAU (moderate quality evidence). At follow-up, no benefit for individual therapy in bipolar depression; CBT may worsen bipolar depression at follow-up vs active control treatment; very low-quality evidence of benefit for individual psychotherapy vs TAU for manic symptoms at follow-up, i.e. not during acute episode effect size 0.38.	Oud et al., 2016

CT = Cognitive Therapy, CBT = Cognitive Behavioural Therapy, DBT = Dialectical Behavioural Therapy, MBCT = Mindfulness-Based Cognitive Therapy, IPT = Interpersonal Therapy, PDT = Psychodynamic Therapy, ST = Supportive Therapy/Counselling

PP = pill placebo control WL = waiting control TAU= treatment as usual control

GAD= generalized anxiety disorder, OCD = obsessive compulsive disorder, PD= panic disorder, PTSD = post-traumatic stress disorder, SAD = social anxiety disorder

Psychotherapy interventions can be helpful for conditions where there is no recommended medication, such as borderline personality disorder. Conversely, there are conditions where medication can be beneficial but psychotherapy has little benefit, such as mania in the acute phase. Combination of antidepressants with psychotherapy is more effective than either treatment alone for depression and some anxiety conditions.

There is slight benefit for CBT for psychosis symptom-rating scale scores. Synthesis of qualitative studies suggests CBT helps with coping with symptoms (as antipsychotics do) but not enough to make as much reduction of psychosis symptom-rating scales as antipsychotics. There may be benefit for more existential issues and personal growth. Most participants in CBT for psychosis trials were on antipsychotics, so the medication may have reduced the scope for CBT to improve psychosis symptom-rating scales. A large CBT for psychosis RCT (Klingberg et al., 2010) should have completed data collection and analysis. but to date has not published results. It is unlikely that a large RCT with positive results demonstrating efficacy would not be submitted for publication, which suggests either an unanticipated problem with the study or negative results.

An RCT randomizing participants who met broad criteria for psychosis and did not wish antipsychotics to either cognitive therapy for up to 26 sessions or TAU (often very little help or support) found statistically significant benefit for cognitive therapy (Morrison et al., 2014). The participants had mild to moderate severity psychosis, that is, less severe symptoms than usual antipsychotic RCT participants (Lepping et al., 2011). There were several methodological problems with the study and the size of benefit from cognitive therapy was less than antipsychotics (Bera and Sarkar, 2014; Coyne and van Linschoten, 2014; Laws and McKenna, 2014). The study found an average difference of 6.52 points lower on PANNS scale for cognitive therapy compared to TAU whereas meta-analysis of second generation antipsychotics reported superiority of 10 points for these antipsychotics compared to placebo in participants meeting schizophrenia criteria (Leucht et al., 2009). This is an indirect comparison so caveats apply.

It is impossible to decide definitively about relative efficacy of antipsychotics versus CBT in psychosis in the absence of RCTs comparing the two. A small RCT comparing antipsychotics with CBT has started and will act as a pilot study for a larger RCT as it is underpowered to detect any differences except large ones (Law et al., 2017).

Psychotherapy has similar effectiveness to psychiatric medications for anxiety conditions and depression, but for some treatment goals and some conditions there is evidence of superior effectiveness for psychotherapy. CBT is the type of psychotherapy with most evidence of effectiveness. For psychosis, the balance of evidence indicates antipsychotics are more effective in reducing symptoms, particularly in more severe psychosis. Antipsychotics are superior to individual psychotherapy in preventing psychosis relapse but family intervention complements relapse reduction. Cognitive remediation, especially if combined with rehabilitation of social functioning, has the best evidence for improving impaired cognition in schizophrenia. Psychiatric medication is more effective in reduction of manic symptoms and preventing relapse of bipolar disorder than psychotherapy, and may be more effective in reducing bipolar depressive symptoms. Psychotherapy, particularly Dialectical Behaviour Therapy or psychodynamic therapy, is the best-evidenced treatment for people meeting borderline personality disorder criteria. Psychotherapy may be more helpful in achieving broader treatment goals such as existential issues and personal growth in a variety of conditions including psychosis.

Frequency and nature of adverse effects resulting from psychotherapy is poorly monitored and reported in research trials; perhaps 14–60% (usually less than 50%) of psychotherapy trial reports mention them (Jonsson et al., 2014; Duggan et al., 2014) and significantly less frequently than in medication trials (Vaughan et al., 2014). Lack of standardized definitions hinders monitoring and reporting adverse effects of psychotherapy. One suggestion for standardizing definitions (Parry et al., 2016) offers the following: adverse events (for harm or serious harm such as suicide or self-harm attempt); clinically significant deterioration (i.e. worsening of symptoms or development of new symptoms); and negative experience of therapy with lasting bad effects (as experienced by the client or those around them). A more detailed classification from the same group (Duggan et al., 2014) defines harm as 'sustained deterioration that is caused directly' by psychotherapy, identifies if client or others were harmed, if subjective or objective measures of harm used, and relationship to treatment (inappropriate treatment, inappropriate application of treatment, and patient characteristics).

In one survey, 76,950 clients of UK psychotherapy services were asked to complete anonymous questionnaires and 15,078 responded. Harm (defined as 'lasting bad effects from treatment') was experienced by 5.2% of respondents and was significantly more common in ethnic minority clients (Crawford et al., 2016). It is likely that transient harm from therapy is more common than this but there is a lack of reliable data. Sexual abuse of client by therapists is amongst the more severe harms possible from psychotherapy but the frequency of this is hard to measure reliably (Sarkar, 2004). Any sexual contact between psychiatrists/psychotherapists and their clients constitutes sexual abuse (Sarkar, 2004). Rates of sexual abuse of their clients is similar between psychologists, social workers, and psychiatrists (Borys and Pope, 1989).

A survey of 1,000 randomly selected clinical psychologists received 581 useable responses on the topic of sexual abuse of clients (Garrett and Davis, 1998). This study's background review reported rates of sexual abuse by therapists and psychiatrists of between 1.9–8.7%. Of the survey respondents, 3.5% admitted to sexual abuse of current or former clients, 22.7% reported seeing clients who reported sexual abuse from another therapist, and 38% reported knowing of clinical psychologists who had sexually abused clients.

Taking into account the paucity of research evidence, my clinical experience suggests that adverse effects of psychotherapy are probably less severe on average than for psychiatric medication, but I may not have noticed harmful effects of psychotherapy. Clearly, more research is needed on the frequency and nature of harmful effects of psychotherapy, who is most vulnerable, and how to prevent harm.

How psychotherapy achieves its benefits is entwined with the 'dodo' hypothesis that all psychotherapy types have equivalent effectiveness (Smith and Glass, 1977). One view is that most of psychotherapy's effectiveness is due to 'common factors' across all types of psychotherapy and that features specific to a type of psychotherapy have little additional effect (Wampold, 2015). These common factors include: the therapeutic alliance (the bond between therapist and client bond, their agreement about psychotherapy's goals and tasks); therapist empathy and other positive therapist attributes; expectations of success generated by the plausibility of therapists' explanations of the client's problems and ability of psychotherapy to help; cultural adaptation of therapy to the client and therapist effects such as degree of interpersonal skills (Wampold, 2015).

This social contextual theory posits that psychotherapy works not by correcting dysfunctional psychological mechanisms but instead by three pathways: the real therapeutic relationship, expectations (see earlier), and encouraging activities that promote health (Wampold, 2015). Others have argued that most evidence for mechanism of change in psychotherapy, often correlational, is limited, including for common factors

Chapter 16

Final conclusions

This chapter summarizes the description of the medical model and the degree of similarity between psychiatry and general medicine. It will then discuss a system for describing the nature of diagnostic constructs and offer a brief comparison of different mental health classifications' utility for different purposes before concluding with potential future developments.

The medical model

Doctors are consulted by patients to help with their problems and they are employed by third parties for this purpose, in part because of their sapiental role—their knowledge of health, medical conditions, and treatment—which requires a model of practice and explanation of causes of conditions (although explanation is not always possible). The concepts of health, disease, and illness are not clear-cut so condition may be a better term to use. 'Medical model' describes both a model of practice of how doctors assess patients and help their health problems as well as explain (if possible) and conceptualize problems often using a biopsychosocial model. The medical model as described in this book is based on the orthodox version (Chapter 1).

Doctors need to learn both procedural skills, such as how to assess patients, and knowledge of usual functioning and structure of humans and conditions that they may encounter. Organizing knowledge of conditions into diagnostic construct categories helps doctors acquire, pass on, and retain knowledge. Doctors often use rapid pattern recognition to identify diagnostic constructs in situations with time and cognitive resource pressures. Diagnostic constructs contain information on presenting clinical picture, prognosis, complications, co-occurring conditions, treatment, and differential diagnosis. Diagnosis is always provisional and should be changed if another diagnosis seems more likely. Diagnosis has other social roles such as permitting access to benefits, and has an administrative function as well, for example, activity recording for third parties and statistical roles (Chapter 2).

Classification of the problems that patients present with is essential for clinical practice, to acquire and recall knowledge to inform clinical care and to allow communication between professionals. Diagnostic constructs are usually prototypical concepts. Diagnostic constructs are used to identify various types of conditions including diseases and syndromes, spectrums of health, spectrums of illness/condition, spectrums of illnesses/conditions, injuries and conditions/situations of interest to healthcare professionals (Chapter 3).

The assessment of patients by professionals, influenced by interpersonal and cultural factors amongst others, produces a clinical picture. Conditions are classified into diagnostic constructs based on sharing similarities of clinical picture or underlying mechanisms (differences of structure or process) or causes. Diagnostic constructs based on similarity of clinical picture are often heterogeneous and may include several different causes or differences in structure/process leading to similar clinical pictures. Deciding on causation is complex; usually more than one causative factor is involved in an individual. Social factors are important in the causation of medical conditions (Chapter 4).

There are multiple ways of helping patients, often complementary to each other, in order to meet a large variety of patient needs and the medical model can be practised by non-doctors. There may be other models that meet a patient's needs as well as or better than the medical model. The sapiental role requires evidence from good-quality research, for example, randomized controlled trials with assessments blind to treatment group for evidence of treatment effectiveness. Research can reduce uncertainty but not eliminate it. The medical model of rapid assessment and using treatments such as medications that work in between assessments allows doctors to see large number of patients and work overnight or in emergency situations. Treatment objectives should be decided jointly between doctor and patient, and it is important to note that medications often do not effect a cure (Chapter 5).

Criticisms of psychiatric diagnosis and treatments were examined to generate a set of questions to compare mainstream psychiatry—the use of the medical model in mental health—with general medicine. This is the best comparison as the use of the medical model in general medicine is usually accepted. Many criticisms focus on validity of diagnostic constructs (such as identifying categories clearly separate from each other and from health and objective evidence of their existence). Doctors use diagnostic constructs mainly for clinical utility (e.g. information on prognosis or treatments). Other ways of helping patients or researchers may find other types of classification more useful. Critiques of psychiatric treatment often wrongly assume psychiatrists think they are curing diseases and state that psychiatric treatments are ineffective and harmful (Chapters 6 and 7).

Comparison of psychiatry with general medicine

The results of the evaluation of the evidence comparing psychiatry with general medicine are in Table 16.1

The evidence strongly indicates that psychiatry is not separate from the rest of medicine in terms of the nature and utility of its diagnostic constructs and effectiveness of treatments. Its diagnostic constructs, the utility, validity, and effectiveness of treatments are not at the 'core' of medical specialties but neither are they detached from them. The criticisms outlined in Chapters 6 and 7, that psychiatry is different from the rest of medicine, rely on idealized views of scientifically near-perfect pure disease diagnostic constructs and of highly effective general medical treatments usually acting to reverse diseases.

Table 16.1 Comparing diagnosis and treatment in psychiatry and general medicine.

	No Overlap	Some Overlap	Near Total Overlap
What is the reliability of the diagnosis when compared to a relevant reference criterion?		X	
What is the reliability of discriminating between different diagnoses?		X	
Is the condition clearly separated from normality?		X	
Is the condition associated with variable clinical pictures?		X	
Is the condition diagnosed with polythetic criteria?		X	
Is the condition described by a diagnosis clearly separated from other conditions in terms of clinical features?		X	
Is there little co-occurrence of conditions, i.e. conditions are separate clinical entities?		X	
Is the condition clearly identified with a causal mechanism (aetiology)?		X	
Is the condition clearly associated with a proven and detectable difference in structure or process?		X	
Is the condition caused by social difficulties and/or traumatic events?		X	
Is the diagnosis associated with stigma?		X	
Is the diagnosis associated with a restriction of liberty such as treatment without valid consent?		X	
Does the condition have uniform prognosis?		X	
Does the condition have different outcomes from other conditions?		X	
Does the condition predict differences in treatments given and their effectiveness?		X	

(*continued*)

Table 16.1 Continued

	No Overlap	Some Overlap	Near Total Overlap
Is the use of the diagnosis justified due to some utilitarian reason such as relieving distress or risk?		X	
Is there a need for clinical information beyond the diagnosis in clinical decision making?		X	
How effective are the treatments used?		X	
How harmful are the treatments used?		X	
Does the treatment used have a disease-reversing mechanism of action that produces clinical benefit?		X	

Diagnostic constructs in both general medicine and psychiatry often identify areas of spectrums (e.g. of symptoms) rather than distinctive categorical entities (Chapters 3, 9, and 11) and are not always reliable in clinical practice (Chapter 8) or may have variable clinical pictures (Chapter 10). Biological mechanisms and/or causes are often unknown in psychiatric diagnostic constructs but this can also occur in general medicine's diagnostic constructs (Chapter 12), and social factors are particularly important causes for both psychiatric and general medicine conditions (Chapter 14). Investigations to confirm diagnosis or guide clinical decision-making are rarer in psychiatry than general medicine but this is explained by the lack of objective measurements of mental processes such as thoughts, emotions, or perceptions (Chapter 12). Treatments in both general medicine and psychiatry may not aim for cure or to reverse a disease process and have overlapping effectiveness (Chapter 15).

Diagnostic constructs in psychiatry are used to describe states usually without assumptions of cause being made, except if specific causes are named as part of the construct (e.g. drug-induced psychosis or post-traumatic stress disorder), with no assumptions of conditions being caused by diseases or other biological causes in the absence of any such being demonstrated in the individual (WHO, 1992), or that they represent neatly defined categories separate from each other or from health (WHO, 1992; APA, 1994). The DSM system assumes that there must be a dysfunction of behaviour, psychology, or biology in the individual; that is, no assumption that biological factors are always the cause (APA, 1994). I disagree with location of dysfunction within the individual as the dysfunction may be located within their environment, including social network, or the actions of others causing an appropriate response but individual factors may modify this response. There is a parallel with infectious diseases such as TB where social environmental factors are important as to whether an individual experiences illness, affecting both likelihood of exposure to infection and the ability to prevent infection progressing to severe illness and access to effective help but individual vulnerability factors may also apply (see Chapters 4 and 13).

There is clear evidence that the common assumption that diagnostic constructs should always represent categorically distinct diseases or syndromes is false. Another common false assumption is that a diagnosis automatically means a biological cause for the condition. A suggested system classifying the nature of diagnostic constructs using the basis of classification and the nature of the condition that the construct is used for is outlined in Table 16.2. The basis of classification refers to what examples of the diagnostic construct category have in common (see Chapter 4).

Table 16.2 Classifying the nature of diagnostic constructs.

Basis of classification	**Examples**
A. Clinical picture including polythetic symptoms/signs	Depression, schizophrenia, type 2 diabetes, hypertension, chronic fatigue syndrome/ME
B. Mechanisms—differences in structures/processes or functions	Alzheimer's disease, multiple sclerosis, type 1 diabetes, idiopathic Parkinson's disease
C. Causes	Hypothyroidism causing depression; temporal lobe tumour causing psychosis; tuberculosis, perforating injury, drug-induced liver failure; type of psychosocial stressor
Nature of condition	**Examples**
1. Disease/syndrome	Alzheimer's disease, melancholia, organic psychosis, tuberculosis, myocardial infarction, type 1 diabetes, multiple sclerosis
2. Spectrum of health	Depression, anxiety, personality traits, type 2 diabetes, features of personality disorder categories, hypertension, hyperlipidaemia acne vulgaris. Some have argued psychosis may be on a continuum with health
3. Spectrums of illness/ condition	Schizophrenia/bipolar, motor neurone disease/ frontotemporal dementia, acute coronary syndromes, inflammatory bowel disease—either one single spectrum or two spectrums of ulcerative colitis/Crohn's disease, tuberculosis
4. Spectrums of illnesses/ conditions	Depression/anxiety disorders, dementias (can be mixtures of Alzheimer's, vascular and Lewy body pathologies), metabolic syndrome (hypertension, type 2 diabetes, obesity and other conditions), autoimmune and inflammatory disorders (e.g. inflammatory bowel diseases, type 1 diabetes, rheumatoid arthritis)
5. Injuries (trauma)	Acute and chronic trauma responses such as PTSD and 'complex trauma'/borderline personality disorder, fractures, crush injuries
6. Other conditions/situations of interest to healthcare	Psychosocial crisis that may benefit from support, grief reaction, termination of pregnancy, cosmetic procedures

This alphanumeric system summarizes the nature of diagnostic constructs. A diagnostic construct may qualify for more than one coding for basis of classification and nature of condition. An organic psychosis caused by a tumour could be coded as AC13 (the cause is known but not intermediate mechanisms; the psychosis is both a disease and a spectrum of illness/condition). Someone presenting with anxiety/depression symptoms that does not have an obvious cause and does not resemble melancholia may be coded as A24. Type 2 diabetes and hypertension would be coded as A24, urinary tract infection as ABC1, inflammatory bowel diseases AB34, and psychosocial stressor (e.g. marital problems) with need for counselling C6. Question marks can be used after a code to indicate uncertainty over nosological status, for example some people regard psychosis as on a spectrum with health but others are not convinced (Chapter 9), so schizophrenia may be coded as A2?3.

Utility of different mental health classification systems

The benefits and drawbacks of different classification systems for a variety of purposes are summarized in Table 16.3. Clinical utility is based on the probabilistic predictive characteristics described in Chapter 2 (e.g. prognosis, complications, treatment), and Chapters 3–15 that help the clinicians perform their role. The secondary beneficiary is the patient as this information allows the clinician to perform their task of helping the patient more effectively. Social purposes are described in Chapters 2, 3, and 4. Judgements on utility for understanding and for research are based on Chapters 4, 5, and 8–15. Utility often varies, depending on the presenting condition.

No classification system dominates the others for all purposes. 'No classification' is clearly the worst option (see Chapter 3). It may be useful for clinical work using long appointments focused on psychosocial issues and for offering some explanation of the situation but has little use for other purposes of classification. Psychological formulation is excellent for some clinical situations and explanation purposes but less so for emergency work, and it has little use for administrative or statistical purposes. It is incompatible with the rest of healthcare and needs to include thresholds/binary statements to be of use for social or research purposes. Diagnostic constructs, especially if enhanced by a formulation including relevant psychosocial information, is probably the best 'all-rounder' for doctors with superior clinical utility for the medical model way of working (Chapter 5)—short appointments or emergency work—with good compatibility with the health sector and usefulness for administrative/statistical/social purposes. There are negative utilities—diagnostic constructs in general medicine and psychiatry can be more easily associated with stigma than other types of classifications (Chapter 13). Dimensional classifications placing mental health problems on a continuum with health may be less stigmatizing (Corrigan et al., 2016).

To make an accurate diagnosis the doctor has to ask the patient what has happened (to identify any triggers or causes or other factors that influence health) as well as about symptoms and their fluctuations, the patient's personal details, their social situation, observe the patient, examine them for signs, and order any relevant investigations. Diagnostic constructs are based on identifying similarities between people of these details (Chapters 3 and 4). Therefore, diagnostic constructs cannot convey the

Table 16.3 Utility of classification systems in mental health.

	No classification ('distress')	Psychological formulation (excluding diagnosis)	Diagnosis	Diagnostic formulation (incorporating broader information including psychosocial)	Symptoms based classification	Dimensions
Clinical utility for short appointments/emergencies (including at night)	–	– to +	++ to +++	++ to +++	+	+ (can be ++ to +++ if added to diagnosis as time allows)
Clinical utility for psychotherapy/long appointments with focus on psychosocial issues	+ to ++	++ to +++	+ to ++	+ to ++	+ to +++	+ to +++
Explanation of clinical picture/situation	+ to ++	+ to +++	+ to ++	+ to +++	+ to +++	+ to +++
Administration codes	–	–	++ to +++	++ to +++ (may just use diagnostic construct)	– to +	– to +
Compatibility with rest of health sector	–	–	++ to +++	++ to +++	– to +	– to +

(*continued*)

Table 16.3 Continued

	No classification ('distress')	**Psychological formulation (excluding diagnosis)**	**Diagnosis**	**Diagnostic formulation (incorporating broader information including psychosocial)**	**Symptoms based classification**	**Dimensions**
Ability to recognize and manage medical problems that may co-occur	– (except if uses medical diagnosis, not necessarily psychiatric diagnosis)	– (except if uses medical diagnosis, not necessarily psychiatric diagnosis)	++ to +++	++ to +++	– (except if uses medical diagnosis, not necessarily psychiatric diagnosis)	– (except if uses medical diagnosis, not necessarily psychiatric diagnosis)
Health statistics	–	–	++ to +++	++ to +++ (may just use diagnostic construct)	+	+
Research for outcomes, e.g. prognosis/treatment response	–	– (Can be used as a technique in treatments but not to classify participants)	+ to +++	+ to +++ (can include additional factors with diagnostic construct)	+ (lot of categorical choices implied and relationship between symptoms)	++ to +++
Research for mechanisms/ causes/ epidemiology	–	– (can be + if incorporates thresholds and makes binary statements)	+ to ++	+ to ++ (can include additional factors with diagnostic construct)	++ to +++	++ to +++

Social purposes requiring binary decisions for eligibility or other decisions such as welfare/legal	–	– (can be + if incorporates thresholds and makes binary statements)	+ to +++	+ to +++	+ (if incorporates thresholds and makes binary statements)	+ (if incorporates thresholds and makes binary statements)
Social purposes such as identity label for charities, public information	–	–	+ t +++	+ to +++ (may just uses diagnostic constructs)	– to +	– to +

- No/very little utility, + small utility, + moderate utility, +++ large utility

uniqueness of an individual, their situation, and context as the construct is based on similarities between others. This can be conveyed in a broader diagnostic formulation but may only include what is thought to be clinically relevant. It is useful to add an idiographic formulation containing biopsychosocial information to integrate this unique meaningful information into a shared understanding (IGDA Working Group, 2003); this information also includes relevant information on social contexts, including immediate social network (e.g. family). It should also be noted that social contexts can be very important for medical conditions, such as TB, but are not explicitly named in the diagnostic construct's label.

Is it feasible to eliminate diagnostic constructs for mental health problems? First, psychiatry as a specialty would have to be eliminated or would have to change its working practices completely to seeing very few patients during office hours. It would have to rethink how it could provide emergency cover because of the advantages of diagnosis for brief appointments, large caseloads, and emergency work compared to other classification systems. Conditions such as dementia or ADHD would have to become the sole preserve of neurology, so more neurologists would be needed. The question of who will provide effective care for patients with mental health problems if psychiatrists are eliminated, especially if patients are a risk to themselves or others, and who are unable or unwilling to engage in psychosocial interventions or for whom there are no effective psychosocial interventions available (such as people meeting mania criteria), will have to be ignored for this scenario. Even this would not see the end of psychiatric diagnostic constructs.

This is because all doctors in clinical practice will encounter patients with mental health problems. Some general medical illnesses may directly cause psychiatric symptoms and they may be the dominating feature at presentation (such as hormonal illnesses causing mood disorders). It is important to recognize these situations when a medical illness is the cause in order to treat this rather than only the psychiatric symptoms. Other patients may have mental health problems caused by unpleasant experiences or consequences of medical problems (such as pain) or of its treatment (such as medication side effects). Some medical patients will also have mental health problems for other reasons than their medical illness or its treatment (such as childhood trauma). Finally, mental health problems can affect the outcome of medical illnesses such as depression and acute coronary syndrome (Lichtman et al., 2014).

For all these reasons, doctors in clinical practice will need to know how to recognize mental health problems, including when to recognize a general medical illness is the cause of them and how to recognize and reduce mental health problems caused by medical interventions. They will also need to know the appropriate treatments or interventions for such mental health problems even if medications for psychiatric treatments are largely abandoned and psychosocial interventions are the main interventions offered. It is unlikely that these non-psychiatric doctors will want to learn classification systems different from their usual diagnostic system, or will have sufficient time to learn such systems when mental health is not their primary focus. Therefore, psychiatric diagnostic constructs are likely always to be needed (but not necessarily the current diagnostic constructs), even if only for doctors whose main area of practice is not mental health.

Classification systems for research

Mental health diagnostic constructs usually identify 'practical' kinds not 'natural' kinds; they often pinpoint spectrums rather than separate categorical entities and are not necessarily optimally configured, but they have useful attached information to help in clinical practice such as prognosis and treatment choices (Zachar, 2015). One of the main barriers to applying the medical model to maximum effect in mental health is lack of understanding of mechanisms on several levels (e.g. interactions of thoughts or neurotransmitter actions) in unproblematic everyday mental states, let alone conditions of medical interest, as well as lack of knowledge of how identified and unidentified causes produce changes in mechanisms. This limits the ability to develop new treatments and laboratory tests to guide clinical decision-making.

Forty years of research since DSM-III and the earlier research diagnostic criteria with improved reliability of diagnostic constructs have provided useful clinical information, for example on prognosis and treatment responses, but have also failed to provide sufficient progress on mechanisms and causes. Are there new classification systems that may help gain this knowledge and lead to improved diagnostic constructs based on mechanisms or causes?

Two promising systems for research are symptom and dimensional classifications. They demonstrate weaknesses, particularly for administration, statistical, and short appointments/emergency clinical utility (Chapter 14), but the more precise descriptions of symptoms and dimensional classifications may make research identifying underlying mechanisms more possible than heterogeneous diagnostic constructs (Bentall, 2014; Hengartner and Lehmann, 2017).

Two forms of these types of classifications are complementary for research: HiTOP and RDOC (Kotov et al., 2017). Hierarchical Taxonomy of Psychopathology (HiTOP) is derived from empirical research into the structure of mental health symptoms organized in a hierarchical system, beginning with symptoms then moving onto various higher levels including 11 syndromes (equivalent to diagnostic constructs) and 6 spectra (e.g. internalizing) (Kotov et al., 2017). HiTOP is not currently suitable for emergency work or short appointments because it is very complex. It is suggested HiTOP's dimensions are measured by use of multiple questionnaires completed by the patient before the appointment with the results analysed to guide how they are classified (Kotov et al., 2017). This is clearly hard to do in emergency situations, and whilst it may be possible for patients to complete lengthy questionnaires in a first, longer appointment, doing so is impractical in brief follow-up appointments. The complexity of HiTOP also strains cognitive resources in these situations. It may be more appropriate for use in research.

Research domain criteria (RDOC) is a matrix constructed by expert opinion. The rows are broad, 'fundamental behavioural components' comprising domains with subsidiary constructs (e.g. 'negative valence' domain with constructs such as 'acute threat (fear) or 'potential threat (anxiety)'), and the columns are 'units of analysis' such as genes, cellular mechanisms, brain circuit activity, and behaviour (Insel et al., 2010; Cuthbert and Insel, 2013). The columns represent potential psychobiological mechanisms which could be tested to see if they showed differences between participants with different ratings for the constructs. RDOC has been criticized, for example for its behavioural domains and constructs being hard to translate into clinical practice (Peterson, 2015), conceptual confusion (Wakefield, 2014; Peterson, 2015), and for focusing on biomarkers not conditions (Carroll, 2015).

These two systems are measuring opposite 'poles' of the clinical picture (HiTOP) and mechanisms/causes with a psychobiological focus (RDoC), and so research using these systems will, hopefully, meet in the middle, linking clinical picture to underlying biopsychosocial mechanisms/causes (Hengartner and Lehmann, 2017; Kotov et al., 2017). This is equivalent to the clinical and pathological correlation that occurs in general medicine (Chapter 13 in Ghaemi, 2007; Chapter 3 in Bynum, 2008). This will, hopefully, lead to new, more scientifically valid homogenous psychiatric diagnostic constructs based on similarity of mechanisms or causes, not just on the clinical picture (Chapters 2, 3, and 4).

Other potential avenues of research that may lead to improved understanding of mechanisms of mental health symptoms include research based on network relationships between symptoms (Borsboom, 2017), or viewing mental health problems as complex dynamic systems rather than categories (Nelson et al., 2017a). Another more biologically orientated form of network research involves analysing networks of interacting biological processes to identify pathways causing symptoms (Silbersweig and Loscalzo, 2017), but this can be extended to analysing networks of psychological processes as described above. Once networks of whatever type, whether purely biological/social/psychological or mixtures of these types, are identified, then mechanistic property clusters of prototypes with fuzzy boundaries can be created as new diagnostic constructs based on mechanisms which should allow superior research and clinical utility (Kendler et al., 2011b).

In general medicine, 'disease modules' of networks of interacting molecules driving fundamental pathological processes such as inflammation or thrombosis have been shown to display significant overlap and are linked to disease-associated genes (Ghiassian et al., 2016). Despite incomplete knowledge of these molecular interactions, it is possible to demonstrate overlap in disease modules between phenotypically diverse diseases such as multiple sclerosis and rheumatoid arthritis (Menche et al., 2015). This is easier in general medicine than psychiatry but HiTOP or similar classifications may identify better phenotypes as well as interacting mechanisms to use for this type of research. For both general medicine and psychiatry, network-focused research may lead to better understanding why co-occurrence of conditions in spectrums occurs (Chapter 11). Research linking biological states to mental health symptoms may still find it hard to achieve valid results (Berrios, 2013; Markova and Berrios, 2015).

Identifying mechanisms and/or causes should lead to research improving knowledge of prognosis and complications and treatments addressing these mechanisms/causes directly, and hence superior effectiveness. Improving diagnostic constructs so that they are based on mechanisms or causes should lead to increased clinical utility by being able to match this research information, including on treatment, to the patients seen by clinicians. We have had many false dawns in psychiatry before and improved diagnostic constructs in the future are not inevitable.

Final words

The medical model as described in this book is one based on the practice of most doctors in clinical practice. It is the ethical use of knowledge and skills to benefit patients. The method of learning and applying this knowledge is based on learning about diagnostic constructs with attached useful probabilistic clinical information (e.g. range of likely prognosis and the chances of success with different treatments) and recognizing which diagnostic construct(s) best match the patient's presenting problems.

A careful history should be taken of the patient's account of what has happened to them, and examination and relevant investigations provide further relevant information. A diagnosis is the professional's opinion about which diagnostic construct best fits this information; it is not an objective truth and is provisional and should be revised if another construct best fits the current or new information. Treatments used in the medical model should be chosen based on the evidence of which is most likely to achieve the patient's treatment objectives and often are not based on achieving cure or reversing disease. Diagnostic constructs themselves are based on similarity of the clinical picture, differences in structure/process, or causes.

The medical model applied to mental health is not completely separate from the medical model used in other medical specialties. There is an overlap in the nature of conditions and diagnostic constructs used to describe them between psychiatry and general medicine. Diagnostic constructs in general medicine and psychiatry are often used to identify conditions that are not diseases or separate categorical entities. They often describe areas of spectrums with no hard boundaries between neighbouring diagnostic constructs. They often lack scientific validity but still retain enough clinical utility for the medical model way of working. In both general medicine and psychiatry, additional important biopsychosocial information is incorporated into diagnostic formulations to guide clinical decision-making. There is an overlap between treatments used in general medicine and psychiatry for effectiveness and harmfulness.

It is important to bear in mind that a classification system (such as diagnosis) is separate from that which is classified (the range of problems that doctors see)—'the map is not the territory'. Doctors do not create a fake reality but try to enable a pragmatic mapping of diverse phenomena ('making sense of chaos'). Given the overlap between psychiatry's diagnostic constructs and treatments and those of general medicine's for many relevant qualities (utility, validity, effectiveness of treatments), it is wrong to talk about psychiatry's (or general medicine's) diagnostic constructs or treatments as a whole. It is better to discuss specific examples of diagnostic constructs and treatments and to reject the notion that psychiatry is not a part of medicine.

There is room for improvement in psychiatry's often heterogeneous diagnostic constructs based usually on clinical picture not underlying mechanisms or causes; that is, they are often descriptive rather than explanatory. Better understanding of mechanisms and/or causes may lead to improvements in psychiatric treatments which currently often do not seem to affect the mechanisms or causes underlying the clinical picture directly. This better understanding may need to be achieved by research using more complex classification systems such as dimensional systems. Even if psychiatry did not exist as a specialty then doctors in other specialties (including GPs) would still encounter mental health problems in patients and would use the medical model of their normal clinical practice in the recognition and management of these problems. Therefore, the medical model will always have a part to play in mental health.

The medical model often allows a greater number of people to be seen and therefore more can be helped, is well suited to emergency (including night-time work), and has high compatibility with the rest of the healthcare sector. This is part of the reason why the medical model is a prominent method used in helping people with mental health problems, although other reasons exist, such as continuity with historical models of delivering care. The medical model is not a disease-based model but a pattern recognition model for diagnostic constructs with attached clinically useful information. Diagnostic constructs in general medicine and psychiatry may also carry costs as well as benefits for patients such as stigma and restrictions of liberty, especially with regard to psychiatric diagnostic constructs.

Other models/methods of helping people and classification systems are often complementary to achieving patients' desired objectives and have varying comparative effectiveness depending on the condition and treatment objective. Patients often require the use of these other models and classification systems, sometimes in conjunction with the medical model, to achieve their desired objectives. The different parties involved in mental healthcare—patients, their carers, and the various mental health professionals—should use whichever classification system (or no classification) that helps them best achieve patients' treatment objectives and perform their roles and duties. They should also recognize that other parties may use different classification systems for good reasons.

The medical model alone is insufficient to help everybody with mental health problems to meet all their needs. Psychology and sociology are still vital both to understand people and the effects of social factors on them as well as to help develop interventions affecting psychosocial factors to both prevent and treat mental health problems. It is also necessary for healthcare professionals to ensure that the knowledge and viewpoints of patients are incorporated in healthcare if their experience of care and its outcomes are to be improved.

References

Aas, M., **Dazzan, P.**, **Mondelli, V.**, **Melle, I.**, **Murray, R.M.**, and **Pariante, C.M.** (2014). 'A systematic review of cognitive function in first-episode psychosis, including a discussion on childhood trauma, stress, and inflammation'. Frontiers in Psychiatry, **4**: 182.

Abel, K.M., **Drake, R.**, and **Goldstein, J.M.** (2010). 'Sex differences in schizophrenia'. International Review of Psychiatry, **22**: 417–28.

Ackner, B., **Harris, A.**, and **Oldham, A. J.** (1957). 'Insulin treatment of schizophrenia: A controlled study'. Lancet, **269**: 607–11.

Adhikari, A., **Topiwala, M.A.**, and **Gordon, J.A.** (2011). 'Single units in the medial prefrontal cortex with anxiety-related firing patterns are preferentially influenced by ventral hippocampal activity'. Neuron, **71**: 898–910.

Adolphs, R. (2015). 'The unsolved problems of neuroscience'. Trends in Cognitive Sciences, **19**: 173–5.

Ahn, R., **Woodbridge, A.**, **Abraham, A.**, **Saba, S.**, **Korenstein, D.**, **Madden, E.**, **Boscardin, W.J.**, and **Keyhani, S.** (2017). 'Financial ties of principal investigators and randomized controlled trial outcomes: cross sectional study'. British Medical Journal, **356**: i6770.

Ajnakina, O., **Trotta, A.**, **Oakley-Hannibal, E.**, **Di Forti, M.**, **Stilo, S.A.**, **Kolliakou, A.**, **Gardner-Sood, P.**, **Gaughran, F.**, **David, A.S.**, **Dazzan, P.**, and **Pariante, C.** (2016). 'Impact of childhood adversities on specific symptom dimensions in first-episode psychosis'. Psychological Medicine, **46**: 317–326.

Akiskal, H.S., **Maser, J.D.**, **Zeller, P.J.**, **Endicott, J.**, **Coryell, W.**, **Keller, M.**, **Warshaw, M.**, **Clayton, P.**, and **Goodwin, F.** (1995). 'Switching from "unipolar" to bipolar II: An 11-year prospective study of clinical and temperamental predictors in 559 patients'. Archives of General Psychiatry, **52**: 114–123.

Alberti, K.G., **Eckel, R.H.**, **Grundy, S.M.**, **Zimmet, P.Z.**, **Cleeman, J.**, **Donato, K.**, **Fruchart, J.C.**, **James, W.P.**, **Loria, C.M.**, and **Smith Jr, S.C.** (2009). 'A joint interim statement of the International Diabetes Federation Task Force on Epidemiology and Prevention; National Heart, Lung, and Blood Institute; American Heart Association; World Heart Federation; International Atherosclerosis Society; and International Association for the Study of Obesity'. Circulation, **120**: 1640–5.

Alemany, S., **Moya, J.**, **Ibáñez, M.I.**, **Villa, H.**, **Mezquita, L.**, **Ortet, G.**, **Gastó, C.**, **Fananas, L.**, and **Arias, B.** (2016). 'Research Letter: Childhood trauma and the rs1360780 SNP of FKBP5 gene in psychosis: A replication in two general population samples'. Psychological Medicine, **46**: 221–3.

Allardyce, J., **McCreadie, R.G.**, **Morrison, G.**, and **van Os, J.** (2007). 'Do symptom dimensions or categorical diagnoses best discriminate between known risk factors for psychosis?' Social Psychiatry and Psychiatric Epidemiology, **42**: 429–37.

ALLHAT Officers and Coordinators for the ALLHAT Collaborative Research Group (2002). 'The Antihypertensive and Lipid-Lowering Treatment to Prevent Heart Attack Trial. Major outcomes in high-risk hypertensive patients randomized to angiotensin-converting enzyme inhibitor or calcium channel blocker vs diuretic: The Antihypertensive and Lipid-Lowering

Treatment to Prevent Heart Attack Trial (ALLHAT)'. Journal of the American Medical Association, **288**: 2981–99.

Alonzo, A.A. and **Reynolds, N.R.** (1995). 'Stigma, HIV and AIDS: An exploration and elaboration of a stigma trajectory'. Social Science & Medicine, **41**: 303–15.

Alvarez-Jimenez, M., Priede, A., Hetrick, S.E., Bendall, S., Killackey, E., Parker, A.G., McGorry, P.D., and **Gleeson, J.F.** (2012). 'Risk factors for relapse following treatment for first episode psychosis: A systematic review and meta-analysis of longitudinal studies'. Schizophrenia Research, **139**: 116–28.

Amad, A., Ramoz, N., Thomas, P., Jardri, R., and **Gorwood, P.** (2014). 'Genetics of borderline personality disorder: Systematic review and proposal of an integrative model', Neuroscience & Biobehavioral Reviews, **40**: 6–19.

Amin, S., Singh, S.P., Brewin, J., Jones, P.B., Medley, I., and **Harrison, G.** (1999). 'Diagnostic stability of first-episode psychosis. Comparison of ICD-10 and DSM-III-R systems'. British Journal of Psychiatry, **175**: 537–43.

Amann, B., Born, C., Crespo, J.M., Pomarol-Clotet, E., and **McKenna, P.** (2011). 'Lamotrigine: When and where does it act in affective disorders? A systematic review'. Journal of Psychopharmacology, **25**: 1289–94.

Amick, H.R., Gartlehner, G., Gaynes, B.N., Forneris, C., Asher, G.N., Morgan, L.C., Coker-Schwimmer, E., Boland, E., Lux, L.J., Gaylord, S., and **Bann, C.** (2015). 'Comparative benefits and harms of second generation antidepressants and cognitive behavioral therapies in initial treatment of major depressive disorder: Systematic review and meta-analysis'. British Medical Journal, **351**: h6019.

Anderson, I.M. and **Tomenson, B.M.** (1995). 'Treatment discontinuation with selective serotonin reuptake inhibitors compared with tricyclic antidepressants: A meta-analysis'. British Medical Journal, **310**: 1433–8.

Anderson, I.M. (1998). 'SSRIs versus tricyclic antidepressants in depressed inpatients: A meta-analysis of efficacy and tolerability'. Depression and Anxiety, **7**(S1): 11–17.

Anderson, I.M. (2000). 'Selective serotonin reuptake inhibitors versus tricyclic antidepressants: A meta-analysis of efficacy and tolerability'. Journal of Affective Disorders, **58**: 19–36.

Anderson, I.M. and **McAllister-Williams, R.H.** (eds) (2016). *Fundamentals of Clinical Psychopharmacology, 4th edn*. Boca Raton, FL: CRC Press.

Andreasen, N.C. and **Flaum, M.** (1991). 'Schizophrenia: The characteristic symptoms'. Schizophrenia Bulletin, **17**: 27–49.

Andreasen, N.C., Liu, D., Ziebell, S., Vora, A., and **Ho, B.C.** (2013). 'Relapse duration, treatment intensity, and brain tissue loss in schizophrenia: A prospective longitudinal MRI study', American Journal of Psychiatry, **170**: 609–15.

Andreassen, O.A., Harbo, H.F., Wang, Y., Thompson, W.K., Schork, A.J., Mattingsdal, M., Zuber, V., Bettella, F., Ripke, S., Kelsoe, J.R., and **Kendler, K.S.** (2015). 'Genetic pleiotropy between multiple sclerosis and schizophrenia but not bipolar disorder: Differential involvement of immune-related gene loci'. Molecular Psychiatry, **20**: 207–14.

Andrews, P.W., Bharwani, A., Lee, K.R., Fox, M., and **Thomson, J.A.** (2015). 'Is serotonin an upper or a downer? The evolution of the serotonergic system and its role in depression and the antidepressant response'. Neuroscience & Biobehavioral Reviews, **51**: 164–88.

Andrion A., Magnani C., Betta P.G., Donna A., Mollo F., Scelsi M., Bernardi P., Botta M., and **Terracini B.** (1995). 'Malignant mesothelioma of the pleura: Interobserver variability'. Journal of Clinical Pathology, **48**: 856–60.

Anglin, D.M., Greenspoon, M., Lighty, Q., and **Ellman, L.M.** (2016). 'Race-based rejection sensitivity partially accounts for the relationship between racial discrimination and distressing attenuated positive psychotic symptoms'. Early Intervention in Psychiatry, **10**: 411–18.

Angst, J. (1985). 'Switch from depression to mania–a record study over decades between 1920 and 1982'. Psychopathology, **18**: 140–54.

Angst, J. (1986). 'The course of affective disorders'. Psychopathology, **19**(Suppl. 2): 47–52.

Angst, J., Gamma, A., Sellaro, R., Lavori, P., and **Zhang, H.** (2003). 'Recurrence of bipolar disorders and major depression'. European Archives of Psychiatry and Clinical Neuroscience, **253**: 236–40.

Angst, J. (1988). 'European long-term followup studies of schizophrenia'. Schizophrenia Bulletin, **14**: 501–13.

Anttila, V., Bulik-Sullivan, B., Finucane, H.K., Bras, J., Duncan, L., Escott-Price, V., Falcone, G., Gormley, P., Malik, R., Patsopoulos, N., and **Ripke, S.** (2016). 'Analysis of shared heritability in common disorders of the brain'. **bioRxiv**, 048991.

Anstee, Q.M., McPherson, S., and **Day, C.P.** (2011). 'How big a problem is non-alcoholic fatty liver disease?' British Medical Journal, **343**(8): d3897.

Aoki, A., Aoki, Y., Goulden, R., Kasai, K., Thornicroft, G., and **Henderson, C.** (2016). 'Change in newspaper coverage of schizophrenia in Japan over 20-year period'. Schizophrenia Research, **175**: 193–7.

Appelbaum, P.S. and **Grisso, T.** (1995). 'The MacArthur Treatment Competence Study. I: Mental illness and competence to consent to treatment'. Law and Human Behavior, **19**: 105–26.

APA American Psychiatric Association (1980). 'Diagnostic and Statistical Manual of Mental Disorders 3rd Edition' (DSM-III). Arlington, VA: American Psychiatric Association Publishing.

APA American Psychiatric Association (1994). 'Diagnostic and Statistical Manual of Mental Disorders 4th Edition' (DSM-IV). Arlington, VA: American Psychiatric Association Publishing.

APA American Psychiatric Association (2013). Diagnostic and Statistical Manual of Mental Disorders, 5th edn (DSM-5). Arlington, VA: American Psychiatric Association Publishing.

Arana, G.W., Baldessarini, R.J., and **Ornsteen, M.** (1985). 'The dexamethasone suppression test for diagnosis and prognosis in psychiatry: Commentary and review'. Archives of General Psychiatry, **42**: 1193–204.

Arroll, B., Macgillivray, S., Ogston, S., Reid, I., Sullivan, F., Williams, B., and **Crombie, I.** (2005). 'Efficacy and tolerability of tricyclic antidepressants and SSRIs compared with placebo for treatment of depression in primary care: A meta-analysis'. Annals of Family Medicine, **3**: 449–56.

Arroll, B., Chin, W.Y., Martis, W., Goodyear-Smith, F., Mount, V., Kingsford, D., Humm, S., Blashki, G., and **MacGillivray, S.** (2016). Antidepressants for treatment of depression in primary care: A systematic review and meta-analysis'. Journal of Primary Health Care, **8**: 325–34.

Asherson, P., Buitelaar, J., Faraone, S.V., and **Rohde, L.A.** (2016). Attention-deficit hyperactivity disorder 2: Adult attention-deficit hyperactivity disorder: key conceptual issues'. Lancet Psychiatry, **3**: 568–78.

Ashton, J. R. (2006). 'Virchow misquoted, part-quoted, and the real McCoy'. Journal of Epidemiology and Community Health, **60**: 671.

Arana, G.W., **Baldessarini, R.J.**, and **Ornsteen, M.** (1985). 'The dexamethasone suppression test for diagnosis and prognosis in psychiatry: Commentary and review'. Archives of General Psychiatry, **42**: 1193–204.

Asnaani A., **Chelminski I.**, **Young D.**, and **Zimmerman M.** (2007). 'Heterogeneity of borderline personality disorder: Do the number of criteria met make a difference?' Journal of Personality Disorders, **21**: 615–25.

Baastrup, P.C., **Poulsen, J.C.**, **Schou, M.**, **Thomsen, K.**, and **Amdisen, A.** (1970). 'Prophylactic lithium: Double blind discontinuation in manic-depressive and recurrent-depressive disorders'. Lancet, **296**: 326–30.

Baca-Garcia, E., **Perez-Rodriguez, M.M.**, **Basurte-Villamor, I.**, **Del Moral, A.L.F.**, **Jimenez-Arriero, M.A.**, **De Rivera, J.L.G.**, **Saiz-Ruiz, J.**, and **Oquendo, M.A.** (2007). 'Diagnostic stability of psychiatric disorders in clinical practice'. The British Journal of Psychiatry, **190**: 210–16.

Bagby, R.M., **Ryder, A.G.**, **Schuller, D.R.**, and **Marshall, M.B.** (2004). 'The Hamilton Depression Rating Scale: Has the gold standard become a lead weight?' American Journal of Psychiatry, **161**: 2163–77.

Baldessarini, R.J., **Tondo, L.**, **Davis, P.**, **Pompili, M.**, **Goodwin, F.K.**, and **Hennen, J.** (2006). Decreased risk of suicides and attempts during long-term lithium treatment: A meta-analytic review'. Bipolar Disorders, **8**: 625–39.

Ball, C.A. and **Barnes, M.** (1994). 'Public health and individual rights: Tuberculosis control and detention procedures in New York City'. Yale Law & Policy Review, **12**: 38–67.

Ballard, E.D., **Van Eck, K.**, **Musci, R.J.**, **Hart, S.R.**, **Storr, C.L.**, **Breslau, N.**, and **Wilcox, H.C.** (2015). 'Latent classes of childhood trauma exposure predict the development of behavioral health outcomes in adolescence and young adulthood'. Psychological Medicine, **45**: 3305–16.

Bally, M., **Dendukuri, N.**, **Rich, B.**, **Nadeau, L.**, **Helin-Salmivaara, A.**, **Garbe, E.**, and **Brophy, J.M.** (2017). 'Risk of acute myocardial infarction with NSAIDs in real world use: Bayesian meta-analysis of individual patient data'. British Medical Journal, **357**: j1909.

Bandelow, B., **Krause, J.**, **Wedekind, D.**, **Broocks, A.**, **Hajak, G.**, and **Rüther, E.** (2005). 'Early traumatic life events, parental attitudes, family history, and birth risk factors in patients with borderline personality disorder and healthy controls'. Psychiatry Research, **134**: 169–79.

Bandelow, B., **Baldwin, D.**, **Abelli, M.**, **Altamura, C.**, **Dell'Osso, B.**, **Domschke, K.**, **Fineberg, N.A.**, **Grünblatt, E.**, **Jarema, M.**, **Maron, E.**, and **Nutt, D.** (2016a). 'Biological markers for anxiety disorders, OCD and PTSD—a consensus statement. Part I: Neuroimaging and genetics'. World Journal of Biological Psychiatry, **17**: 321–65.

Bandelow, B., **Baldwin, D.**, **Abelli, M.**, **Bolea-Alamanac, B.**, **Bourin, M.**, **Chamberlain, S.R.**, **Cinosi, E.**, **Davies, S.**, **Domschke, K.**, **Fineberg, N.**, and **Grünblatt, E.** (2016b). 'Biological markers for anxiety disorders, OCD and PTSD–A consensus statement–Part II: Neurochemistry, neurophysiology and neurocognition'. World Journal of Biological Psychiatry, **18**: 162–214.

Bang, J., **Spina, S.**, and **Miller, B.L.** (2015). 'Frontotemporal dementia'. Lancet, **386**: 1672–82.

Barakat, K., **Wells, Z.**, **Ramdhany, S.**, **Mills, P.G.**, and **Timmis, A.D.** (2003). 'Bangladeshi patients present with non-classic features of acute myocardial infarction and are treated less aggressively in east London, UK'. Heart, **89**: 276–9.

Barch, D.M., **Bustillo, J.**, **Gaebel, W.**, **Gur, R.**, **Heckers, S.**, **Malaspina, D.**, **Owen, M.J.**, **Schultz, S.**, **Tandon, R.**, **Tsuang, M.**, and **Van Os, J.** (2013). 'Logic and justification for dimensional assessment of symptoms and related clinical phenomena in psychosis: relevance to DSM-5'. Schizophrenia Research, **150**: 15–20.

Barrows H.S., **Norman G.R.**, **Neufeld V.R.**, and **Feightner J.W.** (1982). 'The clinical reasoning of randomly selected physicians in general medical practice'. Clinical and Investigative Medicine, **5**: 49–55.

Barth, M., **Kriston, L.**, **Klostermann, S.**, **Barbui, C.**, **Cipriani, A.**, and **Linde, K.** (2016). 'Efficacy of selective serotonin reuptake inhibitors and adverse events: Meta-regression and mediation analysis of placebo-controlled trials'. British Journal of Psychiatry, **208**: 114–19.

Barth, J., **Munder, T.**, **Gerger, H.**, **Nüesch, E.**, **Trelle, S.**, **Znoj, H.**, **Jüni, P.**, and **Cuijpers, P.** (2013). 'Comparative efficacy of seven psychotherapeutic interventions for patients with depression: A network meta-analysis'. PLoS Medicine, **10**: e1001454.

Bate L., **Hutchinson A.**, **Underhill J.**, and **Maskrey N.** (2012). 'How clinical decisions are made'. British Journal of Clinical Pharmacology, **74**: 614–20.

Baumeister, D., **Akhtar, R.**, **Ciufolini, S.**, **Pariante, C.M.**, and **Mondelli, V.** (2016). 'Childhood trauma and adulthood inflammation: A meta-analysis of peripheral C-reactive protein, interleukin-6 and tumour necrosis factor-α'. Molecular Psychiatry, **21**: 642–9.

Baxter, A.J., **Harris, M.G.**, **Khatib, Y.**, **Brugha, T.S.**, **Bien, H.**, and **Bhui, K.** (2016). 'Reducing excess mortality due to chronic disease in people with severe mental illness: Meta-review of health interventions'. British Journal of Psychiatry, **208**: 322–9.

Beards, S., **Gayer-Anderson, C.**, **Borges, S.**, **Dewey, M.E.**, **Fisher, H.L.**, and **Morgan, C.** (2013). 'Life events and psychosis: a review and meta-analysis'. Schizophrenia Bulletin, **39**: 740–7.

Bebbington, P.E., **McBride, O.**, **Steel, C.**, **Kuipers, E.**, **Radovanovič, M.**, **Brugha, T.**, **Jenkins, R.**, **Meltzer, H.I.**, and **Freeman, D.** (2013). 'The structure of paranoia in the general population'. British Journal of Psychiatry, **202**: 419–27.

Beck, A.T. (1964). 'Thinking and depression: II. Theory and therapy'. Archives of General Psychiatry, **10**: 561–71.

Beck A.T., **Rush A.J.**, **Shaw B.E.**, and **Emery G.** (1987). *Cognitive Therapy of Depression.* New York, NY: Guilford Press.

Beck, A.T. (2008). 'The evolution of the cognitive model of depression and its neurobiological correlates'. American Journal of Psychiatry, **165**: 969–77.

Becker, K.G. (2001). 'The common genetic hypothesis of autoimmune/inflammatory disease'. Current Opinion in Allergy and Clinical Immunology, **1**: 399–405.

Bellis, M.A., **Lowey, H.**, **Leckenby, N.**, **Hughes, K.**, and **Harrison, D.** (2014). 'Adverse childhood experiences: retrospective study to determine their impact on adult health behaviours and health outcomes in a UK population'. Journal of Public Health, **36**: 81–91.

Bellis, M.A., **Ashton, K.**, and **Hughes, K.** (2015). 'Adverse Childhood Experiences and their impact on health-harming behaviours in the Welsh adult population'. Liverpool: Centre for Public Health, John Moores University.

Belsher, G. and **Costello, C.G.** (1988). 'Relapse after recovery from unipolar depression: a critical review'. Psychological Bulletin, **104**: 84–96.

Bennell, K.L., **Hunter, D.J.**, and **Hinman, R.S.** (2012). 'Management of osteoarthritis of the knee'. British Medical Journal, **345**: e4934.

Bentall, R.P. (2006). Madness explained: Why we must reject the Kraepelinian paradigm and replace it with a 'complaint-orientated'approach to understanding mental illness'. Medical Hypotheses, **66**: 220–33.

Bentall, R.P., Wickham, S., Shevlin, M., and **Varese, F.** (2012). 'Do specific early-life adversities lead to specific symptoms of psychosis? A study from the 2007 the Adult Psychiatric Morbidity Survey'. Schizophrenia Bulletin, **38**: 734–40.

Bentall, R.P. (2014). 'The search for elusive structure: A promiscuous realist case for researching specific psychotic experiences such as hallucinations'. Schizophrenia Bulletin, **40**(Suppl 40): S198–S201.

Ben-Zeev, D., Young, M.A., and **Corrigan, P.W.** (2010). 'DSM-V and the stigma of mental illness'. Journal of Mental Health, **19**: 318–27.

Bera, S.C., and **Sarkar, S.S.** (2014). 'Cognitive therapy for patients with schizophrenia'. Lancet, **384**: 400.

Bergink, V., Rasgon, N., and **Wisner, K.L.** (2016). 'Postpartum psychosis: Madness, mania, and melancholia in motherhood'. American Journal of Psychiatry, **173**: 1179–88.

Berrios, G.E. and **Chen, E.H.Y.** (1993). 'Recognising psychiatric symptoms relevance to the diagnostic process'. British Journal of Psychiatry, **163**: 308–31.

Berrios G.E. (2013). 'Formation and meaning of mental symptoms: History and epistemology'. Dialogues in Philosophy, Philosophy, Mental and Neurosciences, **6**: 39–48.

Bernadt, M. and **Stein, G.** (1997). 'Lithium: Evidence reconsidered'. British Journal of Psychiatry, **171**: 484.

Berlim, M.T., Eynde, F., and **Daskalakis, Z.J.** (2013). 'Efficacy and acceptability of high frequency repetitive transcranial magnetic stimulation (rtms) versus electroconvulsive therapy (ECT) for major depression: A systematic review and meta-analysis of randomized trials'. Depression and Anxiety, **30**: 614–23.

Berlim, M.T., Van den Eynde, F., Tovar-Perdomo, S., and **Daskalakis, Z.J.** (2014). 'Response, remission and drop-out rates following high-frequency repetitive transcranial magnetic stimulation (rTMS) for treating major depression: A systematic review and meta-analysis of randomized, double-blind and sham-controlled trials'. Psychological Medicine, **44**: 225–39.

Berner E.S. and **Graber M.L.** (2008). 'Overconfidence as a cause of diagnostic error in medicine'. American Journal of Medicine, **121**(5A): S2–23.

Berry, C. and **Hayward, M.** (2011). 'What can qualitative research tell us about service user perspectives of CBT for psychosis? A synthesis of current evidence'. Behavioural and Cognitive Psychotherapy, **39**: 487–94.

Bhagwagar, Z. and **Goodwin, G.M.** (2002). 'The role of lithium in the treatment of bipolar depression'. Clinical Neuroscience Research, **2**: 222–7.

Bhugra, D., Leff, J., Mallett, R., Der, G., Corridan, B., and **Rudge, S.** (1997). 'Incidence and outcome of schizophrenia in whites, African-Caribbeans and Asians in London'. Psychological Medicine, **27**: 791–8.

Biesheuvel-Leliefeld, K.E., Kok, G.D., Bockting, C.L., Cuijpers, P., Hollon, S.D., van Marwijk, H.W., and **Smit, F.** (2015). 'Effectiveness of psychological interventions in preventing recurrence of depressive disorder: Meta-analysis and meta-regression'. Journal of Affective Disorders, **174**: 400–10.

Björkenstam, E., Björkenstam, C., Holm, H., Gerdin, B., and **Ekselius, L.** (2015). 'Excess cause-specific mortality in in-patient-treated individuals with personality disorder: 25-year nationwide population-based study'. British Journal of Psychiatry, **207**: 339–45.

Bjornestad, J., Davidson, L., Joa, I., Larsen, T.K., Hegelstad, W.T.V., Langeveld, J., Veseth, M., Melle, I., Johannessen, J.O., and **Bronnick, K.** (2017). 'Antipsychotic treatment: Experiences of fully recovered service users'. Journal of Mental Health, **26**: 264–70.

Blatchford, O., **Murray, W.R.**, and **Blatchford, M.** (2000). 'A risk score to predict need for treatment for uppergastrointestinal haemorrhage'. Lancet, **356**: 1318–21.

Bloomfield, P.S., **Selvaraj, S.**, **Veronese, M.**, **Rizzo, G.**, **Bertoldo, A.**, **Owen, D.R.**, **Bloomfield, M.A.**, **Bonoldi, I.**, **Kalk, N.**, **Turkheimer, F.**, and **McGuire, P.** (2015). 'Microglial activity in people at ultra high risk of psychosis and in schizophrenia: an [11C] PBR28 PET brain imaging study'. American Journal of Psychiatry, **173**: 44–52.

Bloomgarden, Z.T. (2004). 'Definitions of the insulin resistance syndrome: The 1st World Congress on the insulin resistance syndrome'. Diabetes Care, **27**: 824–30.

Boardman J., **Dogra, N.**, and **Hindley, P.** (2015). 'Mental health and poverty in the UK: Time for change?' British Journal of Psychiatry Interntional, **12**: 27–8.

Bollini, P., **Pampallona, S.**, **Orza, M.J.**, **Adams, M.E.**, and **Chalmers, T.C.** (1994). 'Antipsychotic drugs: is more worse? A meta-analysis of the published randomized control trials'. Psychological Medicine, **24**: 307–16.

Bora, E., **Yucel, M.**, and **Pantelis, C.** (2009). 'Cognitive functioning in schizophrenia, schizoaffective disorder and affective psychoses: Meta-analytic study'. British Journal of Psychiatry, **195**: 475–82.

Bora, E. and **Pantelis, C.** (2015). 'Meta-analysis of cognitive impairment in first-episode bipolar disorder: Comparison with first-episode schizophrenia and healthy controls'. Schizophrenia Bulletin, **41**: 1095–104.

Borsboom, D., **Cramer, A.O.**, **Schmittmann, V.D.**, **Epskamp, S.**, and **Waldorp, L.J.** (2011). 'The small world of psychopathology'. PloS One, **6**: e27407.

Borsboom, D. and **Cramer, A.O.** (2013). 'Network analysis: An integrative approach to the structure of psychopathology'. Annual Review of Clinical Psychology, **9**: 91–121.

Borsboom, D. (2017). 'A network theory of mental disorders'. World Psychiatry, **16**: 5–13.

Borys, D.S. and **Pope, K.S.** (1989). 'Dual relationships between therapist and client: A national study of psychologists, psychiatrists, and social workers'. Professional Psychology: Research and Practice, **20**: 283–93.

Boussageon, R., **Gueyffier, F. Cornu, C.** (2016). 'Metformin as firstline treatment for type 2 diabetes: are we sure?' British Medical Journal, **352**: h6748.

Bowden C.L., **Brugger A.M.**, **Swann A.C.**, **Calabrese J.R.**, **Janicak P.G.**, **Petty F.**, **Dilsaver S.C.**, **Davis J.M.**, **Rush A.J.**, **Small J.G.**, and **Garza-Treviño E.S.** (1994). 'Efficacy of divalproex vs lithium and placebo in the treatment of mania'. Journal of the American Medical Association, **271**: 918–24.

Bowden, C.L., **Grunze, H.**, **Mullen, J.**, **Brecher, M.**, **Paulsson, B.**, **Jones, M.**, **Vagero, M.**, and **Svensson, K.** (2005). 'A randomized, double-blind, placebo-controlled efficacy and safety study of quetiapine or lithium as monotherapy for mania in bipolar disorder'. Journal of Clinical Psychiatry, **66**: 111–21.

Boyle M. (2007). 'The problem with diagnosis'. The Psychologist, **20**: 290–2.

Brewin, C.R., **Andrews, B.**, and **Valentine, J.D.** (2000). 'Meta-analysis of risk factors for posttraumatic stress disorder in trauma-exposed adults'. Journal of Consulting and Clinical Psychology, **68**: 748–66.

Brockington, I.F., **Kendell, R.E.**, **Wainwright, S.**, **Hillier, V.F.**, and **Walker, J.** (1979). 'The distinction between the affective psychoses and schizophrenia'. British Journal of Psychiatry, **135**: 243–8.

Brockington, I.F., **Roper, A.**, **Copas, J.**, **Buckley, M.**, **Andrade, C.E.**, **Wigg, P.**, **Farmer, A.**, **Kaufman, C.**, and **Hawley, R.** (1991). 'Schizophrenia, bipolar disorder and depression.

A discriminant analysis, using "lifetime" psychopathology ratings'. British Journal of Psychiatry, **159**: 4485–94.

Brooks, R. (2000). 'The reliability and validity of the Health of the Nation Outcome Scales: validation in relation to patient derived measures'. Australian and New Zealand Journal of Psychiatry, **34**: 504–11.

Brown, D.W., Anda, R.F., Felitti, V.J., Edwards, V.J., Malarcher, A.M., Croft, J.B., and **Giles, W.H.** (2010a). 'Adverse childhood experiences are associated with the risk of lung cancer: A prospective cohort study'. BMC Public Health, **10**: 20.

Brown G.W. and **Harris T.** (1978). *Social Origins of Depression: A Study of Psychiatric Disorder in Women*. London: Tavistock.

Brown, G.W., Bifulco, A., and **Harris, T.O.** (1987). 'Life events, vulnerability and onset of depression: some refinements'. British Journal of Psychiatry, **150**: 30–42.

Brown, G.W., Harris, T.O., and **Hepworth, C.** (1994). 'Life events and endogenous depression: a puzzle re-examined'. Archives of General Psychiatry, **51**: 525–34.

Brown, S., Barraclough, B., and **Inskip, H.** (2000). 'Causes of the excess mortality of schizophrenia'. British Journal of Psychiatry, **177**: 212–17.

Brown, S., Kim, M., Mitchell, C., and **Inskip, H.** (2010b). 'Twenty-five year mortality of a community cohort with schizophrenia'. British Journal of Psychiatry, **196**: 116–21.

Brown, T.A., Campbell, L.A., Lehman, C.L., Grisham, J.R., and **Mancill, R.B.** (2001). 'Current and lifetime comorbidity of the DSM-IV anxiety and mood disorders in a large clinical sample'. Journal of Abnormal Psychology, **110**: 585–99.

Brown, T.A. and **Barlow, D.H.** (2009). 'A proposal for a dimensional classification system based on the shared features of the DSM-IV anxiety and mood disorders: Implications for assessment and treatment'. Psychological Assessment, **21**: 256–71.

Brown, W.A. (2007). 'Treatment response in melancholia'. Acta Psychiatrica Scandinavica, **115** (Suppl **4330)**: 125–9.

Brunoni, A.R., Chaimani, A., Moffa, A.H., Razza, L.B., Gattaz, W.F., Daskalakis, Z.J., and **Carvalho, A.F.** (2017). 'Repetitive transcranial magnetic stimulation for the acute treatment of major depressive episodes: A systematic review with network meta-analysis'. JAMA Psychiatry, **74**: 143–52.

Brush J.E. (2015). *The Science of the Art of Medicine*. Manakin-Sabot, VA: Dementi Milestone Publishing.

Budd, R. and **Hughes, I.** (2009). 'The Dodo bird verdict—controversial, inevitable and important: A commentary on 30 years of meta-analyses'. Clinical Psychology & Psychotherapy, **16**: 510–22.

Bukh, J.D., Andersen, P.K., and **Kessing, L.V.** (2016). 'Rates and predictors of remission, recurrence and conversion to bipolar disorder after the first lifetime episode of depression: A prospective 5-year follow-up study'. Psychological Medicine, **46**: 1151–61.

Bulik, C.M., Prescott, C.A., and **Kendler, K.S.** (2001). 'Features of childhood sexual abuse and the development of psychiatric and substance use disorders'. British Journal of Psychiatry, **179**: 444–9.

Bulik-Sullivan, B., Finucane, H.K., Anttila, V., Gusev, A., Day, F.R., Loh, P.R., Duncan, L., Perry, J.R., Patterson, N., Robinson, E.B., and **Daly, M.J.** (2015). 'An atlas of genetic correlations across human diseases and traits'. Nature Genetics, **47**: 1236–41.

Bunker, J.P., Frazier, H.S., and **Mosteller, F.** (1995). 'The role of medical care in determining health: Creating an inventory of benefits.' In: B.C. Amick III, S. Levine, A.R. Tarlov, and T.C. Walsh (eds), *Society and Health*. New York, NY: Oxford University Press, pp. 305–41.

Burnam, M.A., Stein, J.A., Golding, J.M., Siegel, J.M., Sorenson, S.B., Forsythe, A.B. and **Telles, C.A.** (1988). 'Sexual assault and mental disorders in a community population'. Journal of Consulting and Clinical Psychology, **56**: 843–50.

Burcusa, S.L. and **Iacono, W.G.** (2007). 'Risk for recurrence in depression'. Clinical Psychology Review, **27**: 959–85.

Burgess, S.S., Geddes, J., Hawton, K.K., Taylor, M.J., Townsend, E., Jamison, K., and **Goodwin, G.** (2001). 'Lithium for maintenance treatment of mood disorders'. Cochrane Database Systematic Reviews, **3**: CD003013.

Burns, J. (2009). 'Dispelling a myth: Developing world poverty, inequality, violence and social fragmentation are not good for outcome in schizophrenia'. African Journal of Psychiatry, **12**: 200–5.

Burns, J.K., Tomita, A., and **Kapadia, A.S.** (2014). 'Income inequality and schizophrenia: Increased schizophrenia incidence in countries with high levels of income inequality'. International Journal of Social Psychiatry, **60**: 185–96.

Burns T. (2006). *Psychiatry A Very Short Introduction*. Oxford: Oxford University Press.

Burrell, J.R., Halliday, G.M., Kril, J.J., Ittner, L.M., Götz, J., Kiernan, M.C., and **Hodges, J.R.** (2016). 'The frontotemporal dementia-motor neuron disease continuum'. Lancet, **388**: 919–31.

Burstein, M., Beesdo-Baum, K., He, J.P., and **Merikangas, K.R.** (2014). 'Threshold and subthreshold generalized anxiety disorder among US adolescents: Prevalence, sociodemographic, and clinical characteristics'. Psychological Medicine, **44**: 2351–62.

Bush, W.S. and **Moore, J.H.** (2012). 'Genome-wide association studies'. PLoS Computational Biology, **8**: e1002822.

Burton, C.Z., Ryan, K.A., Kamali, M., Marshall, D.F., Harrington, G., McInnis, M.G., and **Tso, I.F.** (2019). 'Psychosis in bipolar disorder: Does it represent a more "severe" illness?' **20**: 18–26.

Bynum W. (2008). *The History of Medicine A Very Short Introduction*. Oxford: Oxford University Press.

Cairns, M.J. (2015). 'Circulating miRNA Biomarkers for Schizophrenia?' American Journal of Psychiatry, **172**: 1059–61.

Campbell E.J.M., Scadding J.G., and **Roberts R.S.** (1979). 'The concept of disease'. British Medical Journal, **2**: 757–62.

Canadian Institute for Advanced Research, Health Canada, Population and Public Health Branch AB/NWT 2002, cited in **Kuznetsova D.** (2012). 'Healthy places: Councils leading on public health'. London: New Local Government Network.

Coughlan, H. and **Cannon, M.** (2017). 'Does childhood trauma play a role in the aetiology of psychosis? A review of recent evidence'. British Journal of Psychiatric Advances, **23**: 307–15.

Cantor-Graae, E. and **Selten, J.P.** (2005). 'Schizophrenia and migration: A meta-analysis and review'. American Journal of Psychiatry, **162**: 12–24.

Cardno, A.G., Rijsdijk, F.V., Sham, P.C., Murray, R.M., and **McGuffin, P.** (2002). 'A twin study of genetic relationships between psychotic symptoms'. American Journal of Psychiatry, **159**(4): 539–45.

Care Quality Commision (2016). 'Monitoring the Mental Health Act in 2015/16'. Available at: <http://www.cqc.org.uk/sites/default/files/20161122_mhareport1516_web.pdf>.

Carney, M.W.P., Roth, M., and **Garside, R.F.** (1965). 'The diagnosis of depressive syndromes and the prediction of ECT response'. British Journal of Psychiatry, **111**: 659–74.

Carpenter, W.T., **Bustillo, J.R.**, **Thaker, G.K.**, **Van Os, J.**, **Krueger, R.F.**, and **Green, M.J.** (2009). 'The psychoses: Cluster 3 of the proposed meta-structure for DSM-V and ICD-11'. Psychological Medicine, **39**: 2025–42.

Carroll, B.J. (2012). 'Bringing back melancholia'. Bipolar Disorders, **14**: 1–5.

Carroll, B.J. (2015). 'Clinical science and biomarkers: Against RDoC'. Acta Psychiatrica Scandinavica, **6**: 423–24.

Carvalho, A.F., **Köhler, C.A.**, **Fernandes, B.S.**, **Quevedo, J.**, **Miskowiak, K.W.**, **Brunoni, A.R.**, **Machado-Vieira, R.**, **Maes, M.**, **Vieta, E.**, and **Berk, M.** (2016). 'Bias in emerging biomarkers for bipolar disorder'. Psychological Medicine, **46**: 2287–97.

Casadevall, A. and **Pirofski, L.A.** (1999). 'Host-pathogen interactions: Redefining the basic concepts of virulence and pathogenicity'. Infection and Immunity, **67**: 3703–13.

Casey, J.F., **Bennett, I.F.**, **Lindley, C.J.**, **Hollister, L.E.**, **Gordon, M.H.**, and **Springer, N.N.** (1960). 'Drug therapy in schizophrenia: A controlled study of the relative effectiveness of chlorpromazine, promazine, phenobarbital, and placebo'. Archives of General Psychiatry, **2**: 210–20.

Caspi, A., **Houts, R.M.**, **Belsky, D.W.**, **Goldman-Mellor, S.J.**, **Harrington, H.**, **Israel, S.**, **Meier, M.H.**, **Ramrakha, S.**, **Shalev, I.**, **Poulton, R.**, and **Moffitt, T.E.** (2014). 'The p factor: One general psychopathology factor in the structure of psychiatric disorders?' Clinical Psychological Science, **2**: 119–37.

Castagnini, A. and **Galeazzi, G.M.** (2016). 'Acute and transient psychoses: clinical and nosological issues'. British Journal of Psychiatric Advances, **22**: 292–300.

Castrén, E. and **Rantamäki, T.** (2010). 'The role of BDNF and its receptors in depression and antidepressant drug action: Reactivation of developmental plasticity'. Developmental Neurobiology, 70: 289–97.

CDC (2016). 'National Vital Statistics Reports Deaths: Leading Causes for 2014'. Available at: <https://www.cdc.gov/nchs/data/nvsr/nvsr65/nvsr65_05.pdf>.

Chambers, L.A., **Rueda, S.**, **Baker, D.N.**, **Wilson, M.G.**, **Deutsch, R.**, **Raeifar, E.**, and **Rourke, S.B.** (2015). 'Stigma, HIV and health: A qualitative synthesis'. BMC Public Health, **15**: 848.

Chang, S.M., **Cho, S.J.**, **Jeon, H.J.**, **Hahm, B.J.**, **Lee, H.J.**, **Park, J.I.**, and **Cho, M.J.** (2008). 'Economic burden of schizophrenia in South Korea'. Journal of Korean Medical Science, **23**: 167–75.

Chekroud, A.M., **Gueorguieva, R.**, **Krumholz, H.M.**, **Trivedi, M.H.**, **Krystal, J.H.**, and **McCarthy, G.** (2017). 'Reevaluating the efficacy and predictability of antidepressant treatments: A symptom clustering approach'. JAMA Psychiatry, **74**: 370–8.

Chen, E., **Turiano, N.A.**, **Mroczek, D.K.**, and **Miller, G.E.** (2016). 'Association of reports of childhood abuse and all-cause mortality rates in women'. JAMA Psychiatry, **73**: 920–7.

Chesney, E., **Goodwin, G.M.**, and **Fazel, S.** (2014). 'Risks of all-cause and suicide mortality in mental disorders: A meta-review'. World Psychiatry, **13**: 153–60.

Chetri, S.K., **Mills, R.J.**, **Shaunak, S.**, and **Emsley, H.C.A.** (2014). 'Copper deficiency'. British Medical Journal, **348**: g3691.

Chiang, S.K., **Ni, C.H.**, **Tsai, C.P.**, and **Lin, K.C.** (2016). 'Validation of the cognitively normal range and below normal range subtypes in chronically hospitalized patients with schizophrenia'. Schizophrenia Research: Cognition, **5**: 28–34.

Cho, J.H. (2008). 'The genetics and immunopathogenesis of inflammatory bowel disease'. Nature Reviews Immunology, **8**: 458–66.

Chou, I.C., **Wang, C.H.**, **Lin, W.D.**, **Tsai, F.J.**, **Lin, C.C.**, and **Kao, C.H.** (2016a). 'Risk of epilepsy in type 1 diabetes mellitus: A population-based cohort study'. Diabetologia, **59**: 1196–203.

Chou, R., **Tracy Dana, M.L.S.**, **Blazina, I.**, **Daeges, M.**, and **Jeanne, T.L**, (2016b). 'Statins for prevention of cardiovascular disease in adults evidence report and systematic review for the US Preventive Services Task Force'. Journal of the American Medical Association, **316**: 2008–24.

Cicchetti, D.V. (1994). 'Guidelines, criteria, and rules of thumb for evaluating normed and standardized assessment instruments in psychology'. Psychological Assessment, **6**: 284–90.

Chouinard G. and **Jones B.D.** (1980). 'Neuroleptic-induced supersensitivity psychosis: Clinical and pharmacologic characteristics'. American Journal of Psychiatry, **137**: 16–21.

Chouinard, G., **Samaha, A.N.**, **Chouinard, V.A.**, **Peretti, C.S.**, **Kanahara, N.**, **Takase, M.**, and **Iyo, M.** (2017). 'Antipsychotic-induced dopamine supersensitivity psychosis: Pharmacology, criteria, and therapy'. Psychotherapy and Psychosomatics, **86**: 189–219.

Cipriani A, **Rendell J.M.**, and **Geddes J.** (2006). 'Haloperidol alone or in combination for acute mania'. Cochrane Database of Systematic Reviews, **3**: CD004362.

Cipriani, A., **Hawton, K.**, **Stockton, S.**, and **Geddes, J.R.** (2013). 'Lithium in the prevention of suicide in mood disorders: Updated systematic review and meta-analysis'. British Medical Journal, **346**: f3646.

Clare A. (2011). *Psychiatry in Dissent. Controversial Issues in Thought and Practice*, 2nd edn. Abingdon: Routledge.

Clark, D.M. (1986). 'A cognitive approach to panic'. Behaviour Research and Therapy, **24**: 461–70.

Clayton, E.W. (2015). 'Beyond myalgic encephalomyelitis/chronic fatigue syndrome: An IOM report on redefining an illness'. Journal of the American Medical Association, **313**: 1101–2.

Cleynen, I., **Boucher, G.**, **Jostins, L.**, **Schumm, L.P.**, **Zeissig, S.**, **Ahmad, T.**, **Andersen, V.**, **Andrews, J.M.**, **Annese, V.**, **Brand, S.**, and **Brant, S.R.** (2016). 'Inherited determinants of Crohn's disease and ulcerative colitis phenotypes: A genetic association study'. Lancet, **387**: 156–67.

Close, R.J., **Sachs, C.J.**, and **Dyne, P.L.** (2001). 'Reliability of bimanual pelvic examinations performed in emergency departments'. Western Journal of Medicine, **175**: 240–4.

Coburn, D. (2015). 'Income inequality, welfare, class and health: A comment on Pickett and Wilkinson, 2015'. Social Science Medicine, **146**: 228–32.

Cohen, A., **Patel, V.**, **Thara, R.**, and **Gureje, O.** (2008). 'Questioning an axiom: better prognosis for schizophrenia in the developing world?' Schizophrenia Bulletin, **34**: 229–44.

Cohen, B.L. and **Sachar, D.B.** (2017). 'Update on anti-tumor necrosis factor agents and other new drugs for inflammatory bowel disease'. British Medical Journal, **357**: j2505.

Cohen, J. (1992). 'A power primer'. Psychological Bulletin, **11**: 155–9.

Cole, J., **McGuffin, P.**, and **Farmer, A.E.** (2008). 'The classification of depression: Are we still confused?' British Journal of Psychiatry, **192**: 83–5.

Collins, R., **Reith, C.**, **Emberson, J.**, **Armitage, J.**, **Baigent, C.**, **Blackwell, L.**, **Blumenthal, R.**, **Danesh, J.**, **Smith, G.D.**, **DeMets, D.**, and **Evans, S.** (2016). 'Interpretation of the evidence for the efficacy and safety of statin therapy'. Lancet, **388**: 2532–61.

Collip, D., **Myin-Germeys, I.**, **Wichers, M.**, **Jacobs, N.**, **Derom, C.**, **Thiery, E.**, **Lataster, T.**, **Simons, C.**, **Delespaul, P.**, **Marcelis, M.**, and **van Os, J.** (2013). 'FKBP5 as a possible moderator of the psychosis-inducing effects of childhood trauma'. British Journal of Psychiatry, **202**: 261–8.

Colquhoun, D. (2014). 'An investigation of the false discovery rate and the misinterpretation of p-values'. Royal Society Open Science, **1**: 140216.

Conley, D., Rauscher, E., Dawes, C., Magnusson, P.K., and **Siegal, M.L.** (2013). 'Heritability and the equal environments assumption: Evidence from multiple samples of misclassified twins'. Behavior Genetics, **43**: 415–26.

Conus, P., Cotton, S., Schimmelmann, B.G., McGorry, P.D., and **Lambert, M.** (2010). 'Pretreatment and outcome correlates of sexual and physical trauma in an epidemiological cohort of first-episode psychosis patients'. Schizophrenia Bulletin, **36**: 1105–14.

Conway, F., Majeed, A., and **Easton, G.** (2015). 'Diagnosing chronic obstructive pulmonary disease'. British Medical Journal, **351**: h6171.

Cookson J.O. (1997). 'Lithium: Balancing risks and benefits'. British Journal of Psychiatry, **171**: 120–4.

Cookson J., Taylor D., and **Katona C.** (2002). *Use of Drugs in Psychiatry*, 5th edn. London: Gaskell.

Cooper (1983). Diagnosis and the diagnostic process. In: M. Shepherd and O.L. Zangwill (eds), *Handbook of Psychiatry 1: General Psychopathology*. Cambridge: Cambridge University Press, pp. 199–209.

Cooper J.E. and **Sartorius N.** (2013). *A Companion to The Classification of Mental Disorders*. Oxford: Oxford University Press.

Cooper R. (2007). *Psychiatry and the Philosophy of Science*. Stocksfield: Acumen.

Cooper, R. (2015). 'Why is the Diagnostic and Statistical Manual of Mental Disorders so hard to revise? Path-dependence and "lock-in" in classification'. Studies in History and Philosophy of Science Part C: Studies in History and Philosophy of Biological and Biomedical Sciences, **51**: 1–10.

Coppen, A., Noguera, R., Bailey, J., Burns, B.H., Swani, M.S., Hare, E.H., Gardner, R., and **Maggs, R.** (1971). 'Prophylactic lithium in affective disorders: controlled trial'. Lancet, **298**: 275–9.

Correll, C.U., Detraux, J., De Lepeleire, J., and **De Hert, M.** (2015). 'Effects of antipsychotics, antidepressants and mood stabilizers on risk for physical diseases in people with schizophrenia, depression and bipolar disorder'. World Psychiatry, **14**: 119–36.

Correll, C.U., Solmi, M., Veronese, N., Bortolato, B., Rosson, S., Santonastaso, P., Thapa-Chhetri, N., Fornaro, M., Gallicchio, D., Collantoni, E., and **Pigato, G.** (2017). 'Prevalence, incidence and mortality from cardiovascular disease in patients with pooled and specific severe mental illness: A large-scale meta-analysis of 3,211,768 patients and 113,383,368 controls'. World Psychiatry, **16**: 163–80.

Corrigan P.W. and **Bink A.B.** (2016). 'The stigma of mental illness'. Encyclopaedia of Mental Health, **4**: 230–4.

Corrigan, P.W., Schmidt, A., Bink, A.B., Nieweglowski, K., Al-Khouja, M.A., Qin, S., and **Discont, S.** (2017). 'Changing public stigma with continuum beliefs'. Journal of Mental Health, **26**: 411–18.

Cosgrove, V.E. and **Suppes, T.** (2013). 'Informing DSM-5: Biological boundaries between bipolar I disorder, schizoaffective disorder, and schizophrenia'. BMC Medicine, **11**: 127.

Costain, G., Lionel, A.C., Merico, D., Forsythe, P., Russell, K., Lowther, C., Yuen, T., Husted, J., Stavropoulos, D.J., Speevak, M., and **Chow, E.W.** (2013). 'Pathogenic rare copy number variants in community-based schizophrenia suggest a potential role for clinical microarrays'. Human Molecular Genetics, **22**: 4485–501.

Courtwright, A. and **Turner, A.N.** (2010). 'Tuberculosis and stigmatization: Pathways and interventions'. Public Health Reports, **125**(Suppl 4): 34–42.

Cowen, P.J. (2008). 'Serotonin and depression: Pathophysiological mechanism or marketing myth?' Trends in Pharmacological Sciences, **29**: 433–6.

Cowen, P.J. and **Browning, M.** (2015). 'What has serotonin to do with depression?' World Psychiatry, **14**: 158–60.

Coyne, J.C., **Fechner-Bates, S.**, and **Schwenk, T.L.** (1994). 'Prevalence, nature, and comorbidity of depressive disorders in primary care'. General Hospital Psychiatry, **16**: 267–76.

Coyne, J.C. and **Kok, R.N.** (2014). 'Salvaging psychotherapy research: A manifesto'. Journal of Evidence-Based Psychotherapies, **14**: 105–24.

Coyne, J.C. and **van Linschoten, H.S.** (2014). 'Cognitive therapy for patients with schizophrenia'. Lancet, **384**: 400.

Craddock, N. and **Owen, M.J.** (2010). 'The Kraepelinian dichotomy–going, going . . . but still not gone'. British Journal of Psychiatry, **196**: 92–5.

Crawford, M.J., **Thana, L.**, **Farquharson, L.**, **Palmer, L.**, **Hancock, E.**, **Bassett, P.**, **Clarke, J.**, and **Parry, G.D.** (2016). 'Patient experience of negative effects of psychological treatment: results of a national survey'. British Journal of Psychiatry, **208**: 260–5.

Creed F. (1995). 'How consultants manage their time'. Advances in Psychiatric Treatment, **1**: 65–70.

Creed, F. and **Gureje, O.** (2012). 'Emerging themes in the revision of the classification of somatoform disorders'. International Review of Psychiatry, **24**: 556–67.

Crisp, A.H., **Gelder, M.G.**, **Rix, S.**, **Meltzer, H.I.** and **Rowlands, O.J.** (2000). 'Stigmatisation of people with mental illnesses'. British Journal of Psychiatry, **177**(1): 4–7.

Cristea, I.A., **Gentili, C.**, **Cotet, C.D.**, **Palomba, D.**, **Barbui, C.**, and **Cuijpers, P.** (2017a). 'Efficacy of Psychotherapies for Borderline Personality Disorder: A Systematic Review and Meta-analysis'. JAMA Psychiatry, **74**: 319–28.

Cristea, I.A., **Gentili, C.**, **Pietrini, P.**, and **Cuijpers, P.** (2017b). 'Sponsorship bias in the comparative efficacy of psychotherapy and pharmacotherapy for adult depression: Meta-analysis'. British Journal of Psychiatry, **210**: 16–23.

Cristea, I.A. and **Cuijpers, P.** (2017C). 'In the pursuit of truth, we should not prioritize correlational over causal evidence'. Psychotherapy Research, **27**: 36–7.

Criswell, L.A., **Pfeiffer, K.A.**, **Lum, R.F.**, **Gonzales, B.**, **Novitzke, J.**, **Kern, M.**, **Moser, K.L.**, **Begovich, A.B.**, **Carlton, V.E.**, **Li, W.**, and **Lee, A.T.** (2005). 'Analysis of families in the multiple autoimmune disease genetics consortium (MADGC) collection: The PTPN22 620W allele associates with multiple autoimmune phenotypes'. American Journal of Human Genetics, **76**: 561–71.

Cromby, J. and **Harper, D.J.** (2009). 'Paranoia: A social account'. Theory & Psychology, **19**: 335–61.

Croskerry P. (2002). 'Achieving quality in clinical decision making: Cognitive strategies and detection of bias'. Academic Emergency Medicine, **9**: 1184–204.

Croskerry P. (2003). 'The importance of cognitive errors in diagnosis and strategies to minimize them'. Academic Medicine, **78**: 775–80.

Croskerry P. (2009). 'A universal model of diagnostic reasoning'. Academic Medicine, **84**: 1022–8.

Cross-Disorder Group of the Psychiatric Genomics Consortium (2013a). 'Genetic relationship between five psychiatric disorders estimated from genome-wide SNPs'. Nature Genetics, **45**: 984–94.

Cross-Disorder Group of the Psychiatric Genomics Consortium (2013b). 'Identification of risk loci with shared effects on five major psychiatric disorders: A genome-wide analysis'. Lancet, **381**: 1371–9.

Crow, T.J. (1990). 'The continuum of psychosis and its genetic origins. The sixty-fifth Maudsley lecture'. British Journal of Psychiatry, **156**: 788–97.

Cuijpers, P., Berking, M., Andersson, G., Quigley, L., Kleiboer, A., and **Dobson, K.S.** (2013a). 'A meta-analysis of cognitive-behavioural therapy for adult depression, alone and in comparison with other treatments'. Canadian Journal of Psychiatry, **58**: 376–85.

Cuijpers, P., Sijbrandij, M., Koole, S.L., Andersson, G., Beekman, A.T., and **Reynolds, C.F.** (2013b). 'The efficacy of psychotherapy and pharmacotherapy in treating depressive and anxiety disorders: A meta-analysis of direct comparisons'. World Psychiatry, **12**: 37–148.

Cuijpers, P., Sijbrandij, M., Koole, S.L., Andersson, G., Beekman, A.T., and **Reynolds, C.F.** (2014a). 'Adding psychotherapy to antidepressant medication in depression and anxiety disorders: a meta-analysis'. World Psychiatry, **13**: 56–67.

Cuijpers, P., Turner, E.H., Mohr, D.C., Hofmann, S.G., Andersson, G., Berking, M., and **Coyne, J.** (2014). 'Comparison of psychotherapies for adult depression to pill placebo control groups: A meta-analysis'. Psychological Medicine, **44**: 685–95.

Cuijpers, P. and **Cristea, I.A.** (2015). 'What if a placebo effect explained all the activity of depression treatments?' World Psychiatry, **14**: 310–11.

Cuijpers, P., Karyotaki, E., Andersson, G., Li, J., Mergl, R., and **Hegerl, U.** (2015). 'The effects of blinding on the outcomes of psychotherapy and pharmacotherapy for adult depression: A meta-analysis'. European Psychiatry, **30**: 685–93.

Cuijpers, P. (2016). 'Are all psychotherapies equally effective in the treatment of adult depression? The lack of statistical power of comparative outcome studies'. Evidence-Based Mental Health, **19**: 39–42.

Cuijpers, P., Cristea, I.A., Karyotaki, E., Reijnders, M., and **Huibers, M.J.** (2016). 'How effective are cognitive behavior therapies for major depression and anxiety disorders? A meta-analytic update of the evidence'. World Psychiatry, **15**: 245–58.

Cullen, B.A., McGinty, E.E., Zhang, Y., Dosreis, S.C., Steinwachs, D.M., Guallar, E., and **Daumit, G.L.** (2012). 'Guideline-concordant antipsychotic use and mortality in schizophrenia'. Schizophrenia Bulletin, **39**: 1159–68.

Cuthbert, B.N. Insel, T.R. (2013). 'Toward the future of psychiatric diagnosis: The seven pillars of RDoC'. BMC Medicine, **11**: 126.

Cutcliffe, J.R., Santos, J.C., Kozel, B., Taylor, P. Lees, D. (2015). 'Raiders of the Lost Art: A review of published evaluations of inpatient mental health care experiences emanating from the United Kingdom, Portugal, Canada, Switzerland, Germany and Australia'. International Journal of Mental Health Nursing, **24**: 375–85.

Danaei, G., Vander Hoorn, S., Lopez, A.D., Murray, C.J., Ezzati, M., Comparative Risk Assessment collaborating group (Cancers, 2005. Causes of cancer in the world: comparative risk assessment of nine behavioural and environmental risk factors. Lancet, **366**(9499): 1784–93.

David, A.S. (2010). 'Why we need more debate on whether psychotic symptoms lie on a continuum with normality'. Psychological Medicine, **40**: 1935–42.

Davies, E.C., Green, C.F., Taylor, S., Williamson, P.R., Mottram, D.R., and **Pirmohamed, M.** (2009). 'Adverse drug reactions in hospital in-patients: a prospective analysis of 3695 patient-episodes'. PLoS One, **4**: e4439.

Davis, J., Maes, M., Andreazza, A., McGrath, J.J., Tye, S.J., and **Berk, M.** (2015). 'Towards a classification of biomarkers of neuropsychiatric disease: From encompass to compass'. Molecular Psychiatry, **20**: 152–3.

Davis, J.M., Wang, Z., and **Janicak, P.G.** (1993). 'A quantitative analysis of clinical drug trials for the treatment of affective disorders'. Psychopharmacology Bulletin, **29**: 175–81.

Davies, L.M., Lewis, S., Jones, P.B., Barnes, T.R., Gaughran, F., Hayhurst, K., Markwick, A., and **Lloyd, H., on behalf of the CUtLASS team** (2007). 'Cost-effectiveness of first- v. second-generation antipsychotic drugs: results from a randomised controlled trial in schizophrenia responding poorly to previous therapy'. British Journal of Psychiatry, **191**: 14–22.

Dawson, J. and **Szmukler, G.** (2006). 'Fusion of mental health and incapacity legislation'. British Journal of Psychiatry, **188**: 504–9.

Deber R.B., Kraetschmer N., Urowitz S., and **Sharpe N.** (2005). 'Patient, consumer, client, or customer: What do people want to be called?' Health Expectations, **8**: 345–51.

De Hert, M., Sermon, J., Geerts, P., Vansteelandt, K., Peuskens, J., and **Detraux, J.** (2015). 'The use of continuous treatment versus placebo or intermittent treatment strategies in stabilized patients with schizophrenia: A systematic review and meta-analysis of randomized controlled trials with first-and second-generation antipsychotics'. CNS Drugs, **29**: 637–58.

De Hert, M., Correll, C.U., and **Cohen, D.** (2010). 'Do antipsychotic medications reduce or increase mortality in schizophrenia? A critical appraisal of the FIN-11 study'. Schizophrenia Research, **117**: 68–74.

Dell Osso L. and **Pini S.** (2012). 'What did we learn from research on comorbidity in psychiatry? Advantages and limitations in the forthcoming DSM-V era'. Clinical Practice & Epidemiology in Mental Health, **8**: 180–4.

De Mello, M.F., de Jesus Mari, J., Bacaltchuk, J., Verdeli, H., and **Neugebauer, R.** (2005). 'A systematic review of research findings on the efficacy of interpersonal therapy for depressive disorders'. European Archives of sychiatry and Clinical Neuroscience, **255**: 75–82.

Demjaha, A., Morgan, K., Morgan, C., Landau, S., Dean, K., Reichenberg, A., Sham, P., Fearon, P., Hutchinson, G., Jones, P.B., and **Murray, R.M.** (2009). 'Combining dimensional and categorical representation of psychosis: The way forward for DSM-V and ICD-11?' Psychological Medicine, **39**: 1943–55.

Demjaha, A., Murray, R.M., McGuire, P.K., Kapur, S. and **Howes, O.D.** (2012). 'Dopamine synthesis capacity in patients with treatment-resistant schizophrenia'. American Journal of Psychiatry, **169**: 1203–10.

Demjaha, A., Egerton, A., Murray, R.M., Kapur, S., Howes, O.D., Stone, J.M., and **McGuire, P.K.** (2014). 'Antipsychotic treatment resistance in schizophrenia associated with elevated glutamate levels but normal dopamine function'. Biological Psychiatry, **75**: e11–e13.

De Moor, M.H., Van Den Berg, S.M., Verweij, K.J., Krueger, R.F., Luciano, M., Vasquez, A.A., Matteson, L.K., Derringer, J., Esko, T., Amin, N., and **Gordon, S.D.** (2015). 'Meta-analysis of genome-wide association studies for neuroticism, and the polygenic association with major depressive disorder'. JAMA Psychiatry, **72**: 642–50.

De Vries, Y.A., Roest, A.M., Franzen, M., Munafò, M.R., and **Bastiaansen, J.A.** (2016a). 'Citation bias and selective focus on positive findings in the literature on the serotonin transporter gene (5-HTTLPR), life stress and depression'. Psychological Medicine, **46**: 2971–9.

De Vries, Y.A., de Jonge, P., van den Heuvel, E., Turner, E.H., and **Roest, A.M.** (2016b). 'Influence of baseline severity on antidepressant efficacy for anxiety disorders: Meta-analysis and meta-regression'. British Journal of Psychiatry, **208**: 515–21.

Derry, S. and **Moore, R.A.** (2007). 'Atypical antipsychotics in bipolar disorder: Systematic review of randomised trials'. BMC Psychiatry, **7**: 40.

Detre K.M, **Wright E.**, **Murphy M.L.**, and **Takaro T.** **(1975)**. 'Observer agreement in evaluating coronary angiograms'. Circulation, **52**: 979–86.

Dibben, C.R.M., **Rice, C.**, **Laws, K.**, and **McKenna, P.J.** (2009). 'Is executive impairment associated with schizophrenic syndromes? A meta-analysis'. Psychological Medicine, **39**: 381–92.

Dikeos, D.G., **Wickham, H.**, **McDonald, C.**, **Walshe, M.**, **Sigmundsson, T.**, **Bramon, E.**, **Grech, A.**, **Toulopoulou, T.**, **Murray, R.**, and **Sham, P.C.** (2006). 'Distribution of symptom dimensions across Kraepelinian divisions'. British Journal of Psychiatry, **189**: 346–53.

Di Forti, M., **Iyegbe, C.**, **Sallis, H.**, **Kolliakou, A.**, **Falcone, M.A.**, **Paparelli, A.**, **Sirianni, M.**, **La Cascia, C.**, **Stilo, S.A.**, **Marques, T.R.** and **Handley, R.**, 2012. Confirmation that the AKT1 (rs2494732) genotype influences the risk of psychosis in cannabis users. Biological Psychiatry, **72**(10): 811–16.

Di Forti, M., **Marconi, A.**, **Carra, E.**, **Fraietta, S.**, **Trotta, A.**, **Bonomo, M.**, **Bianconi, F.**, **Gardner-Sood, P.**, **O'Connor, J.**, **Russo, M.**, and **Stilo, S.A.** (2015). 'Proportion of patients in south London with first-episode psychosis attributable to use of high potency cannabis: A case-control study'. Lancet Psychiatry, **2**: 233–8.

Division of Clinical Psychology (2010). *The Core Purpose and Philosophy of the Profession*. Leicester: British Psychological Society.

Division of Clinical Psychology (2011). *Good Practice Guidelines on the Use of Psychological Formulation*. Leicester: British Psychological Society.

Division of Clinical Psychology (2013). *Classification of Behaviour and Experience in Relation to Functional Psychiatric Diagnoses: Time for a Paradigm Shift. DCP Position Statement*. Leicester: British Psychological Society.

Dong, M., **Dube, S.R.**, **Felitti, V.J.**, **Giles, W.H.**, and **Anda, R.F.** (2003). 'Adverse childhood experiences and self-reported liver disease: New insights into the causal pathway'. Archives of Internal Medicine, **163**: 1949–56.

Dong M., **Giles W.H.**, **Felitti V.J.**, **Dube S.R.**, **Williams J.E.**, **Chapman D.P.**, and **Anda R.F.** (2004). 'Insights into causal pathways for ischemic heart diseaseadverse childhood experiences study'. Circulation, **110**: 1761–6.

Douglas G., **Nicol F.**, and **Robertson C.** (2009). *Macleod's Clinical Examination*, 12th edn. Edinburgh: Churchill Livingstone (Elsevier).

Driessen, E., **Hollon, S.D.**, **Bockting, C.L.**, **Cuijpers, P.**, and **Turner, E.H.** (2015). 'Does publication bias inflate the apparent efficacy of psychological treatment for major depressive disorder? A systematic review and meta-analysis of US National Institutes of Health-funded trials'. PLoS One, **10**: e0137864.

Dubos, R. J. (1965). *Man Adapting*. New Haven, CT: Yale University Press.

Dupré, J. (1996). 'Metaphysical disorder and scientific disunity'. In: P. Galison and D.J. Stump (eds), *The Disunity of Science: Boundaries, Contexts, and Power*. Redwood City, CA: Stanford University Press, pp. 101–17.

Dupre J. (2001). 'In defence of classification'. Studies in History and Philosophy of Biological & Biomedical Sciences, **32**: 203–19.

Durham, J., **Newton-John, T.R.**, and **Zakrzewska, J.M.** (2015). 'Temporomandibular disorders'. British Medical Journal, **350**: h1154.

Eisman, S. and **Sinclair, R.** (2015). 'Pityriasis rosea'. British Medical Journal, **351**: h5233.

Eklund, A., **Nichols, T.E.**, and **Knutsson, H.** (2016). 'Cluster failure: Why fMRI inferences for spatial extent have inflated false-positive rates'. Proceedings of the National Academy of Sciences, **113**: 7900–5.

Elkes, J. and **Elkes, C.** (1954). 'Effect of chlorpromazine on the behaviour of chronically overactive psychotic patients'. British Medical Journal, **2**(4887).: 560–6.

Ellam, T., **Twohig, H.**, and **Khwaja, A.** (2016). 'Chronic kidney disease in elderly people: disease or disease label?' British Medical Journal, **352**: h6559.

Ellingson, J.M., **Richmond-Rakerd, L.S.**, **Statham, D.J.**, **Martin, N.G.**, and **Slutske, W.S.** (2016). 'Most of the genetic covariation between major depressive and alcohol use disorders is explained by trait measures of negative emotionality and behavioral control'. Psychological Medicine, **46**: 2919–30.

Elsaesser, A. and **Hamm, C.W.** (2004). 'Acute coronary syndrome the risk of being female'. Circulation, **109**: 565–7.

Emdin, C.A., **Anderson, S.G.**, **Woodward, M.**, and **Rahimi, K.** (2015a). 'Usual blood pressure and risk of new-onset diabetes: Evidence from 4.1 million adults and a meta-analysis of prospective studies'. Journal of the American College of Cardiology, **66**: 1552–62.

Emdin, C.A., **Anderson, S.G.**, **Callender, T.**, **Conrad, N.**, **Salimi-Khorshidi, G.**, **Mohseni, H.**, **Woodward, M.**, and **Rahimi, K.** (2015b). 'Usual blood pressure, peripheral arterial disease, and vascular risk: Cohort study of 4.2 million adults'. British Medical Journal, **351**: h4865.

Enck P., **Bingel U.**, **Schedlowski M.**, and **Rief W.** (2013). 'Opinion: The placebo response in medicine: minimize, maximize or personalize?' Nature Reviews Drug Discovery, **12**: 191–204.

Engel G.L. (1981). 'The clinical application of the biopsychosocial model'. Journal of Medicine and Philosophy, **6**: 101–24.

Enhorn v Sweden (2006). 'The exercise of public health powers in cases of infectious disease: Human rights implications'. Medical Law Review, **14**: 132–43.

Ereshefsky, M. (2009). 'Defining "health"and "disease"'. Studies in History and Philosophy of Science Part C: Studies in History and Philosophy of Biological and Biomedical Sciences, **40**: 221–7.

Fatouros-Bergman, H., **Cervenka, S.**, **Flyckt, L.**, **Edman, G.**, and **Farde, L.** (2014). 'Meta-analysis of cognitive performance in drug-naive patients with schizophrenia'. Schizophrenia Research, **158**: 156–62.

Faulkner A. (2015). 'Talking Point Papers 1: Randomised controlled trials : The straitjacket of mental health'. McPin Foundation. Available at: <http://mcpin.org/wp-content/uploads/talking-point-paper-1.pdf>.

Fava, G.A., **Gatti, A.**, **Belaise, C.**, **Guidi, J.**, and **Offidani, E.** (2015). 'Withdrawal symptoms after selective serotonin reuptake inhibitor discontinuation: A systematic review'. Psychotherapy and Psychosomatics, **84**: 72–81.

FDA Food and Drug Administration (2011). 'Meeting to discuss the classification of electroconvulsive therapy devices (ECT). Executive summary'. Available at: <http://www.fda.gov/downloads/AdvisoryCommittees/CommitteesMeetingMaterials/MedicalDevices/MedicalDevicesAdvisoryCommittee/NeurologicalDevicesPanel/UCM240933.pdf>.

Feinberg, M. and **Carroll, B.J.** (1982). 'Separation of subtypes of depression using discriminant analysis. I. Separation of unipolar endogenous depression from non-endogenous depression'. The British Journal of Psychiatry, **140**: 384–91.

Feinstein, A.R. (1970). 'The pre-therapeutic classification of co-morbidity in chronic disease'. Journal of Chronic Diseases, **23**: 455–68.

Fell B. and **Hewstone M.** (2015). 'Psychological Perspectives On Poverty'. Joseph Rowntree Foundation. Available at: <https://www.jrf.org.uk/file/47481/download?token=2wsFnOis>.

Felitti, V.J., **Anda, R.F.**, **Nordenberg, D.**, **Williamson, D.F.**, **Spitz, A.M.**, **Edwards, V.**, **Koss, M.P.** and **Marks, J.S.** (1998). 'Relationship of childhood abuse and household dysfunction to many of the leading causes of death in adults: The Adverse Childhood Experiences (ACE) Study'. American Journal of Preventive Medicine, **14**: 245–58.

Fernando, M.M., **Stevens, C.R.**, **Walsh, E.C.**, **De Jager, P.L.**, **Goyette, P.**, **Plenge, R.M.**, **Vyse, T.J.**, and **Rioux, J.D.** (2008). 'Defining the role of the MHC in autoimmunity: A review and pooled analysis'. PLoS Genetics, **4**: e1000024.

Fink, M. and **Taylor, M.A.** (2007). 'Resurrecting melancholia'. Acta Psychiatrica Scandinavica, **115** (s433): 14–20.

Fink, W., **Lipatov, V.**, and **Konitzer, M.** (2009). 'Diagnoses by general practitioners: Accuracy and reliability'. International Journal of Forecasting, **25**: 784–93.

Finlay-Jones, R. and **Brown, G.W.** (1981). 'Types of stressful life event and the onset of anxiety and depressive disorders'. Psychological Medicine, **11**: .803–15.

First, M.B. (2005a). 'Mutually exclusive versus co-occurring diagnostic categories: The challenge of diagnostic comorbidity'. Psychopathology, **38**: 206–10.

First, M.B. (2005b). 'Clinical utility: A prerequisite for the adoption of a dimensional approach in DSM'. Journal of Abnormal Psychology, **114**: 560–4.

First M.B., **Pincus H.A.**, **Levine J.B.**, **Williams J.B.W.**, **Ustun B.**, and **Peele R.** (2004). 'Clinical utility as a criterion for revising psychiatric diagnoses'. American Journal of Psychiatry, **161**: 946–54.

Fisher, H.L., **Jones, P.B.**, **Fearon, P.**, **Craig, T.K.**, **Dazzan, P.**, **Morgan, K.**, **Hutchinson, G.**, **Doody, G.A.**, **McGuffin, P.**, **Leff, J.**, and **Murray, R.M.** (2010). 'The varying impact of type, timing and frequency of exposure to childhood adversity on its association with adult psychotic disorder'. Psychological Medicine, **40**: 1967–78.

Fitch, C., **Hamilton, S.**, **Bassett, P.**, and **Davey, R.** (2011). 'The relationship between personal debt and mental health: A systematic review'. Mental Health Review Journal, **16**: 153–66.

Fleiss J.L. (1971). 'Measuring nominal scale agreement among many raters'. Psychological Bulletin, **76**: 378–82.

Flinn, L., **Braham, L.**, and **Nair, R.** (2015). 'How reliable are case formulations? A systematic literature review'. British Journal of Clinical Psychology, **54**: 266–90.

Flint, J. and **Kendler, K.S.** (2014). 'The genetics of major depression'. Neuron, **81**: 484–503.

Flint, J., **Cuijpers, P.**, **Horder, J.**, **Koole, S.L.**, and **Munafò, M.R.** (2015). 'Is there an excess of significant findings in published studies of psychotherapy for depression?' Psychological Medicine, **45**: 439–46.

Fonagy, P. (2015). 'The effectiveness of psychodynamic psychotherapies: An update'. World Psychiatry, **14**: 137–50.

Fosse, R., **Joseph, J.**, and **Richardson, K.** (2015). 'A critical assessment of the equal-environment assumption of the twin method for schizophrenia'. Frontiers in Psychiatry, **6**: 62.

Fone, D., **Greene, G.**, **Farewell, D.**, **White, J.**, **Kelly, M.**, and **Dunstan, F.** (2013). 'Common mental disorders, neighbourhood income inequality and income deprivation: small-area multilevel analysis'. British Journal of Psychiatry, **202**: 286–93.

Ford, J.D. and **Courtois, C.A.** (2014). 'Complex PTSD, affect dysregulation, and borderline personality disorder'. Borderline Personality Disorder and Emotion Dysregulation, **1**: p9.

Fortenberry, J.D., **McFarlane, M.**, **Bleakley, A.**, **Bull, S.**, **Fishbein, M.**, **Grimley, D.M.**, **Malotte, C.K.**, and **Stoner, B.P.** (2002). 'Relationships of stigma and shame to gonorrhea and HIV screening'. American Journal of Public Health, **92**: 378–81.

Fox, K.A., **Dabbous, O.H.**, **Goldberg, R.J.**, **Pieper, K.S.**, **Eagle, K.A.**, **Van de Werf, F.**, **Avezum, Á.**, **Goodman, S.G.**, **Flather, M.D.**, **Anderson, F.A.**, and **Granger, C.B.** (2006). 'Prediction of risk of death and myocardial infarction in the six months after presentation with acute coronary syndrome: Prospective multinational observational study (GRACE)'. British Medical Journal, **333**(7578): 1091–4.

Fournier, J.C., **DeRubeis, R.J.**, **Hollon, S.D.**, **Dimidjian, S.**, **Amsterdam, J.D.**, **Shelton, R.C.**, and **Fawcett, J.** (2010). 'Antidepressant drug effects and depression severity: a patient-level meta-analysis'. Journal of the American Medical Association, **303**: 47–53.

Frances, A. (2016). 'A report card on the utility of psychiatric diagnosis'. World Psychiatry, **15**: 32–3.

Freeman, D., **Garety, P.A.**, **Bebbington, P.E.**, **Smith, B.**, **Rollinson, R.**, **Fowler, D.**, **Kuipers, E.**, **Ray, K.**, and **Dunn, G.** (2005). 'Psychological investigation of the structure of paranoia in a non-clinical population'. British Journal of Psychiatry, **186**: 427–35.

Frueh, B.C., **Knapp, R.G.**, **Cusack, K.J.**, **Grubaugh, A.L.**, **Sauvageot, J.A.**, **Cousins, V.C.**, **Yim, E.**, **Robins, C.S.**, **Monnier, J.**, and **Hiers, T.G.** (2005). 'Special section on seclusion and restraint: Patients' reports of traumatic or harmful experiences within the psychiatric setting'. Psychiatric Services, **56**: 1123–33.

Fryers, T., **Melzer, D.**, and **Jenkins, R.** (2003). 'Social inequalities and the common mental disorders'. Social Psychiatry and Psychiatric Epidemiology, **38**: 229–37.

Fryers, T., **Melzer, D.**, **Jenkins, R.**, and **Brugha, T.** (2005). 'The distribution of the common mental disorders: Social inequalities in Europe'. Clinical Practice and Epidemiology in Mental Health, **1**: 14.

Furukawa, T.A. (1999). 'From effect size into number needed to treat'. Lancet, **353**: 1680.

Furukawa, T.A. and **Leucht, S.** (2011). 'How to obtain NNT from Cohen's d: Comparison of two methods'. PloS One, **6**: e19070.

Furukawa, T.A., **Noma, H.**, **Caldwell, D.M.**, **Honyashiki, M.**, **Shinohara, K.**, **Imai, H.**, **Chen, P.**, **Hunot, V.**, and **Churchill, R.** (2014). 'Waiting list may be a nocebo condition in psychotherapy trials: A contribution from network meta-analysis'. Acta Psychiatrica Scandinavica, **130**: 181–92.

Furukawa, T.A., **Levine, S.Z.**, **Tanaka, S.**, **Goldberg, Y.**, **Samara, M.**, **Davis, J.M.**, **Cipriani, A.**, and **Leucht, S.** (2015). 'Initial severity of schizophrenia and efficacy of antipsychotics: Participant-level meta-analysis of 6 placebo-controlled studies'. JAMA Psychiatry, **72**: 14–21.

Fusar-Poli, P., **Radua, J.**, **McGuire, P.**, and **Borgwardt, S.** (2011). 'Neuroanatomical maps of psychosis onset: Voxel-wise meta-analysis of antipsychotic-naive VBM studies'. Schizophrenia Bulletin, **38**: 1297–307.

Fusar-Poli, P. and **Meyer-Lindenberg, A.** (2013a). 'Striatal presynaptic dopamine in schizophrenia, part I: Meta-analysis of dopamine active transporter (DAT) density'. Schizophrenia Bulletin, **39**: 22–32.

Fusar-Poli, P. and **Meyer-Lindenberg, A.** (2013b). 'Striatal presynaptic dopamine in schizophrenia, Part II: Meta-analysis of [18F/11C]-DOPA PET studies'. Schizophrenia Bulletin, **39**: 33–42.

Fusar-Poli, P., **Cappucciati, M.**, **Rutigliano, G.**, **Heslin, M.**, **Stahl, D.**, **Brittenden, Z.**, **Caverzasi, E.**, **McGuire, P.**, and **Carpenter, W.T.** (2016a). 'Diagnostic stability of ICD/DSM first episode psychosis diagnoses: Meta-analysis'. Schizophrenia Bulletin, **42**: 1395–406.

Fusar-Poli, P., Cappucciati, M., Bonoldi, I., Hui, L.C., Rutigliano, G., Stahl, D.R., Borgwardt, S., Politi, P., Mishara, A.L., Lawrie, S.M., and **Carpenter, W.T.** (2016b). 'Prognosis of brief psychotic episodes: a meta-analysis'. JAMA Psychiatry, **73**: 211–20.

Gabbay J and **Le May A.** (2004). 'Evidence based guidelines or collectively constructed "mindlines"? Ethnographic study of knowledge management in primary care'. British Medical Journal, **329**: 1013.

Galasko, D., Hansen, L.A., Katzman, R., Wiederholt, W., Masliah, E., Terry, R., Hill, L.R., Lessin, P., and **Thal, L.J.** (1994). 'Clinical-neuropathological correlations in Alzheimer's disease and related dementias'. Archives of Neurology, **51**: 888–95.

Galatzer-Levy, I.R. and **Bryant, R.A.** (2013). '636,120 ways to have posttraumatic stress disorder'. Perspectives on Psychological Science, **8**: 651–62.

Gale EA. (2006). 'Declassifying diabetes'. Diabetologia, **49**: 1989–95.**Galea, I., Ward-Abel, N.,** and **Heesen, C.** (2015). 'Relapse in multiple sclerosis'. British Medical Journal, **350**: h1765.

Gao, J., Warren, R., Warren-Forward, H., and **Forbes, J.F.** (2008). 'Reproducibility of visual assessment on mammographic density.".Breast Cancer Research and Treatment, **108**: 121–7.

Garrett, T. and **Davis, J.D.** (1998). 'The prevalence of sexual contact between British clinical psychologists and their patients'. Clinical Psychology and Psychotherapy, **5**: 253–63.

Gauthier, S., Feldman, H.H., Schneider, L.S., Wilcock, G.K., Frisoni, G.B., Hardlund, J.H., Moebius, H.J., Bentham, P., Kook, K.A., Wischik, D.J., and **Schelter, B.O.** (2016). 'Efficacy and safety of tau-aggregation inhibitor therapy in patients with mild or moderate Alzheimer's disease: A randomised, controlled, double-blind, parallel-arm, phase 3 trial'. Lancet, **388**: 2873–84.

Geddes, J.R., Carney, S.M., Davies, C., Furukawa, T.A., Kupfer, D.J., Frank, E., and **Goodwin, G.M.** (2003). 'Relapse prevention with antidepressant drug treatment in depressive disorders: A systematic review'. Lancet, **361**: 653–61.

Geddes, J.R., Calabrese, J.R., and **Goodwin, G.M.** (2009). 'Lamotrigine for treatment of bipolar depression: Independent meta-analysis and meta-regression of individual patient data from five randomised trials'. British Journal of Psychiatry, **194**: 4–9.

Gewitz, M.H., Baltimore, R.S., Tani, L.Y., Sable, C.A., Shulman, S.T., Carapetis, J., Remenyi, B., Taubert, K.A., Bolger, A.F., Beerman, L., and **Mayosi, B.M.** (2015). 'Revision of the Jones criteria for the diagnosis of acute rheumatic fever in the era of doppler echocardiography: A scientific statement from the American Heart Association'. Circulation, **131**: 1806–18.

Ghaemi, S.N. (2007). *The Concepts of Psychiatry: A Pluralistic Approach to the Mind and Mental Illness*. Baltimore, MD: John Hopkins University Press.

Ghiassian, S.D., Menche, J., Chasman, D.I., Giulianini, F., Wang, R., Ricchiuto, P., Aikawa, M., Iwata, H., Müller, C., Zeller, T., and **Sharma, A.** (2016). 'Endophenotype network models: Common core of complex diseases'. Scientific Reports (Nature Publisher Group), **6**: p.27414.

Gibson, L.E., Alloy, L.B., and **Ellman, L.M.** (2016a). 'Trauma and the psychosis spectrum: A review of symptom specificity and explanatory mechanisms'. Clinical Psychology Review, **49**: 92–105.

Gibson, K., Cartwright, C., and **Read, J.** (2016b). '"In my life antidepressants have been . . .": A qualitative analysis of users' diverse experiences with antidepressants'. BMC Psychiatry,16 135.

Gibertini, M., Nations K.R., and **Whitaker J.A.** (2012). 'Obtained effect size as a function of sample size in approved antidepressants: a real-world illustration in support of better trial design'. International Clinical Psychopharmacology, **27**: 100–6.

Gillin, J.C., Lauriello, J., Kelsoe, J.R., Rapaport, M., Golshan, S., Kenny, W.M., and **Sutton, L.** (1995). 'No antidepressant effect of biperiden compared with placebo in depression: a double-blind 6-week clinical trial'. Psychiatry Research, **58**: 99–105.

Glass T.A., Goodman S.N., Hernan M.A., and **Samet J.M.** (2013). 'Causal inference in public health'. Annual Review of Public Health, **34**: 61–75.

Glasziou, P., Chalmers, I., Rawlins, M., and **McCulloch, P.** (2007). 'When are randomised trials unnecessary? Picking signal from noise'. British Medical Journal, **334**: 349–51.

Glen, J., Floros, L., Day, C. and **Pryke, R.** (2016). 'Non-alcoholic fatty liver disease (NAFLD): summary of NICE guidance'. British Medical Journal, **354**: i4428.

Glenn, A. L., and **Raine, A.** (2014). 'Neurocriminology: Implications for the punishment, prediction and prevention of criminal behaviour'. Nature Reviews Neuroscience, **15**: 54–63.

Goff, D.C., Falkai, P., Fleischhacker, W.W., Girgis, R.R., Kahn, R.M., Uchida, H., Zhao, J., and **Lieberman, J.A.** (2017). 'The long-term effects of antipsychotic medication on clinical course in schizophrenia'. American Journal of Psychiatry, **174**: 840–9.

Goffman, E. (1963). *Stigma: Notes on the Management of Spoiled Identity.* Harmondsworth: Penguin.

Goldacre B. (2013). 'Building Evidence into Education'. Available at: <http://media.education.g(ov.uk/assets/files/pdf/b/ben%20goldacre%20paper.pdf>.

Goldacre, B. and **Heneghan, C.** (2015). 'How medicine is broken, and how we can fix it'. British Medical Journal, **350**: h3397.

Goldberg, D. (2000). 'Plato versus Aristotle: Categorical and dimensional models for common mental disorders'. Comprehensive Psychiatry, **41**: 8–13.

Goldberg, D.P., Krueger, R.F., Andrews, G., and **Hobbs, M.J.** (2009). 'Emotional disorders: Cluster 4 of the proposed meta-structure for DSM-V and ICD-11'. Psychological Medicine, **39**: 2043–59.

Goldberg, D. (2010). 'The classification of mental disorder: A simpler system for DSM–V and ICD–11'. Advances in Psychiatric Treatment, **16**: 14–19.

Goldberg, D. (2011). 'The heterogeneity of "major depression"'. World Psychiatry, **10**: 226–8.

Goldberg, J.F. and **Truman, C.J.** (2003). 'Antidepressant-induced mania: An overview of current controversies'. Bipolar Disorders, **5**: 407–20.

Golden, S.K., Harringa, J.B., Pickhardt, P.J., Ebinger, A., Svenson, J.E., Zhao, Y.Q., Li, Z., Westergaard, R.P., Ehlenbach, W.J., Repplinger, and **Jacobs, E.A.** (2016). Emergency Medicine Journal, **33**(7): 458–64

Goodkind, M., Eickhoff, S.B., Oathes, D.J., Jiang, Y., Chang, A., Jones-Hagata, L.B., Ortega, B.N., Zaiko, Y.V., Roach, E.L., Korgaonkar, M.S., and **Grieve, S.M.** (2015). 'Identification of a common neurobiological substrate for mental illness'. JAMA Psychiatry, **72**: 305–15.

Goodwin G.M. (1994). 'Recurrence of mania after lithium withdrawal: Implications for the use of lithium in the treatment of bipolar affective disorder'. British Journal of Psychiatry, **164**: 149–52.

Goodwin G.M. (1995). 'Lithium revisited: A Reply'. British Journal of Psychiatry, **167**: 574–5.

Goodwin, G.M., Haddad, P.M., Ferrier, I.N., Aronson, J.K., Barnes, T.R.H., Cipriani, A., Coghill, D.R., Fazel, S., Geddes, J.R., Grunze, H., and **Holmes, E.A.** (2016). 'Evidence-based guidelines for treating bipolar disorder: Revised third edition recommendations from the British Association for Psychopharmacology'. Journal of Psychopharmacology, **30**: 495–553.

Graber M., Gordon R., and **Franklin, N.** (2002). 'Reducing diagnostic errors in medicine: What's the goal?' Academic Medicine, **77**: 981–92.

Gray, A.J. (2002). 'Stigma in psychiatry'. Journal of the Royal Society of Medicine, **95**: 72–6.

Graber, M.L. (2013). 'The incidence of diagnostic error in medicine'. BMJ Quality & Safety, **22**(Suppl 2): ii21–ii27.

Grant, B.F., Stinson, F.S., Dawson, D.A., Chou, S.P., and **Ruan, W.J.** (2005). 'Co-occurrence of DSM-IV personality disorders in the United States: Results from the National Epidemiologic Survey on alcohol and related conditions'. Comprehensive Psychiatry, **46**: 1–5.

Gray, R. and **Deane, K.** (2016). 'What is it like to take antipsychotic medication? A qualitative study of patients with first-episode psychosis'. Journal of Psychiatric and Mental Health Nursing, **23**: 108–15.

Greenhalgh T. (2010). *How To Read A Paper: The Basics of Evidence Based Medicine.* London: BMJ Books.

Greenway, T. and **Ross, J.S.** (2017). 'US drug marketing: How does promotion correspond with health value?' British Medical Journal, **357**: j1855.

Greenwood, T.A., Swerdlow, N.R., Gur, R.E., Cadenhead, K.S., Calkins, M.E., Dobie, D.J., Freedman, R., Green, M.F., Gur, R.C., Lazzeroni, L.C., and **Nuechterlein, K.H.** (2013). 'Genome-wide linkage analyses of 12 endophenotypes for schizophrenia from the Consortium on the Genetics of Schizophrenia'. American Journal of Psychiatry, **170**: 521–32.

Grof, P., Duffy, A., Cavazzoni, P., Grof, E., Garnham, J., MacDougall, M., O'Donovan, C. and **Alda, M.** (2002). 'Is response to prophylactic lithium a familial trait?' Journal of Clinical Psychiatry, **63**: 942–7.

Gros, D.F., Allan, N.P., and **Szafranski, D.D.** (2016). 'Movement towards transdiagnostic psychotherapeutic practices for the affective disorders'. Evidence-Based Mental Health, **19**: e10–2.

Grove, W.M., Andreasen, N.C., Young, M., Endicott, J., Keller, M.B., Hirschfeld, R.M.A., and **Reich, T.** (1987). Isolation and characterization of a nuclear depressive syndrome. Psychological Medicine, **17**(2): 471–4.

Groves, J.O. (2007). 'Is it time to reassess the BDNF hypothesis of depression?' Molecular Psychiatry, **12**: 1079–88.

Grosse, M. and **Grawe, K.** (2002). 'Bern Inventory of Treatment Goals: Part 1. Development and first application of a taxonomy of treatment goal themes'. Psychotherapy Research, **12**: 79–99.

Grundy, S.M., Brewer, H.B., Cleeman, J.I., Smith, S.C., and **Lenfant, C.** (2004). 'Definition of metabolic syndrome report of the National Heart, Lung, and Blood Institute/American Heart Association Conference on scientific issues related to definition'. Circulation, **109**: 433–8.

Guo, C.C., Hyett, M.P., Nguyen, V.T., Parker, G.B., and **Breakspear, M.J.** (2016). 'Distinct neurobiological signatures of brain connectivity in depression subtypes during natural viewing of emotionally salient films'. Psychological Medicine, **46**: 1535–45.

Gurung, R. and **Prata, D.P.** (2015). 'What is the impact of genome-wide supported risk variants for schizophrenia and bipolar disorder on brain structure and function? A systematic review'. Psychological Medicine, **45**: 2461–80.

Guscott R. and **Taylor L.** (1994). 'Lithium prophylaxis in recurrent affective illness: Efficacy, effectiveness and efficiency'. British Journal of Psychiatry, **164**: 741–6.

Guloksuz, S., van Nierop, M., Lieb, R., van Winkel, R., Wittchen, H.U., and **van Os, J.** (2015). 'Evidence that the presence of psychosis in non-psychotic disorder is environment-dependent and mediated by severity of non-psychotic psychopathology'. Psychological Medicine, **45**: 2389–401.

Guze S.B. (1992). *Why Psychiatry Is A Medical Specialty*. New York, NY: Oxford University Press.

Haddad, P.M. and **Anderson, I.M** (2007). 'Recognising and managing antidepressant discontinuation symptoms'. Advances in Psychiatric Treatment, **13**: 447–57.

Haddad, P.M. and **Sharma, S.G.** (2007). 'Adverse effects of atypical antipsychotics'. CNS Drugs, **21**: 911–36.

Hamani, C., Mayberg, H., Stone, S., Laxton, A., Haber, S., and **Lozano, A.M.** (2011). 'The subcallosal cingulate gyrus in the context of major depression'. Biological Psychiatry, **69**: 301–8.

Hafizi, S., Tseng, H.H., Rao, N., Selvanathan, T., Kenk, M., Bazinet, R.P., Suridjan, I., Wilson, A.A., Meyer, J.H., Remington, G., and **Houle, S.** (2016). 'Imaging microglial activation in untreated first-episode psychosis: A PET study with [18F] FEPPA'. American Journal of Psychiatry, **174**: 118–24.

Hamilton, I. (2017). 'Cannabis, psychosis and schizophrenia: Unravelling a complex interaction'. Addiction, **112**: 1653–57.

Hamilton, J.P., Farmer, M., Fogelman, P., and **Gotlib, I.H.** (2015). 'Depressive rumination, the default-mode network, and the dark matter of clinical neuroscience'. Biological Psychiatry, **78**: 224–30.

Hamilton, M. (1960). 'A rating scale for depression'. Journal of Neurology, Neurosurgery and Psychiatry, **23**: 56–62.

Hampton J. A. (2006). 'Concepts as prototypes'. Psychology of Learning and Motivation, **46**: 79–94.

Hampton J.R., Harrison M.J.G, Mitchell J.R.A., Prichard J.S., and **Seymour C.** (1975). 'Relative contributions of history-taking, physical examination, and laboratory investigation to diagnosis and management of medical outpatients'. British Medical Journal, **2**: 486–9.

Han, B.H., Sutin, D., Williamson, J.D., Davis, B.R., Piller, L.B., Pervin, H., Pressel, S.L., and **Blaum, C.S.** (2017). 'Effect of statin treatment vs usual care on primary cardiovascular prevention among older adults: The ALLHAT-LLT randomized clinical trial'. JAMA Internal Medicine, **177**: 955–65.

Harding, C.M. and **Zahniser, J.H.** (1994). 'Empirical correction of seven myths about schizophrenia with implications for treatment'. Acta Psychiatrica Scandinavica, **90**(s384): 140–6.

Hardy, S., Bastick, L., O'Neill-Kerr, A., Sabesan, P., Lankappa, S., and **Palaniyappan, L.** (2016). 'Transcranial magnetic stimulation in clinical practice'. British Journal of Psychiatric Advances, **22**: 373–9.

Harmer, C.J., Goodwin, G.M., and **Cowen, P.J.** (2009). 'Why do antidepressants take so long to work? A cognitive neuropsychological model of antidepressant drug action'. British Journal of Psychiatry, **195**: 102–8.

Harmer, C.J., Duman, R.S., and **Cowen, P.J.** (2017). 'How do antidepressants work? New perspectives for refining future treatment approaches'. Lancet. Psychiatry, **4**: 409–18.

Haro, J.M., Kamath, S.A., Ochoa, S.O., Novick, D., Rele, K., Fargas, A., Rodriguez, M.J., Rele, R., Orta, J., Kharbeng, A., and **Araya, S.** (2003). 'The Clinical Global Impression-Schizophrenia scale: A simple instrument to measure the diversity of symptoms present in schizophrenia'. Acta Psychiatrica Scandinavica, **107** (Suppl 416): 16–23.

Haro, J.M., Novick, D., Bertsch, J., Karagianis, J., Dossenbach, M., and **Jones, P.B.** (2011). 'Cross-national clinical and functional remission rates: Worldwide Schizophrenia

Outpatient Health Outcomes (W-SOHO) study'. British Journal of Psychiatry, **199**: 194–201.

Harris, E.C. and **Barraclough, B.** (1998). 'Excess mortality of mental disorder'. British Journal of Psychiatry, **173**: 11–53.

Harrison, G., Glazebrook, C., Brewin, J., Cantwell, R., Dalkin, T., Fox, R., Jones, P., and **Medley, I.** (1997). 'Increased incidence of psychotic disorders in migrants from the Caribbean to the United Kingdom'. Psychological Medicine, **27**: 799–806.

Harrison, J.R. and **Owen, M.J.** (2016). 'Alzheimer's disease: The amyloid hypothesis on trial'. British Journal of Psychiatry, **208**: 1–3.

Harrison, P.J. (2015). 'Recent genetic findings in schizophrenia and their therapeutic relevance'. Journal of Psychopharmacology, **29**: 85–96.

Harris, E.C. and **Barraclough, B.** (1997). 'Suicide as an outcome for mental disorders. A meta-analysis'. British Journal of Psychiatry, **170**: 205–28.

Harrow, M., Grossman, L.S., Herbener, E.S., and **Davies, E.W.** (2000). 'Ten-year outcome: Patients with schizoaffective disorders, schizophrenia, affective disorders and mood-incongruent psychotic symptoms'. British Journal of Psychiatry, **177**: 421–6.

Harrow, M., Jobe, T.H., and **Faull, R.N.** (2014). 'Does treatment of schizophrenia with antipsychotic medications eliminate or reduce psychosis? A 20-year multi-follow-up study'. Psychological Medicine, **44**: 3007–16.

Harvey R.A., Clark M.A., Finkel R., Rey J.A., and **Whalen K.** (2011). *Lippincott's Illustrated Reviews: Pharmacology*, 5th edn International edn. Philadelphia, PA: Lippincott, Williams and Wilkins.

Hay, S. and **Barbano, H.** (1972). 'Independent effects of maternal age and birth order on the incidence of selected congenital malformations'. Teratology, **6**: 271–9.

Haslam, N. (2003). 'Categorical versus dimensional models of mental disorder: The taxometric evidence'. Australian and New Zealand Journal of Psychiatry, **37**: 696–704.

Haslam, N., Holland, E., and **Kuppens, P.** (2012). 'Categories versus dimensions in personality and psychopathology: A quantitative review of taxometric research'. Psychological Medicine, **42**: 903–20.

Haslam, N. and **Kvaale, E.P.**, 2015. 'Biogenetic explanations of mental disorder: The mixed-blessings model'. Current Directions in Psychological Science, **24**: 399–404.

Hawton, K. and **Pirkis, J**, (2017). 'Suicide is a complex problem that requires a range of prevention initiatives and methods of evaluation'. British Journal of Psychiatry, **210**: 381–3.

Haynes L., Service O., Goldacre B., and Torgerson B. (2012). 'Developing Public Policy with Randomised Controlled Trials'. Available at: <https://www.gov.uk/government/uploads/system/uploads/attachment_data/file/62529/TLA-1906126.pdf>.

Hawton, K., Bergen, H., Simkin, S., Cooper, J., Waters, K., Gunnell, D., and **Kapur, N.** (2010). 'Toxicity of antidepressants: rates of suicide relative to prescribing and non-fatal overdose'. British Journal of Psychiatry, **196**: 354–8.

Hayes, J.F., Miles, J., Walters, K., King, M., and **Osborn, D.P.J.** (2015). 'A systematic review and meta-analysis of premature mortality in bipolar affective disorder'. Acta Psychiatrica Scandinavica, **13**: 417–25.

Healy D. (2015). 'Serotonin and depression'. British Medical Journal, **350**: h1771.

Hegarty, J.D., Baldessarini, R.J., Tohen, M., Waternaux, C., and **Oepen, G.** (1994). 'One hundred years of schizophrenia: A meta-analysis of the outcome literature'. American Journal of Psychiatry, **151**: 1409–16.

Hemingway, H. and **Marmot, M.** (1999). 'Psychosocial factors in the aetiology and prognosis of coronary heart disease: Systematic review of prospective cohort studies'. British Medical Journal, **318**: 1460–7.

Hengartner, M.P., Ajdacic-Gross, V., Wyss, C., Angst, J., and **Rössler, W.** (2016). 'Relationship between personality and psychopathology in a longitudinal community study: A test of the predisposition model'. Psychological Medicine, **46**: 1693–705.

Hengartner, M.P. and **Lehmann, S.N.** (2017). 'Why psychiatric research must abandon traditional diagnostic classification and adopt a fully dimensional scope: Two solutions to a persistent problem'. Frontiers in Psychiatry, **8**: 101.

Herman, J.L. (1992). 'Complex PTSD: A syndrome in survivors of prolonged and repeated trauma'. Journal of Traumatic Stress, **5**: 377–91.

Herry, C., Ferraguti, F., Singewald, N., Letzkus, J.J., Ehrlich, I. and **Lüthi, A.** (2010). 'Neuronal circuits of fear extinction'. European Journal of Neuroscience, **31**: 599–612.

Hert, M., Correll, C.U., Bobes, J., Cetkovich-Bakmas, M., Cohen, D.A.N., Asai, I., Detraux, J., Gautam, S., Moller, H.J., Ndetei, D.M., and **Newcomer, J.W.** (2011). 'Physical illness in patients with severe mental disorders. I. Prevalence, impact of medications and disparities in health care'. World Psychiatry, **10**: 52–77.

Heslin, M., Lomas, B., Lappin, J.M., Donoghue, K., Reininghaus, U., Onyejiaka, A., Croudace, T., Jones, P.B., Murray, R.M., Fearon, P., and **Dazzan, P.** (2015). 'Diagnostic change 10 years after a first episode of psychosis'. Psychological Medicine, **45**: 2757–69.

Hettema, J.M., Aggen, S.H., Kubarych, T.S., Neale, M.C., and **Kendler, K.S.** (2015). 'Identification and validation of mixed anxiety–depression'. Psychological Medicine, **45**: 3075–84.

Hickman, M., Vickerman, P., Macleod, J., Lewis, G., Zammit, S., Kirkbride, J., and **Jones, P.** (2009). 'If cannabis caused schizophrenia—how many cannabis users may need to be prevented in order to prevent one case of schizophrenia? England and Wales calculations'. Addiction, **104**: 1856–61.

Hieronymus, F., Emilsson, J.F., Nilsson, S., and **Eriksson, E.** (2016). 'Consistent superiority of selective serotonin reuptake inhibitors over placebo in reducing depressed mood in patients with major depression'. Molecular Psychiatry, **21**: 523–30.

Hill A. B. (1951). 'The Clinical Trial'. British Medical Bulletin, **7**: 278–82.

Hill A.B. (1952). 'The Clinical Trial'. New England Journal of Medicine, **247**: 115–19.

Hill A. B. (1965). 'The environment and disease: Association or causation?' Proceedings of the Royal Society of Medicine, **58**: 295–300.

Hill, S.K., Reilly, J.L., Keefe, R.S., Gold, J.M., Bishop, J.R., Gershon, E.S., Tamminga, C.A., Pearlson, G.D., Keshavan, M.S., and **Sweeney, J.A.**, (2013). Neuropsychological impairments in schizophrenia and psychotic bipolar disorder: Findings from the Bipolar-Schizophrenia Network on Intermediate Phenotypes (B-SNIP) study. American Journal of Psychiatry, **170**(11): 1275–84.

Hippisley-Cox, J., Coupland, C., Vinogradova, Y., Robson, J., May, M., and **Brindle, P.** (2007). 'Derivation and validation of QRISK, a new cardiovascular disease risk score for the United Kingdom: Prospective open cohort study'. British Medical Journal, **335**: 136–47.

Hippisley-Cox, J., Coupland, C., Vinogradova, Y., Robson, J., Minhas, R., Sheikh, A., and **Brindle, P.** (2008). 'Predicting cardiovascular risk in England and Wales: prospective derivation and validation of QRISK2'. British Medical Journal, **336**: 1475–82.

Ho, B.C., **Andreasen, N.C.**, **Ziebell, S.**, **Pierson, R.**, and **Magnotta, V.** (2011). 'Long-term antipsychotic treatment and brain volumes: a longitudinal study of first-episode schizophrenia'. Archives of General Psychiatry, **68**: 128–37.

Ho, C.S., **Zhang, M.W.**, **Mak, A.**, and **Ho, R.C.** (2014). 'Metabolic syndrome in psychiatry: advances in understanding and management'. British Journal of Psychiatric Advances, **20**: 101–12.

Hoenig, J. (1983). 'The concept of schizophrenia. Kraepelin–Bleuler–Schneider'. British Journal of Psychiatry, **142**: 547–56.

Hofler M. (2005). 'The Bradford Hill considerations on causality: A counterfactual perspective'. Emerging Themes in Epidemiology, **2**: 11–19.

Hohe-Schram, M., **Cording-T, C.**, **Schmid-Bode, W.**, **Wittchen, H.U.**, **Zaudig, M.**, and **von Zerssen, D.** (1989). 'The classification of functional psychoses and its implications for prognosis'. British Journal of Psychiatry, **154**: 467–72.

Holmes C., **Cairns N.**, **Lantos P.**, and **Mann A.** (1999). 'Validity of current clinical criteria for Alzheimer's disease, vascular dementia and dementia with Lewy bodies'. British Journal of Psychiatry, **174**: 45–50.

Holmes, S.E., **Hinz, R.**, **Drake, R.J.**, **Gregory, C.J.**, **Conen, S.**, **Matthews, J.C.**, **Anton-Rodriguez, J.M.**, **Gerhard, A.**, and **Talbot, P.S.** (2016). 'In vivo imaging of brain microglial activity in antipsychotic-free and medicated schizophrenia: A [11C](R)-PK11195 positron emission tomography study'. Molecular Psychiatry, **21**: 1672–9.

Holtforth, M.G., **Wyss, T.**, **Schulte, D.**, **Trachsel, M.**, and **Michalak, J.** (2009). 'Some like it specific: The difference between treatment goals of anxious and depressed patients'. Psychology and Psychotherapy: Theory, Research and Practice, **82**: 279–90.

Hopwood, C.J., **Thomas, K.M.**, **Markon, K.E.**, **Wright, A.G.**, and **Krueger, R.F.** (2012). 'DSM-5 personality traits and DSM–IV personality disorders'. Journal of Abnormal Psychology, **121**: 424–32.

Hotopf, M., **Hardy, R.**, and **Lewis, G.** (1997). 'Discontinuation rates of SSRIs and tricyclic antidepressants: A meta-analysis and investigation of heterogeneity'. British Journal of Psychiatry, **170**: 120–7.

Howes, O.D. and **Kapur, S.** (2009). 'The dopamine hypothesis of schizophrenia: Version III—the final common pathway'. Schizophrenia Bulletin, **35**: 549–62.

Howes, O.D., **Kambeitz, J.**, **Kim, E.**, **Stahl, D.**, **Slifstein, M.**, **Abi-Dargham, A.**, and **Kapur, S.** (2012). 'The nature of dopamine dysfunction in schizophrenia and what this means for treatment: Meta-analysis of imaging studies'. Archives of General Psychiatry, **69**: 776–86.

Howes, O.D. and **Kapur, S.** (2014). 'A neurobiological hypothesis for the classification of schizophrenia: Type A (hyperdopaminergic) and type B (normodopaminergic)'. British Journal of Psychiatry, **205**: 1–3.

Howick J., **Glasziou P.**, and **Aronson J.K.** (2009). 'The evolution of evidence hierarchies: What can Bradford Hill's "guidelines for causation" contribute?' Journal of Royal Society of Medicine, **102**: 186–94.

Huang, E.S., 2016. 'Management of diabetes mellitus in older people with comorbidities'. British Medical Journal, **353**: i2200.

Hucklenbroich, P. (2014). '"Disease entity" as the key theoretical concept of medicine'. Journal of Medicine and Philosophy, **39**: 609–33.

Hutchinson, G., **Takei, N.**, **Fahy, T.A.**, **Bhugra, D.**, **Gilvarry, C.**, **Moran, P.**, **Mallett, R.**, **Sham, P.**, **Leff, J.**, and **Murray, R.M.** (1996). 'Morbid risk of schizophrenia in first-degree relatives of white and African-Caribbean patients with psychosis'. British Journal of Psychiatry, **169**: 776–80.

Hughes V (2012). 'Microglia, the Constant Gardeners'. Nature, **485**: 570–2.

Hyde, C.L., Nagle, M.W., Tian, C., Chen, X., Paciga, S.A., Wendland, J.R., Tung, J.Y., Hinds, D.A., Perlis, R.H., and **Winslow, A.R.** (2016). 'Identification of 15 genetic loci associated with risk of major depression in individuals of European descent'. Nature Genetics, **48**: 1031–6.

Hyett, M.P., Breakspear, M.J., Friston, K.J., Guo, C.C., and **Parker, G.B.** (2015). 'Disrupted effective connectivity of cortical systems supporting attention and interoception in melancholia'. JAMA Psychiatry, **72**: 350–8.

Hyman S.E. (2010). 'The diagnosis of mental disorders: The problem of reification'. Annual Review Clinical Psychology, **6**: 155–79.

IGDA Workgroup (2003). 'International Guidelines Diagnostic Assessment 8: Idiographic (personalised) diagnostic formulation'. British Journal of Psychiatry, **182** (Suppl 45): s55–s57.

Insel, T.R., Cuthbert, B.N., Garvey, M.A., Heinssen, R.K., Pine, D.S., Quinn, K.J., Sanislow, C.A., and **Wang, P.S.** (2010). 'Research Domain Criteria (RDoC): Toward a new classification framework for research on mental disorders'. American Journal of Psychiatry, **167**: 748–51.

Ivbijaro, G. and **Goldberg, D.** (2013). 'Bodily distress syndrome (BDS): The evolution from medically unexplained symptoms (MUS)'. Mental Health in Family Medicine, **10**: 63–4.

Ivleva, E.I., Bidesi, A.S., Keshavan, M.S., Pearlson, G.D., Meda, S.A., Dodig, D., Moates, A.F., Lu, H., Francis, A.N., Tandon, N., and **Schretlen, D.J.** (2013). 'Gray matter volume as an intermediate phenotype for psychosis: Bipolar-Schizophrenia Network on Intermediate Phenotypes (B-SNIP)'. American Journal of Psychiatry, **170**: 1285–96.

Jääskeläinen, E., Juola, P., Hirvonen, N., McGrath, J.J., Saha, S., Isohanni, M., Veijola, J., and **Miettunen, J.** (2013). 'A systematic review and meta-analysis of recovery in schizophrenia'. Schizophrenia Bulletin, **39**: 1296–306.

Jablensky, A., Sartorius, N., Ernberg, G., Anker, M., Korten, A., Cooper, J.E., Day, R., and **Bertelsen, A.** (1992). 'Schizophrenia: manifestations, incidence and course in different cultures A World Health Organization ten-country study'. Psychological Medicine. Monograph Supplement, **20**: 1–97.

Jakobsen, J.C., Katakam, K.K., Schou, A., Hellmuth, S.G., Stallknecht, S.E., Leth-Møller, K., Iversen, M., Banke, M.B., Petersen, I.J., Klingenberg, S.L., and **Krogh, J.** (2017). 'Selective serotonin reuptake inhibitors versus placebo in patients with major depressive disorder. A systematic review with meta-analysis and trial sequential analysis'. BMC Psychiatry, **17**: 58.

Jacoby, A. and **Austin, J.K.** (2007). 'Social stigma for adults and children with epilepsy'. Epilepsia, **48**(Suppl 9): 6–9.

Jäger, M., Bottlender, R., Strauss, A., and **Möller, H.J.** (2004). 'Fifteen-year follow-up of ICD-10 schizoaffective disorders compared with schizophrenia and affective disorders'. Acta Psychiatrica Scandinavica, **109**: 30–7.

Jakobsen, J.C., Katakam, K.K., Schou, A., Hellmuth, S.G., Stallknecht, S.E., Leth-Møller, K., Iversen, M., Banke, M.B., Petersen, I.J., Klingenberg, S.L., and **Krogh, J.** (2017). 'Selective serotonin reuptake inhibitors versus placebo in patients with major depressive disorder. A systematic review with meta-analysis and trial sequential analysis'. BMC Psychiatry, **17**: 58.

Järvinen, T.L., Michaëlsson, K., Jokihaara, J., Collins, G.S., Perry, T.L., Mintzes, B., Musini, V., Erviti, J., Gorricho, J., Wright, J.M. and **Sievänen, H.** (2015). 'Overdiagnosis of bone fragility in the quest to prevent hip fracture'. British Medical Journal, **350**: h2088.

Jauhar, S., **McKenna, P. J.**, **Radua, J.**, **Fung, E.**, **Salvador, R.**, and **Laws, K. R.** (2014). 'Cognitive-behavioural therapy for the symptoms of schizophrenia: systematic review and meta-analysis with examination of potential bias'. British Journal of Psychiatry, **204**: 20–9.

Jauhar, S., **McKenna, P.J.**, and **Laws, K.R.**, (2016). NICE guidance on psychological treatments for bipolar disorder: Searching for the evidence. Lancet Psychiatry, **3**(4): 386–8.

Jefferson J.W. (1998). 'Effectiveness of lithium'. British Journal of Psychiatry, **172**: 364–5.

Jelovac, A., **Kolshus, E.**, and **McLoughlin, D.M.** (2013). 'Relapse following successful electroconvulsive therapy for major depression: A meta-analysis'. Neuropsychopharmacology, **38**: 2467–74.

Jenkins, R., **Lewis, G.**, **Bebbington, P.**, **Brugha, T.**, **Farrell, M.**, **Gill, B.**, and **Meltzer, H.** (1997). 'The National Psychiatric Morbidity surveys of Great Britain–initial findings from the household survey'. Psychological Medicine, **27**: 775–89.

Jenkins, R., **Bhugra, D.**, **Bebbington, P.**, **Brugha, T.**, **Farrell, M.**, **Coid, J.**, **Fryers, T.**, **Weich, S.**, **Singleton, N.**, and **Meltzer, H.** (2008). 'Debt, income and mental disorder in the general population'. Psychological Medicine, **38**: 1485–93.

Jensen, J.H., **Knorr, U.**, **Vinberg, M.**, **Kessing, L.V.**, and **Miskowiak, K.W.** (2016). 'Discrete neurocognitive subgroups in fully or partially remitted bipolar disorder: Associations with functional abilities'. Journal of Affective Disorders, **205**: 378–86.

Jeronimus, B.F., **Kotov, R.**, **Riese, H.**, and **Ormel, J.** (2016). 'Neuroticism's prospective association with mental disorders halves after adjustment for baseline symptoms and psychiatric history, but the adjusted association hardly decays with time: A meta-analysis on 59 longitudinal/prospective studies with 443 313 participants'. Psychological Medicine, **46**: 2883–906.

Jerrim, J., and **Vignoles, A.** (2015). 'The causal effect of East Asian "mastery" teaching methods on English children's mathematics skills' (Working Paper No. 15-05). Department of Quantitative Social Science–UCL Institute of Education, University College London.

Jin, H., **Shih, P.A.B.**, **Golshan, S.**, **Mudaliar, S.**, **Henry, R.**, **Glorioso, D.K.**, **Arndt, S.**, **Kraemer, H.C.**, and **Jeste, D.V.**, 2013 'Comparison of longer-term safety and effectiveness of four atypical antipsychotics in patients over age 40: A trial using equipoise-stratified randomization'. Journal of Clinical Psychiatry, **74**: 10–18.

Joas, E., **Karanti, A.**, **Song, J.**, **Goodwin, G.M.**, **Lichtenstein, P.**, and **Landén, M.** (2017). 'Pharmacological treatment and risk of psychiatric hospital admission in bipolar disorder'. British Journal of Psychiatry, **210**: 197–202.

Jobe, T.H. and **Harrow, M.** (2005). 'Long-term outcome of patients with schizophrenia: A review'. Canadian Journal of Psychiatry, **50**: 892–900.

Johansen, J.P. (2013). 'Neuroscience: Anxiety is the sum of its parts'. Nature, **496**: 174–5.

Johansson, M., **Jørgensen, K.J.**, **Getz, L.**, and **Moynihan, R.** (2016). '"Informed choice" in a time of too much medicine—no panacea for ethical difficulties'. British Medical Journal, **353**: i2230.

Johns, L.C., **Kompus, K.**, **Connell, M.**, **Humpston, C.**, **Lincoln, T.M.**, **Longden, E.**, **Preti, A.**, **Alderson-Day, B.**, **Badcock, J.C.**, **Cella, M.**, and **Fernyhough, C.** (2014). 'Auditory verbal hallucinations in persons with and without a need for care'. Schizophrenia Bulletin, **40**(Suppl 4): S255–S264.

Johnson, J.G., **Cohen, P.**, **Brown, J.**, **Smailes, E.M.**, and **Bernstein, D.P.** (1999). 'Childhood maltreatment increases risk for personality disorders during early adulthood'. Archives of General Psychiatry, **56**: 600–6.

Jonsson, U., **Alaie, I.**, **Parling, T.** and **Arnberg, F.K.** (2014). 'Reporting of harms in randomized controlled trials of psychological interventions for mental and behavioral disorders: a review of current practice'. Contemporary Clinical Trials, **38**: 1–8.

Johnstone, E.C., **Crow, T.J.**, **Frith, C.D.**, and **Owens, D.G.** (1988). 'The Northwick Park "functional" psychosis study: Diagnosis and treatment response'. Lancet, **332**: 119–25.

Jolley D. (2015). 'Depressive pseudodementia: How "pseudo" is it really?' Old Age Psychiatrist Newsletter of the Old Age Faculty of the Royal College of Psychiatrists Issue, **62**: 30–7.

Jones, N. (2012). 'Antipsychotic medications, psychological side effects and treatment engagement'. Issues in Mental Health Nursing, **33**: 492–3.

Joukamaa, M., **HeliÖvaara, M.**, **Knekt, P.**, **Aromaa, A.**, **Raitasalo, R.**, and **Lehtinen, V.** (2001). 'Mental disorders and cause-specific mortality'. British Journal of Psychiatry, **179**: 498–502.

Judd, L.L. (1997). 'The clinical course of unipolar major depressive disorders'. Archives of General Psychiatry, **54**: 989–91.

Judd, L.L., **Akiskal, H.S.**, **Maser, J.D.**, **Zeller, P.J.**, **Endicott, J.**, **Coryell, W.**, **Paulus, M.P.**, **Kunovac, J.L.**, **Leon, A.C.**, **Mueller, T.I.**, and **Rice, J.A.** (1998). 'A prospective 12-year study of subsyndromal and syndromal depressive symptoms in unipolar major depressive disorders'. Archives of General Psychiatry, **55**: 694–700.

Kahn, R.S., **Fleischhacker, W.W.**, **Boter, H.**, **Davidson, M.**, **Vergouwe, Y.**, **Keet, I.P.**, **Gheorghe, M.D.**, **Rybakowski, J.K.**, **Galderisi, S.**, **Libiger, J.**, and **Hummer, M.** (2008). 'Effectiveness of antipsychotic drugs in first-episode schizophrenia and schizophreniform disorder: An open randomised clinical trial'. Lancet, **371**: 1085–97.

Kales, H.C., **Gitlin, L.N.**, and **Lyketsos, C.G.** (2015). 'State of the art review: Assessment and management of behavioral and psychological symptoms of dementia'. British Medical Journal, **350**: h369.

Kambeitz, J., **Abi-Dargham, A.**, **Kapur, S.**, and **Howes, O.D.** (2014). 'Alterations in cortical and extrastriatal subcortical dopamine function in schizophrenia: Systematic review and meta-analysis of imaging studies'. British Journal of Psychiatry, **204**: 420–9.

Kambeitz, J., **Kambeitz-Ilankovic, L.**, **Leucht, S.**, **Wood, S.**, **Davatzikos, C.**, **Malchow, B.**, **Falkai, P.**, and **Koutsouleris, N.** (2015). 'Detecting neuroimaging biomarkers for schizophrenia: A meta-analysis of multivariate pattern recognition studies'. Neuropsychopharmacology, **40**: 1742–51.

Kamenov, K., **Twomey, C.**, **Cabello, M.**, **Prina, A.M.**, and **Ayuso-Mateos, J.L.** (2017). 'The efficacy of psychotherapy, pharmacotherapy and their combination on functioning and quality of life in depression: A meta-analysis'. Psychological Medicine, **47**: 414–25.

Kanai, T., **Takeuchi, H.**, **Furukawa, T.A.**, **Yoshimura, R.**, **Imaizumi, T.**, **Kitamura, T.** and **Takahashi, K.**, 2003. Time to recurrence after recovery from major depressive episodes and its predictors. Psychological Medicine, **33**(5): 839–45.

Kannel, W.B., **McGee, D.**, and **Gordon, T.** (1976). A general cardiovascular risk profile: the Framingham study'. American Journal of Cardiology, **38**: 46–51.

Kaplan, G.A. and **Keil, J.E.** (1993). 'Socioeconomic factors and cardiovascular disease: a review of the literature'. Circulation, **88**: 1973–98.

Kaplan, M.H. and **Feinstein, A.R.** (1974). 'The importance of classifying initial co-morbidity in evaluating the outcome of diabetes mellitus'. Journal of Chronic Diseases, **27**: 387–404.

Kaplan, R.M. and **Irvin, V.L.** (2015). 'Likelihood of null effects of large NHLBI clinical trials has increased over time'. PLoS One, **10**: e0132382.

Kapur, S. and **Seeman, P.** (2001). 'Does fast dissociation from the dopamine D2 receptor explain the action of atypical antipsychotics?: A new hypothesis'. American Journal of Psychiatry, **158**: 360–9.

Kapur, S. (2003). 'Psychosis as a state of aberrant salience: A framework linking biology, phenomenology, and pharmacology in schizophrenia'. American Journal of Psychiatry, **160**: 13–23.

Kapur, S., Agid, O., Mizrahi, R., and **Li, M.** (2006). 'How antipsychotics work—from receptors to reality'. NeuroRx, **3**: 10–21.

Kapur, S., Phillips, A.G., and **Insel, T.R.** (2012). 'Why has it taken so long for biological psychiatry to develop clinical tests and what to do about it?' Molecular Psychiatry, **17**: 1174–9.

Kasper, S., Moises, H.W., and **Beckmann, H.** (1981). 'The anticholinergic biperiden in depressive disorders'. Pharmacopsychiatry, **14**: 195–8.

Kasper, S. Dold, M. (2015). Factors contributing to the increasing placebo response in antidepressant trials'. World Psychiatry, **14**: 304–6.

Kassi, E., Pervanidou, P., Kaltsas, G., and **Chrousos, G.** (2011). 'Metabolic syndrome: definitions and controversies'. BMC Medicine, **9**: 48–60.

Katon, W.J. and **Walker, E.A.** (1998). 'Medically unexplained symptoms in primary care'. Journal of Clinical Psychiatry, **59**: 15–21.

Katon W.J. (2011). 'Epidemiology and treatment of depression in patients with chronic medical illness'. Dialogues in Clinical Neuroscience, **13**: 7–23.

Kay, S.R., **Flszbein, A.**, and **Opfer, L.A.** (1987). 'The positive and negative syndrome scale (PANSS) for schizophrenia'. Schizophrenia Bulletin, **13**: 261–76.

Kaymaz, N. and **Van Os, J.** (2010). 'Extended psychosis phenotype–yes: single continuum–unlikely', Psychological Medicine, **40**: 1963–6.

Kazanetz, E.P. (1989). 'The delineation of schizophrenia from other psychiatric illnesses'. British Journal of Psychiatry, **155**: 160–5.

Keefe, R.S. and **Fenton, W.S.** (2007). 'How should DSM-V criteria for schizophrenia include cognitive impairment?' Schizophrenia Bulletin, **33**: 912–20.

Keefe, R.S., Haig, G.M., Marder, S.R., Harvey, P.D., Dunayevich, E., Medalia, A., Davidson, M., Lombardo, I., Bowie, C.R., Buchanan, R.W., and **Bugarski-Kirola, D.** (2015). 'Report on ISCTM consensus meeting on clinical assessment of response to treatment of cognitive impairment in schizophrenia'. Schizophrenia Bulletin, **42**: 19–33.

Keeley, J.W. (2015). The background assumptions of psychological assessment and psychiatric diagnosis. In: P. Zachar, D.S. Stoyanov, M. Aragona, and A. Jablensky (eds), *Alternative Perspectives on Psychiatric Validation—DSM, ICD, RDoC, and Beyond*. Oxford: Oxford University Press, pp. 94–111.

Kelly, S., van Velzen, L.S., Hatton, S., Aleman, A., Baune, B.T., Cheng, Y., Dannlowski, U., Deppe, M., Frodl, T., Glahn, D., and **Gotlib, I.H.** (2016). 'White matter differences in major depression: Meta-analytic findings from enigma-MDD DTI'. Bipolar Disorders, **18**: 114–15.

Kellner, C.H., Husain, M.M., Knapp, R.G., McCall, W.V., Petrides, G., Rudorfer, M.V., Young, R.C., Sampson, S., McClintock, S.M., Mueller, M., and **Prudic, J.** (2016). 'A novel strategy for continuation ECT in geriatric depression: Phase 2 of the PRIDE study'. American Journal of Psychiatry, **173**: 1110–18.

Kendell, R.E. and **Gourlay, J.** (1970). 'The clinical distinction between psychotic and neurotic depressions'. British Journal of Psychiatry, **117**: 257–60.

Kendell, R.E., Cooper, J.E., Gourlay, A.J., Copeland, J.R.M., Sharpe, L., and **Gurland, B.J.** (1971). 'Diagnostic criteria of American and British psychiatrists'. Archives of General Psychiatry, **25**: 123–30.

Kendell, R.E. (1976). 'The classification of depression. A review of contemporary confusion'. British Journal of Psychiatry, **129**: 15–28.

Kendell R.E. (1983). Chapter 7 The principles of classification in relation to disease. In: M. Shepherd and O.L. Zangwill (eds), *Handbook of Psychiatry 1: General Psychopathology*. Cambridge: Cambridge University Press, pp. 191–8.

Kendell R.E. and **Jablensky A.** (2003). 'Distinguishing between validity and utility of psychiatric diagnoses'. American Journal of Psychiatry, **160**: 4–12.

Kendler K.S. (1980). 'The nosologic validity of paranoia (simple delusional disorder)'. Archives of General Psychiatry, **37**: 699–706.

Kendler K.S. (1990). 'Towards a scientific psychiatric nosology: Strength and limitations'. Archives of General Psychiatry, **47**: 969–73.

Kendler, K.S., Neale, M.C., Kessler, R.C., Heath, A.C., and **Eaves, L.J.** (1993). 'A test of the equal-environment assumption in twin studies of psychiatric illness'. Behavior Genetics, **23**: 21–7.

Kendler, K.S., Gardner, C.O., Neale, M.C. and **Prescott, C.A.** (2001). 'Genetic risk factors for major depression in men and women: Similar or different heritabilities and same or partly distinct genes?' Psychological Medicine, **31**: 605–16.

Kendler, K.S., Prescott, C.A., Myers, J., and **Neale, M.C.** (2003). 'The structure of genetic and environmental risk factors for common psychiatric and substance use disorders in men and women'. Archives of General Psychiatry, **60**: 929–37.

Kendler, K.S., Kuhn, J. and Prescott, C.A. (2004). 'The interrelationship of neuroticism, sex, and stressful life events in the prediction of episodes of major depression'. American Journal of Psychiatry, **70**: 599–607.

Kendler, K.S., Gatz, M., Gardner, C.O., and **Pedersen, N.L.** (2006). 'A Swedish national twin study of lifetime major depression'. American Journal of Psychiatry, **163**: 109–14.

Kendler, K.S., Aggen, S.H., Knudsen, G.P., Røysamb, E., Neale, M.C., and **Reichborn-Kjennerud, T.** (2011a). 'The structure of genetic and environmental risk factors for syndromal and subsyndromal common DSM-IV axis I and all axis II disorders'. American Journal of Psychiatry, **168**: 29–39.

Kendler, K.S., Zachar, P., and **Craver, C.** (2011b). 'What kinds of things are psychiatric disorders?' Psychological Medicine, **41**: 1143–50.

Kendler K.S. and **Parnas J.** (eds) (2012). *Philosophical Issues in Psychiatry II: Nosology*. Oxford: Oxford University Press.

Kendler, K.S. (2012). 'The dappled nature of causes of psychiatric illness: Replacing the organic–functional/hardware–software dichotomy with empirically based pluralism'. Molecular Psychiatry, **17**: 377–88.

Kendler, K.S., Aggen, S.H., and **Neale, M.C.** (2013). 'Evidence for multiple genetic factors underlying DSM-IV criteria for major depression'. JAMA Psychiatry, **70**: 599–607.

Kendler, K.S. and **Solomon, M.** (2016). 'Expert consensus v. evidence-based approaches in the revision of the DSM'. Psychological Medicine, **46**: 2255–62.

Kendler, K.S. (2016). 'The phenomenology of major depression and the representativeness and nature of DSM criteria'. American Journal of Psychiatry, **178**: 771–80.

Kendler, K.S. (2017). 'DSM disorders and their criteria: How should they inter-relate?' Psychological Medicine, **47**: 2054–60.

Kennard, L. and **O'Shaughnessy, K.M.** (2016). 'Treating hypertension in patients with medical comorbidities'. British Medical Journal, **352**: i101.

Kennedy, N., **Abbott, R.**, and **Paykel, E.S.** (2003). 'Remission and recurrence of depression in the maintenance era: long-term outcome in a Cambridge cohort'. Psychological Medicine, **33**: 827–38.

Kerner, N. and **Prudic, J.** (2014). 'Current electroconvulsive therapy practice and research in the geriatric population'. Neuropsychiatry, **4**: 33–54.

Kessing, L.V. (2004). 'Severity of depressive episodes according to ICD-10: Prediction of risk of relapse and suicide'. British Journal of Psychiatry, **184**: 153–6.

Kessing, L.V., **Hansen, M.G.**, **Andersen, P.K.**, and **Angst, J.** (2004). 'The predictive effect of episodes on the risk of recurrence in depressive and bipolar disorders: A life-long perspective'. Acta Psychiatrica Scandinavica, **109**: 339–44.

Kessing, L.V. (2005). 'Diagnostic stability in depressive disorder as according to ICD-10 in clinical practice'. Psychopathology, **38**: 32–7.

Kessing, L.V., **Gerds, T.A.**, **Feldt-Rasmussen, B.**, **Andersen, P.K.**, and **Licht, R.W.** (2015). 'Use of lithium and anticonvulsants and the rate of chronic kidney disease: A nationwide population-based study'. JAMA Psychiatry, **72**: 1182–91.

Kessler, R.C., **Sonnega, A.**, **Bromet, E.**, **Hughes, M.**, and **Nelson, C.B.** (1995). 'Posttraumatic stress disorder in the National Comorbidity Survey'. Archives of General Psychiatry, **52**: 1048–60.

Kessler, R.C. (1997). 'The effects of stressful life events on depression'. Annual Review of Psychology, **48**: 191–214.

Kessler, R.C., **Berglund, P.**, **Demler, O.**, **Jin, R.**, **Koretz, D.**, **Merikangas, K.R.**, **Rush, A.J.**, **Walters, E.E.**, and **Wang, P.S.** (2003). 'The epidemiology of major depressive disorder: Results from the National Comorbidity Survey Replication (NCS-R)'. Journal of American Medical Association, **289**: 3095–105.

Kessler, R.C., **Chiu, W.T.**, **Demler, O.**, and **Walters, E.E.** (2005). 'Prevalence, severity, and comorbidity of 12-month DSM-IV disorders in the National Comorbidity Survey replication'. Archives of General Psychiatry, **62**: 617–27.

Keyloun, K.R., **Hansen, R.N.**, **Hepp, Z.**, **Gillard, P.**, **Thase, M.E.**, and **Devine, E.B.** (2017). 'Adherence and persistence across antidepressant therapeutic classes: A retrospective claims analysis among insured US patients with major depressive disorder (MDD)'. CNS Drugs, **31**: 421–2.

Khan, A. and **Brown, W.A.** (2015). 'Antidepressants versus placebo in major depression: An overview'. World Psychiatry, **14**: 294–300.

Khan, A., **Fahl Mar, K.**, **Faucett, J.**, **Khan Schilling, S.**, and **Brown, W.A.** (2017). 'Has the rising placebo response impacted antidepressant clinical trial outcome? Data from the US Food and Drug Administration 1987–2013'. World Psychiatry, **16**: 181–92.

Kiecolt-Glaser, J.K., **Derry, H.M.**, and **Fagundes, C.P.** (2015). 'Inflammation: Depression fans the flames and feasts on the heat'. American Journal of Psychiatry, **172**: 1075–91.

Kienle G.S. and **Kiene H.** (1996). "Placebo effect and placebo concept: a critical methodological and conceptual analysis of reports on the magnitude of the placebo effect." Alternative Therapies in Health and Medicine, **2**: 39–54.

Kienle G.S. and **Kiene H.** (1997). 'The powerful placebo effect: Fact or fiction?' Journal of Clinical Epidemiology, **50**: 1311–18.

Kim, W., Woo, Y.S., Chae, J.H., and **Bahk, W.M.** (2011). 'The diagnostic stability of DSM-IV diagnoses: An examination of major depressive disorder, bipolar I disorder, and schizophrenia in Korean patients'. Clinical Psychopharmacology and Neuroscience, **9**: 117–21.

Kinderman P., Read J., Moncrieff J., and **Bentall R.** (2013). 'Drop the language of disorder'. Evidence Based Mental Health, **16**: 2–3.

Kinderman, P., Schwannauer, M., Pontin, E., and **Tai, S.** (2013). 'Psychological processes mediate the impact of familial risk, social circumstances and life events on mental health'. PloS One, **8**: e76564.

Kincaid, H. (2008). 'Do We Need Theory to Study Disease?: Lessons from cancer research and their implications for mental illness'. Perspectives in Biology and Medicine, **51**: 367–78.

Kirkbride, J.B. (2017). 'Migration and psychosis: Our smoking lung?' World Psychiatry, **16**: 119–120.

Kirsch, I. (2005). 'Placebo psychotherapy: synonym or oxymoron?' Journal of Clinical Psychology, **61**: 791–803.

Kirsch, I., Deacon, B.J., Huedo-Medina, T.B., Scoboria, A., Moore, T.J., and **Johnson, B.T.** (2008). 'Initial severity and antidepressant benefits: A meta-analysis of data submitted to the Food and Drug Administration'. PLoS Medicine, **5**: e45.

Kirk, S.A. and Kutchins, H. (1994). 'The myth of the reliability of DSM'. Journal of Mind and Behavior, **15**: 71–86.

Kirkbride, J.B., Barker, D., Cowden, F., Stamps, R., Yang, M., Jones, P.B., and **Coid, J.W.** (2008). 'Psychoses, ethnicity and socio-economic status'. British Journal of Psychiatry, **193**: 18–24.

Kirov, G., Rees, E., and **Walters, J.** (2015). 'What a psychiatrist needs to know about copy number variants'. British Journal of Psychiatric Advances, **2**: 157–63.

Kisely, S., Goldberg, D., and **Simon, G.** (1997). 'A comparison between somatic symptoms with and without clear organic cause: results of an international study'. Psychological Medicine, **27**: 1011–19.

Kleinman, A. (1987). 'Anthropology and psychiatry. The role of culture in cross-cultural research on illness'. British Journal of Psychiatry, **151**: 447–54.

Kleinman, A. (2004). 'Culture and depression'. New England Journal of Medicine, **351**: 951–3.

Klingberg, S., Wittorf, A., Meisner, C., Wölwer, W., Wiedemann, G., Herrlich, J., Bechdolf, A., Müller, B.W., Sartory, G., Wagner, M., and **Kircher, T.** (2010). 'Cognitive behavioural therapy versus supportive therapy for persistent positive symptoms in psychotic disorders: The POSITIVE Study, a multicenter, prospective, single-blind, randomised controlled clinical trial'. Trials, **11**: 123.

Koenigs, M. (2012). 'The role of prefrontal cortex in psychopathy'. Reviews in the Neurosciences, **23**: 253–62.

Kollias, G., Douni, E., Kassiotis, G., and **Kontoyiannis, D.** (1999). 'The function of tumour necrosis factor and receptors in models of multi-organ inflammation, rheumatoid arthritis, multiple sclerosis and inflammatory bowel disease'. Annals of the Rheumatic Diseases, **58**: (Suppl 1): I32–9.

Kolar, D. (2017). 'Current status of electroconvulsive therapy for mood disorders: A clinical review'. Evidence-Based Mental Health, **20**: 12–14.

Kolshus, E., Jelovac, A., and **McLoughlin, D.M.** (2017). 'Bitemporal v. high-dose right unilateral electroconvulsive therapy for depression: A systematic review and meta-analysis of randomized controlled trials'. Psychological Medicine, **47**: 518–30.

Koran, L.M. (1975a). 'The reliability of clinical methods, data and judgments (First of Two Parts)'. New England Journal of Medicine, **293**: 642–6.

Koran, L.M. (1975b). 'The reliability of clinical methods, data and judgments (Second of Two Parts)'. New England Journal of Medicine, **293**: 695–701.

Kotov, R., Gamez, W., Schmidt, F., and **Watson, D.** (2010). 'Linking "big" personality traits to anxiety, depressive, and substance use disorders: A meta-analysis'. Psychological Bulletin, **136**: 768–821.

Kotov, R., Ruggero, C.J., Krueger, R.F., Watson, D., Yuan, Q., and **Zimmerman, M.** (2011). 'New dimensions in the quantitative classification of mental illness'. Archives of General Psychiatry, **68**: 1003–11.

Kotov, R., Leong, S.H., Mojtabai, R., Erlanger, A.C.E., Fochtmann, L.J., Constantino, E., Carlson, G.A., and **Bromet, E.J.** (2013). 'Boundaries of schizoaffective disorder: revisiting Kraepelin'. JAMA Psychiatry, **70**: 1276–86.

Kotov, R., Krueger, R.F., Watson, D., Achenbach, T.M., Althoff, R.R., Bagby, R.M., Brown, T.A., Carpenter, W.T., Caspi, A., Clark, L.A., and **Eaton, N.R.** (2017). 'The Hierarchical Taxonomy of Psychopathology (HiTO): A dimensional alternative to traditional nosologies'. Journal of Abnormal Psychology, **126**: 454–77.

Kraaij, V., Arensman, E., and **Spinhoven, P.** (2002). 'Negative life events and depression in elderly persons a meta-analysis'. Journals of Gerontology Series B: Psychological Sciences and Social Sciences, **57**: 87–94.

Kraemer, H.C., Noda, A., and **O'Hara, R.** (2004). 'Categorical versus dimensional approaches to diagnosis: Methodological challenges'. Journal of Psychiatric Research, **38**: 17–25.

Kraemer, H.C., Kupfer, D.J., Clarke, D.E., Narrow, W.E., and **Regier, D.A.** (2012). 'DSM-5: How reliable is reliable enough?' American Journal of Psychiatry, **169**: 13–15.

Kraepelin, E. and **Diefendorf, A.R.** (1904/1907). *Clinical Psychiatry; A Text-Book for Students and Physicians*, 7th edn. New York, NY: The Macmillan Company.

Kraepelin E. (1921). *Manic Depressive Insanity and Paranoia*. Edinburgh: Livingstone.

Krawiecka, M., Goldberg, D., and **Vaughan, M.** (1977). 'A standardized psychiatric assessment scale for rating chronic psychotic patients'. Acta Psychiatrica Scandinavica, **55**: 299–308.

Krueger, R.F. (1999). 'The structure of common mental disorders'. Archives of General Psychiatry, **56**: 921–6.

Kulhara, P., Shah, R., and **Grover, S.** (2009). 'Is the course and outcome of schizophrenia better in the "developing'world?"' Asian Journal of Psychiatry, **2**: 55–62.

Kulkarni, J. (2017). 'Complex PTSD: A better description for borderline personality disorder?' Australasian Psychiatry, **25**(4): 333–5.

Kunz, M., Cereser, K.M., Goi, P.D., Fries, G.R., Teixeira, A.L., Fernandes, B.S., Belmonte-de-Abreu, P.S., Kauer-Sant'Anna, M., Kapczinski, F., and **Gama, C.S.** (2011). 'Serum levels of IL-6, IL-10 and TNF-α in patients with bipolar disorder and schizophrenia: Differences in pro-and anti-inflammatory balance'. Revista Brasileira de Psiquiatria, **33**: 268–74.

Lahey, B.B., Applegate, B., Hakes, J.K., Zald, D.H., Hariri, A.R., and **Rathouz, P.J.** (2012). 'Is there a general factor of prevalent psychopathology during adulthood?' Journal of Abnormal Psychology, **121**: 971–77.

Lahey, B.B., Zald, D.H., Hakes, J.K., Krueger, R.F., and **Rathouz, P.J.** (2014). 'Patterns of heterotypic continuity associated with the cross-sectional correlational structure of prevalent mental disorders in adults'. JAMA Psychiatry, **71**: 989–96.

Łakuta, P., Marcinkiewicz, K., Bergler-Czop, B., and **Brzezińska-Wcisło, L.** (2017). 'How does stigma affect people with psoriasis?' Advances in Dermatology and Allergology, **34**: 36–41.

Lambert, M., Naber, D., Schacht, A., Wagner, T., Hundemer, H.P., Karow, A., Huber, C.G., Suarez, D., Haro, J.M., Novick, D., and **Dittmann, R.W.** (2008). 'Rates and predictors of remission and recovery during 3 years in 392 never-treated patients with schizophrenia'. Acta Psychiatrica Scandinavica, **118**: 220–9.

Landin-Romero, R., McKenna, P.J., Romaguera, A., Álvarez-Moya, E., Sarró, S., Aguirre, C., Sarri, C., Compte, A., Bosque, C., Salvador, R., and **Pomarol-Clotet, E.** (2016). 'Examining the continuum of psychosis: Frequency and characteristics of psychotic-like symptoms in relatives and non-relatives of patients with schizophrenia'. Schizophrenia Research. Available at: <http://www.sciencedirect.com/science/article/pii/S0920996416303309>.

Laruelle, M. and **Abi-Dargham, A.** (1999). 'Dopamine as the wind of the psychotic fire: New evidence from brain imaging studies'. Journal of Psychopharmacology, **13**: 358–71.

Launer, J., 2005. 'Anna O and the "talking cure"'. Quarterly Journal of Medicine, **98**(6): 465–6.

Laupacis, A., Sackett, D.L., and **Roberts, R.S.** (1988). 'An assessment of clinically useful measures of the consequences of treatment'. New England Journal of Medicine, **318**: 1728–33.

Law, H., Carter, L., Sellers, R., Emsley, R., Byrne, R., Davies, L., French, P., Haddad, P.M., Pitt, E., Pyle, M., and **Shiers, D.** (2017). 'A pilot randomised controlled trial comparing antipsychotic medication, to cognitive behavioural therapy to a combination of both in people with psychosis: Rationale, study design and baseline data of the COMPARE trial'. Psychosis, 1–12.

Lawrie S.M. (2015). 'Patients need reliable facts and figures about antipsychotics'. British Journal of Psychiatric Advances, **21**: 85–7.

Laws, K. and **McKenna, P.** (2014). 'Cognitive therapy for patients with schizophrenia'. Lancet, **384**: 399.

LeDoux, J.E. and **Pine, D.S.** (2016). 'Using neuroscience to help understand fear and anxiety: A two-system framework'. American Journal of Psychiatry, **173**: 1083–93.

Le Fanu, J. (2012). 'Mathematics is bad for you: Population risk reduction medicalises us all'. British Medical Journal, **344**: e2612.

Lenzer, J. and **Brownlee, S.** (2008). 'An untold story?' British Medical Journal, **336**: 532–4.

Lepping, P., Sambhi, R.S., Whittington, R., Lane, S., and **Poole, R.** (2011). 'Clinical relevance of findings in trials of antipsychotics: Systematic review'. British Journal of Psychiatry, **198**: 341–5.

Lesh, T.A., Tanase, C., Geib, B.R., Niendam, T.A., Yoon, J.H., Minzenberg, M.J., Ragland, J.D., Solomon, M., and **Carter, C.S.** (2015). 'A multimodal analysis of antipsychotic effects on brain structure and function in first-episode schizophrenia'. JAMA Psychiatry, **72**: 226–34.

Leucht, S., Kane, J.M., Etschel, E., Kissling, W., Hamann, J., and **Engel, R.R.** (2006). 'Linking the PANSS, BPRS, and CGI: Clinical implications'. Neuropsychopharmacology, **31**: 2318–25.

Leucht, S., Arbter, D., Engel, R.R., Kissling, W., and **Davis, J.M.** (2009). 'How effective are second-generation antipsychotic drugs? A meta-analysis of placebo-controlled trials'. Molecular Psychiatry, **14**: 429–47.

Leucht S., Tardy M., Komossa K., Heres S., Kissling W., Salanti G., and **Davis J.M.** (2012a). 'Antipsychotic drugs versus placebo for relapse prevention in schizophrenia: A systematic review and meta-analysis'. Lancet, **379**: 2063–71.

Leucht, S., **Hierl, S.**, **Kissling, W.**, **Dold, M.**, and **Davis, J.M.** (2012b). 'Putting the efficacy of psychiatric and general medicine medication into perspective: Review of meta-analyses'. British Journal of Psychiatry, **200**: 97–106.

Leucht, S., **Cipriani, A.**, **Spineli, L.**, **Mavridis, D.**, **Örey, D.**, **Richter, F.**, **Samara, M.**, **Barbui, C.**, **Engel, R.R.**, **Geddes, J.R.**, and **Kissling, W.** (2013a). 'Comparative efficacy and tolerability of 15 antipsychotic drugs in schizophrenia: A multiple-treatments meta-analysis'. Lancet, **382**: 951–62.

Leucht, S., **Fennema, H.**, **Engel, R.**, **Kaspers–Janssen, M.**, **Lepping, P.**, and **Szegedi, A.** (2013b). 'What does the HAMD mean?' Journal of Affective Disorders, **148**: 243–8.

Leucht S., **Helfer B.**, **Dold M.**, **Kissling W.**, and **McGrath J.J.** (2015a). 'Lithium for schizophrenia'. Cochrane Database of Systematic Reviews, **10**: CD003834.

Leucht, S., **Helfer, B.**, **Gartlehner, G.**, and **Davis, J.M.** (2015). 'How effective are common medications: a perspective based on meta-analyses of major drugs'. BMC Medicine, **13**: 253.

Leucht, S. and **Davis, J.M.** (2017). 'Do antipsychotic drugs lose their efficacy for relapse prevention over time?' British Journal of Psychiatry, **211**: 127–9.

Leucht, S., **Leucht, C.**, **Huhn, M.**, **Chaimani, A.**, **Mavridis, D.**, **Helfer, B.**, **Samara, M.**, **Rabaioli, M.**, **Bächer, S.**, **Cipriani, A.**, and **Geddes, J.R.** (2017). 'Sixty years of placebo-controlled antipsychotic drug trials in acute schizophrenia: Systematic review, Bayesian meta-analysis, and meta-regression of efficacy predictors'. American Journal of Psychiatry, **174**: 927–42.

Leuchter, A.F., **Hunter, A.M.**, **Tartter, M.**, and **Cook, I.A.** (2014). 'Role of pill-taking, expectation and therapeutic alliance in the placebo response in clinical trials for Its Galatzer-major depression'. British Journal of Psychiatry, **205**: 443–9.

Lewine, R., **Renders, R.O.**, **Kirchhofer, M.A.**, **Monsour, A.**, and **Watt, N.O.** (1982). 'The empirical heterogeneity of first rank symptoms in schizophrenia'. British Journal of Psychiatry, **140**: 498–502.

Lewis, A. (1953). 'Health as a social concept'. British Journal of Sociology, **4**: 109–24. **Lewis, G.**, and **Appleby, L.** (1988). 'Personality disorder: The patients psychiatrists dislike'. British Journal of Psychiatry, **153**: 44–9.

Lewis, S. (1992). 'Sex and schizophrenia: Vive la difference'. British Journal of Psychiatry, **16**: 445–50.

Lewis, S.J. (2016). 'Fifty years of Parkinson's disease: One step forwards, two steps back?' British Journal of Hospital Medicine, 77: 560–4.

Li, L., **Geraghty, O.C.**, **Mehta, Z.**, **Rothwell, P.M.**, and **Study, O.V.** (2017). 'Age-specific risks, severity, time course, and outcome of bleeding on long-term antiplatelet treatment after vascular events: A population-based cohort study'. Lancet, **390**: 490–9.

Li, M., **Fletcher, P.J.**, and **Kapur, S.** (2007). 'Time course of the antipsychotic effect and the underlying behavioral mechanisms'. Neuropsychopharmacology, **32**: 263–72.

Li, M., **D'arcy, C.**, and **Meng, X.** (2016). 'Maltreatment in childhood substantially increases the risk of adult depression and anxiety in prospective cohort studies: Systematic review, meta-analysis, and proportional attributable fractions'. Psychological Medicine, **46**: 717–30.

Li, Z., **Xiang, Y.**, **Chen, J.**, **Li, Q.**, **Shen, J.**, **Liu, Y.**, **Li, W.**, **Xing, Q.**, **Wang, Q.**, **Wang, L.**, and **Feng, G.** (2015). 'Loci with genome-wide associations with schizophrenia in the Han Chinese population'. British Journal of Psychiatry, **207**: 490–4.

Lichtenstein, P., **Yip, B.H.**, **Björk, C.**, **Pawitan, Y.**, **Cannon, T.D.**, **Sullivan, P.F.**, and **Hultman, C.M.** (2009). 'Common genetic determinants of schizophrenia and bipolar disorder in Swedish families: A population-based study'. Lancet, **373**: 234–9.

Lichtman J.H., Froelicher E.S., Blumenthal, J.A., Carney, R.M., Doering, L.V., Frasure-Smith, N., Freedland, K.E., Jaffe, A.S., Leifheit-Limson, E.C., Sheps, D.S., and **Vaccarino, V.** (2014). 'Depression as a risk factor for poor prognosis among patients with acute coronary syndrome: Systematic review and recommendations'. Circulation, **129**: 1350–69.

Lidz, C.W. (1998). 'Coercion in psychiatric care: What have we learned from research?' Journal of the American Academy of Psychiatry and the Law, **26**: 631–7.

Lieb, K., von der Osten-Sacken, J., Stoffers-Winterling, J., Reiss, N., and **Barth, J.** (2016). 'Conflicts of interest and spin in reviews of psychological therapies: A systematic review'. BMJ Open, **6**: e010606.

Lieberman, J.A., Stroup, T.S., McEvoy, J.P., Swartz, M.S., Rosenheck, R.A., Perkins, D.O., Keefe, R.S., Davis, S.M., Davis, C.E., Lebowitz, B.D., and **Severe, J.** (2005). 'Effectiveness of antipsychotic drugs in patients with chronic schizophrenia'. New England Journal of Medicine, **353**: 1209–23.

Leichsenring, F., Abbass, A., Hilsenroth, M.J., Leweke, F., Luyten, P., Keefe, J.R., Midgley, N., Rabung, S., Salzer, S., and **Steinert, C.** (2017). 'Biases in research: Risk factors for non-replicability in psychotherapy and pharmacotherapy research'. Psychological Medicine, **47**: 1000–11.

Lim, W., Qushmaq, I., Cook, D.J., Devereaux, P.J., Heels-Ansdell, D., Crowther, M.A., Tkaczyk, A., Meade, M.O., Cook, R.J., and **Troponin T Study Group** (2006). 'Reliability of electrocardiogram interpretation in critically ill patients'. Critical Care Medicine, **34**: 1338–43.

Linscott, R.J., Allardyce, J., and **van Os, J.** (2009). 'Seeking verisimilitude in a class: a systematic review of evidence that the criterial clinical symptoms of schizophrenia are taxonic'. Schizophrenia Bulletin, **36**: 811–29.

Linscott, R.J. and **Van Os, J.** (2010). 'Systematic reviews of categorical versus continuum models in psychosis: Evidence for discontinuous subpopulations underlying a psychometric continuum. Implications for DSM-V, DSM-VI, and DSM-VII'. Annual Review of Clinical Psychology, **6**: 391–419.

Linscott, R.J. and **Van Os, J.** (2013). 'An updated and conservative systematic review and meta-analysis of epidemiological evidence on psychotic experiences in children and adults: On the pathway from proneness to persistence to dimensional expression across mental disorders'. Psychological Medicine, **43**: 1133–49.

Lipman, M. and **White J.** (2015). 'Collaborative tuberculosis strategy for England'. British Medical Journal, **350**: h810.

Lishman W.A. (1997). *Organic Psychiatry. The Psychological Consequences of Cerebral Disorder*, 3rd edn. Oxford: Blackwell Science.

Liu, H., Petukhova, M.V., Sampson, N.A., Aguilar-Gaxiola, S., Alonso, J., Andrade, L.H., Bromet, E.J., de Girolamo, G., Haro, J.M., Hinkov, H., and **Kawakami, N.** (2017). 'Association of DSM-IV posttraumatic stress disorder with traumatic experience type and history in the World Health Organization World Mental Health Surveys'. JAMA Psychiatry, **74**: 270–81.

Liu, M., Malone, S.M., Vaidyanathan, U., Keller, M.C., Abecasis, G., McGue, M., Iacono, W.G., and **Vrieze, S.I.** (2017). 'Psychophysiological endophenotypes to characterize mechanisms of known schizophrenia genetic loci'. Psychological Medicine, **47**: 1116–25.

Lloyd, C. (1980). 'Life events and depressive disorder reviewed: II. Events as precipitating factors'. Archives of General Psychiatry, **37**: 541–8.

Loken, E.K., Hettema, J.M., Aggen, S.H., and **Kendler, K.S.** (2014). 'The structure of genetic and environmental risk factors for fears and phobias'. Psychological Medicine, **44**: 2375–84.

Lønnberg, A.S., **Skov, L.**, **Skytthe, A.**, **Kyvik, K.O.**, **Pedersen, O.B.**, and **Thomsen, S.F.** (2016). 'Association of psoriasis with the risk for type 2 diabetes mellitus and obesity'. JAMA Dermatology, **152**: 761–7.

Löwe, B., **Spitzer, R.L.**, **Williams, J.B.**, **Mussell, M.**, **Schellberg, D.**, and **Kroenke, K.** (2008). 'Depression, anxiety and somatization in primary care: Syndrome overlap and functional impairment'. General Hospital Psychiatry, **30**: 191–9.

Lubke, G.H. and **Miller, P.J.** (2015). 'Does nature have joints worth carving? A discussion of taxometrics, model-based clustering and latent variable mixture modelling'. Psychological Medicine, **45**: 705–15.

Lund, C., **Breen, A.**, **Flisher, A.J.**, **Kakuma, R.**, **Corrigall, J.**, **Joska, J.A.**, **Swartz, L.**, and **Patel, V.** (2010). 'Poverty and common mental disorders in low and middle income countries: A systematic review'. Social Science and Medicine, **71**: 517–28.

Lynam, D.R. and **Widiger, T.A.** (2001). 'Using the five-factor model to represent the DSM-IV personality disorders: an expert consensus approach'. Journal of Abnormal Psychology, **110**: 401–12.

Lynch, D., **Laws, K.R.**, and **McKenna, P.J.** (2010). 'Cognitive behavioural therapy for major psychiatric disorder: Does it really work? A meta-analytical review of well-controlled trials'. Psychological Medicine, **40**: 9–24.

Lysaker, P.H., **Meyer, P.S.**, **Evans, J.D.**, **Clements, C.A.**, and **Marks, K.A.** (2001). 'Childhood sexual trauma and psychosocial functioning in adults with schizophrenia'. Psychiatric Services, **52**: 1485–8.

Ma, Y. (2015). 'Neuropsychological mechanism underlying antidepressant effect: A systematic meta-analysis'. Molecular Psychiatry, **20**: 311–19.

Mackenbach, J.P., **Kulhánová, I.**, **Artnik, B.**, **Bopp, M.**, **Borrell, C.**, **Clemens, T.**, **Costa, G.**, **Dibben, C.**, **Kalediene, R.**, **Lundberg, O.**, and **Martikainen, P.** (2016). 'Changes in mortality inequalities over two decades: Register based study of European countries'. British Medical Journal, **353**: i1732.

Maj, M. (2005). '"Psychiatric comorbidity": An artefact of current diagnostic systems?' British Journal of Psychiatry, **186**: 182–4.

Maj, M. (2012). When does depression become a mental disorder? In: K.S. Kendler and J. Parnas (eds), *Philosophical Issues in Psychiatry II: Nosology*. Oxford: Oxford University Press, pp. 221–9.

Maj, M. (2013). Introduction: the relevance of Karl Jaspers' General Psychopathology to current psychiatric debate. In: G. Stanghellini and T. Fuchs (eds), *One Century of Karl Jaspers' General Psychopathology*. Oxford: Oxford University Press, pp. xxiv–xxviii.

Malaspina, D., **Owen, M.J.**, **Heckers, S.**, **Tandon, R.**, **Bustillo, J.**, **Schultz, S.**, **Barch, D.M.**, **Gaebel, W.**, **Gur, R.E.**, **Tsuang, M.**, and **Van Os, J.** (2013). 'Schizoaffective disorder in the DSM-5'. Schizophrenia Research, **150**: 21–5.

Mangalore R, **Knapp M** (2007). 'Cost of schizophrenia in England'. Journal of Mental Health Policy and Economics, **109**: 23–41.

Manji, H.K., **Quiroz, J.A.**, **Sporn, J.**, **Payne, J.L.**, **Denicoff, K.**, **Gray, N.A.**, **Zarate, C.A.**, and **Charney, D.S.** (2003). 'Enhancing neuronal plasticity and cellular resilience to develop novel, improved therapeutics for difficult-to-treat depression'. Biological Psychiatry, **53**: 707–42.

Mansell, W., **Harvey, A.**, **Watkins, E.**, and **Shafran, R.** (2009). 'Conceptual foundations of the transdiagnostic approach to CBT'. Journal of Cognitive Psychotherapy, **23**: 6–19.

Marchesi, C., **Affaticati, A.**, **Monici, A.**, **De Panfilis, C.**, **Ossola, P.**, **Ottoni, R.**, and **Tonna, M.** (2015). 'Decrease of functioning in remitted and non-remitted patients 16 years after a first-episode schizophrenia'. Journal of Nervous and Mental Disease, **203**: 406–11.

Marcinkiewcz, C.A., **Mazzone, C.M.**, **D'agostino, G.**, **Halladay, L.R.**, **Hardaway, J.A.**, **Diberto, J.F.**, **Navarro, M.**, **Burnham, N.**, **Cristiano, C.**, **Dorrier, C.E.**, and **Tipton, G.J.** (2016). 'Serotonin engages an anxiety and fear-promoting circuit in the extended amygdala'. Nature, **537**: 97–101.

Marconi, A., **Di Forti, M.**, **Lewis, C.M.**, **Murray, R.M.**, and **Vassos, E.** (2016). 'Meta-analysis of the association between the level of cannabis use and risk of psychosis'. Schizophrenia Bulletin, **42**: 1262–9.

Marcus, D.K., **O'Connell, D.**, **Norris, A.L.**, and **Sawaqdeh, A.** (2014). 'Is the Dodo bird endangered in the 21st century? A meta-analysis of treatment comparison studies'. Clinical Psychology Review, **34**: 519–30.

Maren, S. and **Quirk, G.J.** (2004). 'Neuronal signalling of fear memory'. Nature Reviews Neuroscience, **5**: 844–52.

Margison, F.R., **Barkham, M.**, **Evans, C.**, **McGrath, G.**, **Clark, J.M.**, **Audin, K.**, and **Connell, J.** (2000). 'Measurement and psychotherapy. Evidence-based practice and practice-based evidence'. British Journal of Psychiatry, **177**: 123–30.

Marin, J.R., **Bilker, W.**, **Lautenbach, E.**, and **Alpern, E.R.** (2010). 'Reliability of clinical examinations for pediatric skin and soft-tissue infections'. Pediatrics, **126**: 925–30.

Markar H.R. and **Mander A.J.** (1989). 'Efficacy of lithium prophylaxis in clinical practice'. British Journal of Psychiatry, **155**: 496–500.

Markova I.S. and **Berrios G.E.** (2015). Neuroimaging in psychiatry: epistemological concerns In: P. Zachar, D.S. Stoyanov, M. Aragona, and A. Jablensky (eds), *Alternative Perspectives on Psychiatric Validation—DSM, ICD, RDoC, and Beyond*. Oxford: Oxford University Press, pp.112–27.

Marmot, M. and **Allen, J.J.** (2014). 'Social determinants of health equity'. American Journal of Public Health, **104** (Suppl 4): S517–S519.

Marneros, A., **Deister, A.**, and **Rohde, A.** (1990). 'Psychopathological and social status of patients with affective, schizophrenic and schizoaffective disorders after long-term course'. Acta Psychiatrica Scandinavica, **82**: 352–8.

Marques, T.R., **Arenovich, T.**, **Agid, O.**, **Sajeev, G.**, **Muthen, B.**, **Chen, L.**, **Kinon, B.J.**, and **Kapur, S.** (2011). 'The different trajectories of antipsychotic response: Antipsychotics versus placebo'. Psychological Medicine, **41**: 1481–8.

Marsella, A.J. (1978). 'Thoughts on cross-cultural studies on the epidemiology of depression'. Culture, Medicine and Psychiatry, **2**: 343–57.

Marshall, C., **Howrigan, D.**, **Merico, D.**, **Thiruvahindrapuram, B.**, **Wu, W.**, **Greer, D.**, **Antaki, D.**, **Shetty, A.**, **Holmans, P.**, **Pinto, D.**, and **Gujral, M.** (2016b). 'A contribution of novel CNVs to schizophrenia from a genome-wide study of 41,321 subjects'. BioRxiv: 040493.

Marshall, D.C., **Jackson, M.E.**, and **Hattangadi-Gluth, J.A.** (2016a). 'Disclosure of industry payments to physicians: An epidemiologic analysis of early data from the open payments program'. Mayo Clinic Proceedings, **91**: 84–96.

Marshall, M., **Lewis, S.**, **Lockwood, A.**, **Drake, R.**, **Jones, P.**, and **Croudace, T.** (2005). 'Association between duration of untreated psychosis and outcome in cohorts of first-episode patients: A systematic review'. Archives of General Psychiatry, **62**: 975–83.

Martinelli, C. and **Shergill, S.S.** (2015). 'Everything you wanted to know about neuroimaging and psychiatry, but were afraid to ask'. Britis Journal of Psychiatric Advances, **21**: 251–60.

Maslej M.M., **Bolker B.M.**, **Russell M.J.**, **Eaton K.**, **Durisko Z.**, **Hollon S.D.**, **Swanson G.M.**, **Thomson J.A. Jr**, **Mulsant B.H.**, and **Andrews P.W.** (2017). 'The mortality and myocardial effects of antidepressants are moderated by preexisting cardiovascular disease: A meta-analysis'. Psychotherapy and Psychosomatics, **86**: 268–82.

Matheson, S.L., **Shepherd, A.M.**, **Pinchbeck, R.M.**, **Laurens, K.R.**, and **Carr, V.J.** (2013). 'Childhood adversity in schizophrenia: A systematic meta-analysis'. Psychological Medicine, **43**: 225–38.

Matheson, S.L., **Shepherd, A.M.**, and **Carr, V.J.** (2014). 'How much do we know about schizophrenia and how well do we know it? Evidence from the Schizophrenia Library'. Psychological Medicine, **44**: 3387–405.

Matthews, A., **Herrett, E.**, **Gasparrini, A.**, **Van Staa, T.**, **Goldacre, B.**, **Smeeth, L.**, and **Bhaskaran, K.** (2016). 'Impact of statin related media coverage on use of statins: Interrupted time series analysis with UK primary care data'. British Medical Journal, **353**: i3283.

Matussek, P. and **Nagel, D.** (1981). 'Identification of the endogenous depressive syndrome based on the symptoms and the characteristics of the course'. British Journal of Psychiatry, **138**: 361–72.

Mayo-Wilson, E., **Dias, S.**, **Mavranezouli, I.**, **Kew, K.**, **Clark, D.M.**, **Ades, A.E.**, and **Pilling, S.** (2014). 'Psychological and pharmacological interventions for social anxiety disorder in adults: A systematic review and network meta-analysis'. Lancet Psychiatry, **1**: 68–376.

McCreadie, R.G., **Latha, S.**, **Thara, R.**, **Padmavathi, R.**, and **Ayankaran, J.R.** (1997). 'Poor memory, negative symptoms and abnormal movements in never-treated Indian patients with schizophrenia'. British Journal of Psychiatry, **171**: 360–3.

McCreadie, R.G., **Thara, R.**, **Padmavati, R.**, **Srinivasan, T.N. Jaipurkar, S.D.** (2002a). 'Structural brain differences between never-treated patients with schizophrenia, with and without dyskinesia, and normal control subjects: A magnetic resonance imaging study'. Archives of General Psychiatry, **59**: 332–6.

McCreadie, R.G., **Padmavati, R.**, **Thara, R.**, and **Srinivasan, T.N.** (2002b). 'Spontaneous dyskinesia and parkinsonism in never-medicated, chronically ill patients with schizophrenia: 18-month follow-up'. British Journal of Psychiatry, **181**: 135–7.

McCusker, J., **Cole, M.**, **Dendukuri, N.**, **Han, L.**, and **Belzile, É.** (2003). 'The course of delirium in older medical inpatients'. Journal of General Internal Medicine, **18**: 696–704.

McGinnis, J.M., **Williams-Russo, P.**, and **Knickman, J.R.** (2002). 'The case for more active policy attention to health promotion'. Health Affairs, **21**: 78–93.

McGirr, A., **Vöhringer, P.A.**, **Ghaemi, S.N.**, **Lam, R.W.**, and **Yatham, L.N.** (2016). 'Safety and efficacy of adjunctive second-generation antidepressant therapy with a mood stabiliser or an atypical antipsychotic in acute bipolar depression: A systematic review and meta-analysis of randomised placebo-controlled trials'. Lancet, Psychiatry, **3**: 1138–46.

McGlashan, T.H. (1984). 'The Chestnut Lodge follow-up study: II. Long-term outcome of schizophrenia and the affective disorders'. Archives of General Psychiatry, **41**: 586–601.

McGlashan, T.H. (1986). 'The prediction of outcome in chronic schizophrenia: IV. The Chestnut Lodge follow-up study'. Archives of General Psychiatry, **43**: 167–76.

McGlashan, T.H. (1988). 'A selective review of recent North American long-term followup studies of schizophrenia'. Schizophrenia Bulletin, **14**: 515–42.

McGorry, P., Keshavan, M., Goldstone, S., Amminger, P., Allott, K., Berk, M., Lavoie, S., Pantelis, C., Yung, A., Wood, S., and **Hickie, I.** (2014). 'Biomarkers and clinical staging in psychiatry'. World Psychiatry, **13**: 211–23.

McGrail, K., Lavergne, R. and **Lewis, S.** (2016). 'The chronic disease explosion: Artificial bang or empirical whimper?' British Medical Journal, **352**: i1312.

McGrath, J., Saha, S., Welham, J., El Saadi, O., MacCauley, C., and **Chant, D.** (2004). 'A systematic review of the incidence of schizophrenia: The distribution of rates and the influence of sex, urbanicity, migrant status and methodology'. BMC Medicine, **2**: 13.

McGrath, J., Saha, S., Chant, D., and **Welham, J.** (2008). 'Schizophrenia: A concise overview of incidence, prevalence, and mortality'. Epidemiologic Reviews, **30**: 67–76.

McGrath, J.J., Saha, S., Al-Hamzawi, A., Alonso, J., Bromet, E.J., Bruffaerts, R., Caldas-de-Almeida, J.M., Chiu, W.T., de Jonge, P., Fayyad, J., and **Florescu, S.** (2015). 'Psychotic experiences in the general population: A cross-national analysis based on 31 261 respondents from 18 countries'. JAMA Psychiatry, **72**: 697–705.

McGrath, J.J., McLaughlin, K.A., Saha, S., Aguilar-Gaxiola, S., Al-Hamzawi, A., Alonso, J., Bruffaerts, R., de Girolamo, G., de Jonge, P., Esan, O., and **Florescu, S.** (2017). 'The association between childhood adversities and subsequent first onset of psychotic experiences: A cross-national analysis of 23 998 respondents from 17 countries'. Psychological Medicine, **47**: 1230–45.

McGuffin, P., Farmer, A., and **Harvey, I.** (1991). 'A polydiagnostic application of operational criteria in studies of psychotic illness: Development and reliability of the OPCRIT system'. Archives of General Psychiatry, **48**: 764–70.

McGuire-Snieckus R., McCabe R., and **Priebe S** (2003). 'Patient, client or service user? A survey of patient preferences of dress and address of six mental health professions'. The Psychiatrist, **27**: 305–8.

McHugh P.R. and **Slavney P.R.** (1998). *The Perspectives of Psychiatry*, 2nd edn, Baltimore, MD: John Hopkins University Press.

McKeith, I. (2007). 'Dementia with Lewy bodies and Parkinson's disease with dementia: Where two worlds collide'. Practical Neurology, **7**: 374–82.

McKnight, R.F., Adida, M., Budge, K., Stockton, S., Goodwin, G.M., and **Geddes J.R.** (2012). 'Lithium toxicity profile: A systematic review and meta-analysis'. Lancet, **379**: 721–8.

McManus S., Meltzer H., Brugha T., Bebbington P., and **Jenkins R.** (2009). 'Adult psychiatric morbidity in England, 2007 Results of a household survey'. London: Her Majestey's Stationery Office.

Meehl, P.E. (1962). 'Schizotaxia, schizotypy, schizophrenia'. American Psychologist, **17**: 827–38.

Meehl, P.E. (1973). *Psychodiagnosis: Selected Papers*. Minneapolis, MN: University of Minnesota Press.

Melander, H., Salmonson, T., Abadie, E., and **van Zwieten-Boot, B.** (2008). 'A regulatory Apologia—a review of placebo-controlled studies in regulatory submissions of new-generation antidepressants'. European Neuropsychopharmacology, **18**: 623–7.

Melzer, D., Fryers, T., Jenkins, R., Brugha, T., and **McWilliams, B.** (2003). 'Social position and the common mental disorders with disability'. Social Psychiatry and Psychiatric Epidemiology, **38**: 238–43.

Menche, J., Sharma, A., Kitsak, M., Ghiassian, S.D., Vidal, M., Loscalzo, J., and **Barabási, A.L.** (2015). 'Uncovering disease-disease relationships through the incomplete interactome'. Science, **347**: p1257601.

Mendenhall, E., **Kohrt, B.A.**, **Norris, S.A.**, **Ndetei, D.**, and **Prabhakaran, D.** (2017). 'Non-communicable disease syndemics: Poverty, depression, and diabetes among low-income populations'. Lancet, **389**: 951–63.

Menezes, N.M., **Arenovich, T.**, and **Zipursky, R.B.** (2006). 'A systematic review of longitudinal outcome studies of first-episode psychosis'. Psychological Medicine, **36**: 1349–62.

Mertens, J., **Wang, Q.W.**, **Kim, Y.**, **Diana, X.Y.**, **Pham, S.**, **Yang, B.**, **Zheng, Y.**, **Diffenderfer, K.E.**, **Zhang, J.**, **Soltani, S.**, and **Eames, T.** (2015). 'Differential responses to lithium in hyperexcitable neurons from patients with bipolar disorder'. Nature, **527**: 95–9.

Miettunen, J., **Nordström, T.**, **Kaakinen, M.**, and **Ahmed, A.O.** (2016). 'Latent variable mixture modeling in psychiatric research–a review and application'. Psychological Medicine, **46**: 457–67.

Miller, M.R. and **Levy M.L.** (2015). 'Chronic obstructive pulmonary disease: Missed diagnosis versus misdiagnosis'. British Medical Journal, **351**: h3021.

Miller, P.R., **Dasher, R.**, **Collins, R.**, **Griffiths, P.**, and **Brown, F.** (2001). 'Inpatient diagnostic assessments: 1. Accuracy of structured vs. unstructured interviews'. Psychiatry Research, **105**: 255–64.

Miloyan, B. and **Fried, E. I.** (2017). 'A reassessment of the relationship between depression and all-cause mortality in 3,604,005 participants from 293 studies'. World Psychiatry, **16**: 219–20.

Mindlis, I. and **Boffetta, P.** (2017). 'Mood disorders in first- and second-generation immigrants: Systematic review and meta-analysis'. British Journal of Psychiatry, **210**: 182–9.

Mitchell K.M. (ed.) (2015). *The Genetics of Neurodevelopmental Disorders*. Hoboken, NJ: Wiley-Blackwell.

Mizrahi, R., **Bagby, R.M.**, **Zipursky, R.B.**, and **Kapur, S.** (2005). 'How antipsychotics work: The patients' perspective'. Progress in Neuro-Psychopharmacology and Biological Psychiatry, **29**: 859–64.

Mizrahi, R., **Kiang, M.**, **Mamo, D.C.**, **Arenovich, T.**, **Bagby, R.M.**, **Zipursky, R.B. Kapur, S.** (2006). 'The selective effect of antipsychotics on the different dimensions of the experience of psychosis in schizophrenia spectrum disorders'. Schizophrenia Research, **88**: 111–18.

Mnie-Filali, O., **Abrial, E.**, **Lambás-Señas L.**, and **Haddjeri N.** (2013). 'Long-term adaptive changes induced by antidepressants: From conventional to novel therapies'. In: *Mood Disorders*, Kocabasoglu N. (ed.). InTech. Available at: <https://www.intechopen.com/books/mood-disorders/long-term-adaptive-changes-induced-by-antidepressants-from-conventional-to-novel-therapies>.

Moffitt, T.E., **Harrington, H.**, **Caspi, A.**, **Kim-Cohen, J.**, **Goldberg, D.**, **Gregory, A.M.**, and **Poulton, R.** (2007). 'Depression and generalized anxiety disorder: Cumulative and sequential comorbidity in a birth cohort followed prospectively to age 32 years'. Archives of General Psychiatry, **64**: 651–60.

Moghaddam, B. and **Javitt, D.** (2012). 'From revolution to evolution: The glutamate hypothesis of schizophrenia and its implication for treatment'. Neuropsychopharmacology, **37**: 4–15.

Mohan, C. and **Assassi, S.** (2015). 'Biomarkers in rheumatic diseases: How can they facilitate diagnosis and assessment of disease activity?' British Medical Journal, **351**: h5079.

Mohr, D.C., **Spring, B.**, **Freedland, K.E.**, **Beckner, V.**, **Arean, P.**, **Hollon, S.D.**, **Ockene, J.**, and **Kaplan, R.** (2009). 'The selection and design of control conditions for randomized controlled trials of psychological interventions'. Psychotherapy and Psychosomatics, **78**: 275–84.

Møller, P., Haug, E., Raballo, A., Parnas, J., and **Melle, I.** (2011). 'Examination of anomalous self-experience in first-episode psychosis: Interrater reliability'. Psychopathology, **44**: 386–90.

Moncrieff J. (1995). 'Lithium revisited'. British Journal of Psychiatry, **167**: 569–74.

Moncrieff J. (1997). 'Lithium: Evidence reconsidered'. British Journal of Psychiatry, **171**: 113–19.

Moncrieff J., Wessely S., and **Hardy R.** (1998). 'Meta-analysis of trials comparing antidepressants with active placebos'. British Journal of Psychiatry, **172**: 227–31.

Moncrieff, J. and **Kirsch, I.** (2005). 'Efficacy of antidepressants in adults'. British Medical Journal, **331**: 155–7.

Moncrieff J. (2006). 'Does antipsychotic withdrawal provoke psychosis? Review of the literature on rapid onset psychosis (supersensitivity psychosis) and withdrawal-related relapse'. Acta Psychiatrica Scandinavica, **114**: 3–13.

Moncrieff, J. (2009a). *The Myth of the Chemical Cure: A Critique of Psychiatric Drug Treatment*. London: Palgrave Macmillan.

Moncrieff J. (2009b). 'Changing the balance of psychosis treatment'. Advances in Psychiatric Treatment ,**15**: 221–3.

Moncrieff, J., Cohen, D., and **Mason, J.P.** (2009c). 'The subjective experience of taking antipsychotic medication: a content analysis of Internet data'. Acta Psychiatrica Scandinavica, **120**: 102–11.

Moncrieff, J. and **Leo, J.** (2010). 'A systematic review of the effects of antipsychotic drugs on brain volume'. Psychological Medicine, **40**: 1409–22.

Moncrieff J. (2015a). 'Long term effects of antipsychotics'. British Journal of Psychiatric Advances, **21**: 78–9.

Moncrieff, J. (2015b). 'Antidepressants: Misnamed and misrepresented'. World Psychiatry, **14**: 302–3.

Mondelli, V., Dazzan, P., and **Pariante, C.M.** (2015). 'Immune abnormalities across psychiatric disorders: clinical relevance'. British Journal of Psychiatric Advances, **21**: 150–6.

Montgomery, S.A. (2015). 'Antidepressant or antidepressant plus placebo effect?' World Psychiatry, **14**: 303–4.

Monzani, B., Rijsdijk, F., Harris, J., and **Mataix-Cols, D.** (2014). 'The structure of genetic and environmental risk factors for dimensional representations of DSM-5 obsessive-compulsive spectrum disorders'. JAMA Psychiatry, **71**: 182–9.

Morey, L.C., Hopwood, C.J., Markowitz, J.C., Gunderson, J.G., Grilo, C.M., McGlashan, T.H., Shea, M.T., Yen, S., Sanislow, C.A., Ansell, E.B., and **Skodol, A.E.** (2012). 'Comparison of alternative models for personality disorders, II: 6-, 8- and 10-year follow-up'. Psychological Medicine, **42**: 1705–21.

Morey, L.C., Benson, K.T., Busch, A.J., and **Skodol, A.E.** (2015). 'Personality disorders in DSM-5: Emerging research on the alternative model'. Current Psychiatry Reports, **17**: 1–9.

Morgan, C., Kirkbride, J., Leff, J., Craig, T., Hutchinson, G., McKenzie, K., Morgan, K., Dazzan, P., Doody, G.A., Jones, P., and **Murray, R.** (2007). 'Parental separation, loss and psychosis in different ethnic groups: A case-control study'. Psychological Medicine, **37**(04): 495–503.

Morgan, C., Lappin, J., Heslin, M., Donoghue, K., Lomas, B., Reininghaus, U., Onyejiaka, A., Croudace, T., Jones, P.B., Murray, R.M., and **Fearon, P.** (2014). 'Reappraising the long-term course and outcome of psychotic disorders: The AESOP-10 study'. Psychological Medicine, **44**: 2713–26.

Morrison, A.P., Turkington, D., Pyle, M., Spencer, H., Brabban, A., Dunn, G., Christodoulides, T., Dudley, R., Chapman, N., Callcott, P., and **Grace, T.** (2014). 'Cognitive therapy for people with schizophrenia spectrum disorders not taking antipsychotic drugs: A single-blind randomised controlled trial'. Lancet, **383**: 1395–403.

Mössner, R., Mikova, O., Koutsilieri, E., Saoud, M., Ehlis, A.C., Müller, N., Fallgatter, A.J., and **Riederer, P.** (2007). 'Consensus paper of the WFSBP Task Force on Biological Markers: Biological markers in depression'. World Journal of Biological Psychiatry, **8**: 141–74.

Moynihan, R., Doust, J., and **Henry, D.** (2012). 'Preventing overdiagnosis: How to stop harming the healthy'. British Medical Journal, **344**: e3502.

Müller, V.I., Cieslik, E.C., Serbanescu, I., Laird, A.R., Fox, P.T., and **Eickhoff, S.B.** (2017). 'Altered brain activity in unipolar depression revisited: Meta-analyses of neuroimaging studies'. JAMA Psychiatry, **74**: 47–55.

Mullins, N., Power, R.A., Fisher, H.L., Hanscombe, K.B., Euesden, J., Iniesta, R., Levinson, D.F., Weissman, M.M., Potash, J.B., Shi, J., and **Uher, R.** (2016). 'Polygenic interactions with environmental adversity in the aetiology of major depressive disorder'. Psychological Medicine, **46**: 759–70.

Muntaner, C., Eaton, W.W., Miech, R., and **O'Campo, P.** (2004). 'Socioeconomic position and major mental disorders'. Epidemiologic Reviews, **26**: 53–62.

Murad, M.H., Asi, N., Alsawas, M., and **Alahdab, F.** (2016). 'New evidence pyramid'. Evidence Based Medicine, **21**: 125–7.

Musini, V.M., Nazer, M., Bassett, K. Wright, J.M. (2014). 'Blood pressure-lowering efficacy of monotherapy with thiazide diuretics for primary hypertension'. Cochrane Database of Systematic Reviews, **5**: CD003824.

Muth, C. and **Glasziou P.P.** (2015). 'Guideline recommended treatments in patients with multimorbidity'. British Medical Journal, **351**: h514.

NAMC (2012). 'National Ambulatory Medical Care Survey: 2012 State and National Summary Tables'. Available at: <http://www.cdc.gov/nchs/data/ahcd/namcs_summary/2012_namcs_web_tables.pdf>.

Najjar, S. and **Pearlman, D.M.** (2015). 'Neuroinflammation and white matter pathology in schizophrenia: Systematic review'. Schizophrenia Research, **161**: 102–12.

Nanni, V., Uher, R., and **Danese, A.** (2012). 'Childhood maltreatment predicts unfavorable course of illness and treatment outcome in depression: A meta-analysis'. American Journal of Psychiatry, **16**: 141–51.

Napier, A.D., Ancarno, C., Butler, B., Calabrese, J., Chater, A., Chatterjee, H., Guesnet, F., Horne, R., Jacyna, S., Jadhav, S., and **Macdonald, A.**, 2014 'Culture and health'. Lancet, **384**: 1607–39.

Nelson, B., McGorry, P.D., Wichers, M., Wigman, J.T., and **Hartmann, J.A.** (2017a). 'Moving from static to dynamic models of the onset of mental disorder: A review'. JAMA Psychiatry, **74**: 528–34.

Nelson, J., Klumparendt, A., Doebler, P., and **Ehring, T.** (2017b). 'Childhood maltreatment and characteristics of adult depression: Meta-analysis'. British Journal of Psychiatry, **201**: 96–104.

Newman, S.C., Bland, R.C., and **Thompson, A.H.** (2012). 'Long-term course and outcome in schizophrenia: A 34-year follow-up study in Alberta, Canada'. Psychological Medicine, **42**: 2137–43.

NICE (2009). 'Clinical Guidelines 78. Borderline personality disorder: Recognition and management'. Available at: <https://www.nice.org.uk/guidance/cg78/evidence/bpd-full-guideline-pdf-242147197>.

NICE (2011). 'Clinical Guidelines 127. Hypertension in adults: Diagnosis and management'. Available at: <http://www.nice.org.uk/guidance/cg127/evidence/full-guideline-248588317>.

NICE. (2014a). 'Clinical Guideline 181. Cardiovascular disease: risk assessment and reduction, including lipid modification'. Available at: <https://www.nice.org.uk/Guidance/CG181/Evidence>.

NICE. (2014b). 'Clinical Guidelines 185. The assessment and management of bipolar disorder in adults, children and young people in primary and secondary care'. Available at: <https://www.nice.org.uk/guidance/cg185/evidence/full-guideline-pdf-193212829>.

NICE. (2014c). 'Clinical Guidelines 189. Obesity: dentification, assessment and management'. Available at: <https://www.nice.org.uk/guidance/cg189/resources/obesity-identification-assessment-and-management-35109821097925>.

Nicodemus, K.K., Marenco, S., Batten, A.J., Vakkalanka, R., Egan, M.F., Straub, R.E., and **Weinberger, D.R.** (2008). 'Serious obstetric complications interact with hypoxia-regulated/vascular-expression genes to influence schizophrenia risk'. Molecular Psychiatry, **13**: 873–7.

Nimnuan, C., Hotopf, M., and **Wessely, S.** (2000). 'Medically unexplained symptoms: how often and why are they missed?' Quarterly Journal of Medicine, **93**: 21–8.

Nimnuan, C., Hotopf, M., and **Wessely, S.** (2001). 'Medically unexplained symptoms: An epidemiological study in seven specialities'. Journal of Psychosomatic Research, **51**: 361–7.

Niranjan, U. and Wright, N.P. (2016). 'Should we treat subclinical hypothyroidism in obese children?' British Medical Journal, **352**: i941.

Norman, R.E., Byambaa, M., De, R., Butchart, A., Scott, J., and **Vos, T.**, 2012 'The long-term health consequences of child physical abuse, emotional abuse, and neglect: A systematic review and meta-analysis'. PLoS Medicine, **9**: e1001349.

O'Brien J.T. and **Thomas A.** (2015). 'Vascular dementia'. Lancet, **386**: 1698–706.

O'Donoghue, B., Lyne, J.P., Renwick, L., Lane, A., Madigan, K., Staines, A., O'Callaghan, E., and **Clarke, M.** (2016). 'Neighbourhood characteristics and the incidence of first-episode psychosis and duration of untreated psychosis'. Psychological Medicine, **46**: 1367–78.

Office of National Statistics (2016). 'Abuse during childhood: Findings from the Crime Survey for England and Wales, year ending March 2016'. Available at: <https://www.ons.gov.uk/peoplepopulationandcommunity/crimeandjustice/articles/abuseduringchildhood/findingsfromtheyearendingmarch2016crimesurveyforenglandandwales>.

Olfson, M., Gerhard, T., Huang, C., Crystal, S., and **Stroup, T.S.** (2015). 'Premature mortality among adults with schizophrenia in the United States'. JAMA Psychiatry, **72**(12): 1172–81.

Okai, D., Owen, G., McGuire, H., Singh, S., Churchill, R., and **Hotopf, M.** (2007). 'Mental capacity in psychiatric patients'. British Journal of Psychiatry, **191**: 291–7.

Okkels, N., Trabjerg, B., Arendt, M., and **Pedersen, C.B.** (2017). 'Traumatic stress disorders and risk of subsequent schizophrenia spectrum disorder or bipolar disorder: A nationwide cohort study'. Schizophrenia Bulletin, **43**: 180–6.

Ontaneda D., Thompson A.J., Fox R.J., and **Cohen J.A.** (2017). 'Progressive multiple sclerosis: Prospects for disease therapy, repair, and restoration of function'. Lancet, **389**: 1357–66.

Ortblad, K.F., Salomon, J.A., Bärnighausen, T., and **Atun, R.** (2015). 'Stopping tuberculosis: A biosocial model for sustainable development'. Lancet, **386**: 2354–62.

Orgeta, V., **Tabet, N.**, **Nilforooshan, R.**, and **Howard, R.** (2017). 'Efficacy of antidepressants for depression in Alzheimer's disease: Systematic review and meta-analysis'. Journal of Alzheimer's Disease, **58**: 725–33.

Ossenkoppele, R., **Jansen, W.J.**, **Rabinovici, G.D.**, **Knol, D.L.**, **van der Flier, W.M.**, **van Berckel, B.N.**, **Scheltens, P.**, **Visser, P.J.**, **Verfaillie, S.C.**, **Zwan, M.D.**, and **Adriaanse, S.M.** (2015). 'Prevalence of amyloid PET positivity in dementia syndromes: A meta-analysis'. Journal of the American Medical Association, **313**: 1939–49.

Oxman, A.D. and **GRADE Working Group** (2004). 'Grading quality of evidence and strength of recommendations'. British Medical Journal, **328**: 1490–4.

Oud, M., **Mayo-Wilson, E.**, **Braidwood, R.**, **Schulte, P.**, **Jones, S.H.**, **Morriss, R.**, **Kupka, R.**, **Cuijpers, P. Kendall, T.** (2016). 'Psychological interventions for adults with bipolar disorder: Systematic review and meta-analysis'. British Journal of Psychiatry, **208**: 213–22.

Overall, J.E. and **Gorham, D.R.** (1962). 'The brief psychiatric rating scale'. Psychological Reports, **10**: 799–812.

Owen, G.S., **Szmukler, G.**, **Richardson, G.**, **David, A.S.**, **Raymont, V.**, **Freyenhagen, F.**, **Martin, W.** and **Hotopf, M.** (2013). 'Decision-making capacity for treatment in psychiatric and medical in-patients: Cross-sectional, comparative study'. British Journal of Psychiatry, **203**(6): 461–7.

Owen, M.J. (2012). 'Implications of genetic findings for understanding schizophrenia'. Schizophrenia Bulletin, **38**: 904–7.

Ozer, E.J., **Best, S.R.**, **Lipsey, T.L.**, and **Weiss, D.S.** (2003). 'Predictors of posttraumatic stress disorder and symptoms in adults: a meta-analysis'. Psychological Bulletin, **129**: 52–73.

Pagnin, D., **de Queiroz, V.**, **Pini, S.**, and **Cassano, G.B.** (2004). 'Efficacy of ECT in depression: A meta-analytic review'. Journal of ECT, **20**: 13–20.

Palmier-Claus, J.E., **Berry, K.**, **Bucci, S.**, **Mansell, W.**, and **Varese, F.** (2016). 'Relationship between childhood adversity and bipolar affective disorder: Systematic review and meta-analysis'. British Journal of Psychiatry, **209**: 454–9.

Papadopoulos, F.C., **Ekbom, A.**, **Brandt, L.**, and **Ekselius, L.** (2009). 'Excess mortality, causes of death and prognostic factors in anorexia nervosa'. British Journal of Psychiatry, **194**: 10–17.

Parker, G., **Hadzi-Pavlovic, D.**, **Hickie, I.**, **Boyce, P.**, **Mitchell, P.**, **Wilhelm, K.**, and **Brodaty, H.** (1991). 'Distinguishing psychotic and non-psychotic melancholia'. Journal of Affective Disorders, **22**: 135–48.

Parmar, D., **Stavropoulou, C.**, and **Ioannidis, J.P.** (2016). 'Health outcomes during the 2008 financial crisis in Europe: Systematic literature review'. British Medical Journal, **354**: i4588.

Parnas, J., **Handest, P.**, **Saebye, D.**, and **Jansson, L.** (2003). 'Anomalies of subjective experience in schizophrenia and psychotic bipolar illness'. Acta Psychiatrica Scandinavica, **108**: 126–33.

Parnas, J., **Møller, P.**, **Kircher, T.**, **Thalbitzer, J.**, **Jansson, L.**, **Handest, P.**, and **Zahavi, D.** (2005). 'EASE: Examination of anomalous self-experience'. Psychopathology, **38**: 236–58.

Parnas, J. (2011). 'A disappearing heritage: The clinical core of schizophrenia'. Schizophrenia Bulletin, **37**: 1121–30.

Parnas, J. and **Henriksen, M.G.** (2014). 'Disordered self in the schizophrenia spectrum: A clinical and research perspective'. Harvard Review of Psychiatry, **22**: 251–65.

Parnas J. (2015). 'Differential diagnosis and current polythetic classification'. World Psychiatry, **14**: 284–7.

Parnas, J. and **Henriksen, M.G.** (2016). 'Epistemological error and the illusion of phenomenological continuity'. World Psychiatry, **15**: 126–7.

Parker, G., Anderson, I.M., and **Haddad, P.** (2003). 'Clinical trials of antidepressant medications are producing meaningless results'. British Journal of Psychiatry, **183**: 102–4.

Parker, G., Fink, M., Shorter, E., Taylor, M.A., Akiskal, H., Berrios, G., Bolwig, T., Brown, W.A., Carroll, B., Healy, D., and **Klein, D.F.** (2010). 'Issues for DSM-5: Whither melancholia? The case for its classification as a distinct mood disorder'. American Journal of Psychiatry, **167**: 745–7.

Parry, G.D., Crawford, M.J., and **Duggan, C.** (2016). 'Iatrogenic harm from psychological therapies: Time to move on'. British Journal of Psychiatry, **208**: 210–12.

Paykel, E.S. (1994). 'Life events, social support and depression'. Acta Psychiatrica Scandinavica, **89**(s377): 50–8.

Parsons, T (1951). *The Social System*. Glencoe, IL: The Free Press.

Patel, V. and **Kleinman, A.** (2003). 'Poverty and common mental disorders in developing countries'. Bulletin of the World Health Organization, **81**: 609–15.

Peen, J., Schoevers, R.A., Beekman, A.T., and **Dekker, J.** (2010). 'The current status of urban-rural differences in psychiatric disorders'. Acta Psychiatrica Scandinavica, **121**: 84–93.

Pendleton D., Schofield T., Tate P., and **Havelock P.** (1984). *The Consultation: An Approach to Learning and Teaching*. Oxford: Oxford University Press.

Penttilä, M., Jääskeläinen, E., Hirvonen, N., Isohanni, M., and **Miettunen, J.** (2014). 'Duration of untreated psychosis as predictor of long-term outcome in schizophrenia: Systematic review and meta-analysis'. British Journal of Psychiatry, **205**: 88–94.

Peralta, V. and **Cuesta, M.J.** (2016). 'Delusional disorder and schizophrenia: A comparative study across multiple domains'. Psychological Medicine, **46**: 2829–39.

Perry, D.C., Sturm, V.E., Peterson, M.J., Pieper, C.F., Bullock, T., Boeve, B.F., Miller, B.L., Guskiewicz, K.M., Berger, M.S., Kramer, J.H. and Welsh-Bohmer, K.A. (2016). 'Association of traumatic brain injury with subsequent neurological and psychiatric disease: A meta-analysis'. Journal of Neurosurgery, **124**: 511–26.

Peterson, B.S. (2015). 'Research Domain Criteria (RDoC): A new psychiatric nosology whose time has not yet come'. Journal of Child Psychology and Psychiatry, **56**: 719–22.

Pettersson, E., Larsson, H., and **Lichtenstein, P.** (2016). 'Common psychiatric disorders share the same genetic origin: A multivariate sibling study of the Swedish population'. Molecular Psychiatry, **21**: 717–21.

Petitte, T., Mallow, J., Barnes, E., Petrone, A., Barr, T., and **Theeke, L.** (2015). 'A systematic review of loneliness and common chronic physical conditions in adults'. The Open Psychology Journal, **8**(Suppl 2): 113–32.

Pharoah, F., Mari, J., Rathbone, J., and **Wong, W.** (2010). 'Family intervention for schizophrenia'. Cochrane Database of Systematic Reviews, **12**: CD000088.

Philips, B. (2009). 'Comparing apples and oranges: How do patient characteristics and treatment goals vary between different forms of psychotherapy?' Psychology and Psychotherapy: Theory, Research and Practice, **82**: 323–36.

Phillips, M.R. (2016). 'Would the use of dimensional measures improve the utility of psychiatric diagnoses?' World Psychiatry, **15**: 38–9.

Pickett, K.E., James, O.W., and **Wilkinson, R.G.** (2006). 'Income inequality and the prevalence of mental illness: a preliminary international analysis'. Journal of Epidemiology and Community Health, **60**: 646–7.

Pickett, K.E. and **Wilkinson, R.G.** (2010). 'Inequality: An underacknowledged source of mental illness and distress'. British Journal of Psychiatry, **197**: 426–8.

Pies, R. (2007). 'How "objective" are psychiatric diagnoses? (guess again)'. Psychiatry (Edgmont), **4**: 18–22.

Pillinger, T., Beck, K., Gobjila, C., Donocik, J.G., Jauhar, S., and **Howes, O.D.** (2017). 'Impaired glucose homeostasis in first-episode schizophrenia: A systematic review and meta-analysis'. JAMA Psychiatry, **74**: 261–9.

Pocklington, A.J., Rees, E., Walters, J.T., Han, J., Kavanagh, D.H., Chambert, K.D., Holmans, P., Moran, J.L., McCarroll, S.A., Kirov, G., and **O'Donovan, M.C.** (2015). 'Novel findings from CNVs implicate inhibitory and excitatory signaling complexes in schizophrenia'. Neuron, **86**: 1203–14.

Pope, H.G., Lipinski, J.F., Cohen, B.M., and **Axelrod, D.T.** (1980). 'Schizoaffective disorder: An invalid diagnosis? A comparison of schizoaffective disorder, schizophrenia, and affective disorder'. American Journal of Psychiatry, **137**: 921–7.

Pincus, H.A., Tew, J.D., and **First, M.B.** (2004). 'Psychiatric comorbidity: Is more less?' World Psychiatry, **3**: 18–23.

Plomin, R., DeFries, J.C., Knopik, V.S., and **Neiderhiser, J.M.** (2016). 'Top 10 replicated findings from behavioral genetics'. Perspectives on Psychological Science, **11**: 3–23.

Poels, E.M.P., Kegeles, L.S., Kantrowitz, J.T., Slifstein, M., Javitt, D.C., Lieberman, J.A., Abi-Dargham, A., and **Girgis, R.R.** (2014). 'Imaging glutamate in schizophrenia: Review of findings and implications for drug discovery'. Molecular Psychiatry, **19**: 20–9.

Pollak, T.A., McCormack, R., Peakman, M., Nicholson, T.R., and **David, A.S.** (2014). 'Prevalence of anti-N-methyl-D-aspartate (NMDA) receptor antibodies in patients with schizophrenia and related psychoses: A systematic review and meta-analysis'. Psychological Medicine, **44**: 2475–87.

Polman, C.H., Reingold, S.C., Banwell, B., Clanet, M., Cohen, J.A., Filippi, M., Fujihara, K., Havrdova, E., Hutchinson, M., Kappos, L., and **Lublin, F.D.** (2011). 'Diagnostic criteria for multiple sclerosis: 2010 revisions to the McDonald criteria'. Annals of Neurology, **69**: 292–302.

Polubriaginof, F., Quinnies, K., Vanguri, R., Yahi, A., Simmerling, M., Ionita-Laza, I., Salmasian, H., Bakken, S., Hripcsak, G., Goldstein, D., and **Kiryluk, K.** (2016). 'Estimate of disease heritability using 4.7 million familial relationships inferred from electronic health records'. BioRxiv: 066068.

Posternak, M.A. and **Miller, I.** (2001). 'Untreated short-term course of major depression: A meta-analysis of outcomes from studies using wait-list control groups'. Journal of Affective Disorders, **66**: 139–46.

Priebe, S. (2015). 'The political mission of psychiatry'. World Psychiatry, **14**: 1–2.

Priebe, S. (2016). 'A social paradigm in psychiatry: Themes and perspectives'. Epidemiology and Psychiatric Sciences, **25**: 521–7.

Prien, R.F., Klett, C.J., and **Caffey, E.M.** (1973). 'Lithium carbonate and imipramine in prevention of affective episodes: A comparison in recurrent affective illness'. Archives of General Psychiatry, **28**: 337–41.

Prospective Studies Collaboration (2009). 'Body-mass index and cause-specific mortality in 900 000 adults: Collaborative analyses of 57 prospective studies'. Lancet, **373**: 1083–96.

Puhl, R.M. and **Heuer, C.A.** (2009). 'The stigma of obesity: a review and update'. Obesity, **17**: 941–64.

Prudic, J., Olfson, M., Marcus, S.C., Fuller, R.B., and **Sackeim, H.A.** (2004). 'Effectiveness of electroconvulsive therapy in community settings'. Biological Psychiatry,**55**: 301–312.

Rabinowitz, J., Werbeloff, N., Mandel, F.S., Menard, F., Marangell, L., and **Kapur, S.** (2016). 'Initial depression severity and response to antidepressants v. placebo: Patient-level data analysis from 34 randomised controlled trials'. British Journal of Psychiatry, **209**: 427–8.

Rafferty, J. (2005). 'Curing the stigma of leprosy'. Leprosy Review, **76**: 119–26.**Rai, D., Zitko, P., Jones, K., Lynch, J.,** and **Araya, R.** (2013). 'Country-and individual-level socioeconomic determinants of depression: Multilevel cross-national comparison'. British Journal of Psychiatry, **202**: 195–203.

Rai, D., Zitko, P., Jones, K., Lynch, J., and **Araya, R.** (2013). 'Country-and individual-level socioeconomic determinants of depression: Multilevel cross-national comparison'. British Journal of Psychiatry, **202**: 195–203.

Raleigh, Z.T. (2010). 'A biopsychosocial perspective on the experience of lung cancer'. Journal of Psychosocial Oncology, **28**: 116–25.

Ram, R., Bromet, E.J., Eaton, W.W., Pato, C., and **Schwartz, J.E.** (1992). 'The natural course of schizophrenia: A review of first-admission studies'. Schizophrenia Bulletin, **18**: 185–207.

Ramsey W. (1992). 'Prototypes and conceptual analysis'. Topoi, **11**: 59–70.

Rangaka, M.X., Cavalcante, S.C., Marais, B.J., Thim, S., Martinson, N.A., Swaminathan, S., and **Chaisson, R.E.** (2015). 'Controlling the seedbeds of tuberculosis: Diagnosis and treatment of tuberculosis infection'. Lancet, **386**: 2344–53.

Ravinder, S., Burghardt, N.S., Brodsky, R., Bauer, E.P., and **Chattarji, S,** (2013). 'A role for the extended amygdala in the fear-enhancing effects of acute selective serotonin reuptake inhibitor treatment'. Translational Psychiatry, **3**: e209.

Ravnskov, U., Diamond, D.M., Hama, R., Hamazaki, T., Hammarskjöld, B., Hynes, N., Kendrick, M., Langsjoen, P.H., Malhotra, A., Mascitelli, L., and **McCully, K.S.** (2016). 'Lack of an association or an inverse association between low-density-lipoprotein cholesterol and mortality in the elderly: A systematic review'. BMJ Open, **6**: e010401.

Read, J. and **Bentall, R.** (2010). 'The effectiveness of electroconvulsive therapy: A literature review'. Epidemiologia e Psichiatria Sociale, **19**: 333–47.**Reaven, G.M.,** 1988 'Role of insulin resistance in human disease'. Diabetes, **37**: 1595–607.

Rees, E., Walters, J.T., Georgieva, L., Isles, A.R., Chambert, K.D., Richards, A.L., Mahoney-Davies, G., Legge, S.E., Moran, J.L., McCarroll, S.A., and **O'Donovan, M.C.** (2014). 'Analysis of copy number variations at 15 schizophrenia-associated loci'. British Journal of Psychiatry, **204**: 108–14.

Regier, D.A., Kaelber, C.T., Roper, M.T., Rae, D.S., and **Sartorius, N.** (1994). 'The ICD-10 clinical field trial for mental and behavioral disorders: Results in Canada and the United States'. American Journal of Psychiatry, **151**: 1340–50.

Regier, D.A., Narrow, W.E., Clarke, D.E., Kraemer, H.C., Kuramoto, S.J., Kuhl, E.A., and **Kupfer, D.J.** (2013). 'DSM-5 Field Trials in the United States and Canada, Part II: Test-retest reliability of selected categorical diagnoses'. American Journal of Psychiatry, **170**: 59–70.

Reichborn-Kjennerud, T., Czajkowski, N., Ystrøm, E., Ørstavik, R., Aggen, S.H., Tambs, K., Torgersen, S., Neale, M.C., Røysamb, E., Krueger, R.F., and **Knudsen, G.P.** (2015). 'A longitudinal twin study of borderline and antisocial personality disorder traits in early to middle adulthood'. Psychological Medicine, **45**: 3121–31.

Reid, S., Wessely, S., Crayford, T., and **Hotopf, M.** (2001). 'Medically unexplained symptoms in frequent attenders of secondary health care: retrospective cohort study'. British Medical Journal, **322**: 767–70.

Reininghaus, U, Priebe S and **Bentall, R.P.** (2013). 'Testing the psychopathology of psychosis: Evidence for a general psychosis dimension'. Schizophrenia Bulletin, **39**: 884–95.

Resick, P.A., **Bovin, M.J.**, **Calloway, A.L.**, **Dick, A.M.**, **King, M.W.**, **Mitchell, K.S.**, **Suvak, M.K.**, **Wells, S.Y.**, **Stirman, S.W.**, and **Wolf, E.J.** (2012). 'A critical evaluation of the complex PTSD literature: Implications for DSM-5'. Journal of Traumatic Stress, **25**: 241–51.

Riblet, N.B., **Shiner, B.**, **Young-Xu, Y.**, and **Watts, B.V.** (2017). 'Strategies to prevent death by suicide: Meta-analysis of randomised controlled trials'. British Journal of Psychiatry, **210**: 396–402.

Rickards, H., **Jacob, S.**, **Lennox, B.**, and **Nicholson, T.** (2014). 'Autoimmune encephalitis: A potentially treatable cause of mental disorder'. Advances in Psychiatric Treatment, **20**: 92–100.

Riihimäki, K.A., **Vuorilehto, M.S.**, **Melartin, T.K.**, and **Isometsä, E.T.** (2014). 'Five-year outcome of major depressive disorder in primary health care'. Psychological Medicine, **44**: 1369–79.

Ripke, S., **O'Dushlaine, C.**, **Chambert, K.**, **Moran, J.L.**, **Kähler, A.K.**, **Akterin, S.**, **Bergen, S.E.**, **Collins, A.L.**, **Crowley, J.J.**, **Fromer, M.**, and **Kim, Y.** (2013). 'Genome-wide association analysis identifies 13 new risk loci for schizophrenia'. Nature Genetics, **45**: 1150–9.

Ripke, S., **Neale, B.M.**, **Corvin, A.**, **Walters, J.T.**, **Farh, K.H.**, **Holmans, P.A.**, **Lee, P.**, **Bulik-Sullivan, B.**, **Collier, D.A.**, **Huang, H.** and **Pers, T.H.** (2014). 'Biological insights from 108 schizophrenia-associated genetic loci'. Nature, **511**: 421–7.

Robertson, H. and **Pryor, R.** (2006). 'Memory and cognitive effects of ECT: Informing and assessing patients'. Advances in Psychiatric Treatment, **12**: 228–37.

Robins E. and **Guze S.B.** (1970). 'Establishment of diagnostic validity in psychiatric illness: Its application to schizophrenia'. American Journal of Psychiatry, **126**: 983–7.

Robinson, L., **Tang, E.**, and **Taylor, J.P.** (2015). 'Dementia: Timely diagnosis and early intervention'. British Medical Journal, **350**: h3029.

Rodrigues, A. and **Banzato, C.** (2015). Reality and utility unbound: An argument for dual-track nosologic validation. In: P. Zachar, D.S. Stoyanov, M. Aragona, and A. Jablensky, (eds). *Alternative Perspectives on Psychiatric Validation—DSM, ICD, RDoC, and Beyond.* Oxford: Oxford University Press, pp. 47–59.

Rodriguez-Seijas, C., **Stohl, M.**, **Hasin, D.S.**, and **Eaton, N.R.** (2015). 'Transdiagnostic factors and mediation of the relationship between perceived racial discrimination and mental disorders'. JAMA Psychiatry, **72**: 706–13.

Romanelli, R.J., **Wu, F.M.**, **Gamba, R.**, **Mojtabai, R.**, and **Segal, J.B.** (2014). 'Behavioral therapy and serotonin reuptake inhibitor pharmacotherapy in the treatment of obsessive-compulsive disorder: A systematic review and meta-analysis of head-to-head randomized controlled trials'. Depression and Anxiety, **31**: 641–52.

Roest, A.M., **De Jonge, P.**, **Williams, C.D.**, **de Vries, Y.A.**, **Schoevers, R.A.**, and **Turner, E.H.** (2015). 'Reporting bias in clinical trials investigating the efficacy of second-generation antidepressants in the treatment of anxiety disorders: A report of 2 meta-analyses'. JAMA Psychiatry, **72**: 500–10.

Rosch E. and **Mervis C.B.** (1975). 'Family resemblances: Studies in the internal structure of categories'. Cognitive Psychology, **7**: 573–605.

Rose, N. (2013). 'What is Diagnosis For?' Lecture given at the Institute of Psychiatry (London). Transcript available at: <http://nikolasrose.com/wp-content/uploads/2013/07/Rose-2013-What-is-diagnosis-for-IoP-revised-July-2013.pdf>.

Rosenhan, D.L. (1973). 'On being sane in insane places'. Science, **179**: 250–8.**Rosenman, S.**, **Korten, A.**, **Medway, J.**, and **Evans, M.** (2003). 'Dimensional vs. categorical diagnosis in psychosis'. Acta Psychiatrica Scandinavica, **107**: 378–84.

Rothman K.J. (1976). 'Causes'. American Journal of Epidemiology, **104**: 587–92.

Rothman K.J. (ed.) (1998). *Causal Inference*. Chestnut Hill, MA: Epidemiology Resources, Inc.

Ruderfer, D.M., **Fanous, A.H.**, **Ripke, S.**, **McQuillin, A.**, **Amdur, R.L.**, **Gejman, P.V.**, **O'Donovan, M.C.**, **Andreassen, O.A.**, **Djurovic, S.**, **Hultman, C.M.**, and **Kelsoe, J.R.** (2014). 'Polygenic dissection of diagnosis and clinical dimensions of bipolar disorder and schizophrenia'. Molecular Psychiatry, **19**: 1017–24.

Russo, M., **Levine, S.Z.**, **Demjaha, A.**, **Di Forti, M.**, **Bonaccorso, S.**, **Fearon, P.**, **Dazzan, P.**, **Pariante, C.M.**, **David, A.S.**, **Morgan, C.**, and **Murray, R.M.** (2014). 'Association between symptom dimensions and categorical diagnoses of psychosis: A cross-sectional and longitudinal investigation'. Schizophrenia Bulletin, **40**: 1111–99.

Rutherford, B.R. and **Roose, S.P.** (2013). 'A model of placebo response in antidepressant clinical trials'. American Journal of Psychiatry, **170**: 723–33.

Rutherford, B.R., **Pott, E.**, **Tandler, J.M.**, **Wall, M.M.**, **Roose, S.P.**, and **Lieberman, J.A.** (2014). 'Placebo response in antipsychotic clinical trials: A meta-analysis'. JAMA Psychiatry, **71**: 1409–21.

Ryan, D.J., **O'Regan, N.A.**, **Caoimh, R.Ó.**, **Clare, J.**, **O'Connor, M.**, **Leonard, M.**, **McFarland, J.**, **Tighe, S.**, **O'Sullivan, K.**, **Trzepacz, P.T.**, and **Meagher, D.** (2013). 'Delirium in an adult acute hospital population: Predictors, prevalence and detection'. BMJ Open, **3**: e001772.

Ruscio, J. and **Ruscio, A.M.** (2000). 'Informing the continuity controversy: A taxometric analysis of depression'. Journal of Abnormal Psychology, **109**: 473–87.**Sachar, D.B.** and **Walfish, A.** (2013). 'Inflammatory bowel disease: One or two diseases?' Current Gastroenterology Reports, **15**: 298.

Sackeim, H.A., **Prudic, J.**, **Fuller, R.**, **Keilp, J.**, **Lavori, P.W. Olfson, M.** (2007). 'The cognitive effects of electroconvulsive therapy in community settings'. Neuropsychopharmacology, **32**: 244–54.

Sackett D.L., **Haynes R.B.**, **Guyatt G.H.**, and **Tugwell P.** (1991). *Clinical Epidemiology: A Basic Science for Clinical Medicine*, 2nd edn. Boston, MA: Little, Brown and Company.

Saddichha, S., **Manjunatha, N.**, **Ameen, S.**, and **Akhtar, S.** (2008). 'Metabolic syndrome in first episode schizophrenia—a randomized double-blind controlled, short-term prospective study'. Schizophrenia Research, **101**: 266–72.

Saha, S., **Chant, D.**, **Welham, J.** and **McGrath, J.** (2005). 'A systematic review of the prevalence of schizophrenia'. PLoS Medicine, **2**: e141.

Salkovskis, P.M. (1999). 'Understanding and treating obsessive—compulsive disorder'. Behaviour Research and Therapy, **37**: S29–S52.

Salize, H.J., **Dreßing, H.**, and **Peitz, M.** (2002). 'Compulsory admission and involuntary treatment of mentally ill patients-legislation and practice in EU-member states. Central Institute of Mental Health Research Project Final Report'. Mannheim, Germany. Available at: <http://ec.europa.eu/health/ph_projects/2000/promotion/fp_promotion_2000_frep_08_en.pdf>.

Salize, H.J. and **Dressing, H.** (2004). 'Epidemiology of involuntary placement of mentally ill people across the European Union'. British Journal of Psychiatry, **184**(2): 163–8.

Santelmann, H., **Franklin, J.**, **Bußhoff, J.**, and **Baethge, C.** (2016). 'Interrater reliability of schizoaffective disorder compared with schizophrenia, bipolar disorder, and unipolar depression: A systematic review and meta-analysis'. Available at: <http://www.schres-journal.com/article/S0920-9964(16)30328-0/abstract>.

Sariaslan, A., **Larsson, H.**, **D'Onofrio, B.**, **Långström, N.**, **Fazel, S.**, and **Lichtenstein, P.** (2015). 'Does population density and neighborhood deprivation predict schizophrenia?

A nationwide Swedish family-based study of 2.4 million individuals'. Schizophrenia Bulletin, **41**: 494–502.

Sariaslan, A., Fazel, S., D'onofrio, B.M., Långström, N., Larsson, H., Bergen, S.E., Kuja-Halkola, R., and **Lichtenstein, P.** (2016). 'Schizophrenia and subsequent neighborhood deprivation: Revisiting the social drift hypothesis using population, twin and molecular genetic data'. Translational Psychiatry, **6**:.e796.

Sarkar, S.P. (2004). 'Boundary violation and sexual exploitation in psychiatry and psychotherapy: A review'. Advances in Psychiatric Treatment, **10**: 312–20.

Sartorius, N., Üstün, T.B., Lecrubier, Y., and **Wittchen, H.U.** (1996). 'Depression comorbid with anxiety: Results from the WHO study on Psychological disorders in primary health care'. British Journal of Psychiatry, **168**(Suppl 30): 38–43.

Sartorius N. (2002). 'Iatrogenic stigma of mental illness begins with behaviour and attitudes of medical professionals, especially psychiatrists'. British Medical Journal, **324**: 1470–1.

Scadding, J.G. (1967). 'Diagnosis: The clinician and the computer'. Lancet, **290**: 877–82.

Scarella, T.M., Laferton, J.A., Ahern, D.K., Fallon, B.A., and **Barsky, A.** (2016). 'The relationship of hypochondriasis to anxiety, depressive, and somatoform disorders'. Psychosomatics, **57**: 200–7.

Scheltens P., Blennow K., Breteler M.M.B., de Strooper B., Frisoni G.B., Salloway S., and **Van der Flier W.V.** (2016). 'Alzheimer's disease'. Lancet, **388**: 505–17.**Scherk, H., Pajonk, F.G.**, and **Leucht, S.** (2007). 'Second-generation antipsychotic agents in the treatment of acute mania: A systematic review and meta-analysis of randomized controlled trials'. Archives of General Psychiatry, **64**: 442–55.

Scherrer, J.F., Garfield, L.D., Lustman, P.J., Hauptman, P.J., Chrusciel, T., Zeringue, A., Carney, R.M., Freedland, K.E., Bucholz, K.K., Owen, R., and **Newcomer, J.W.** (2011). 'Antidepressant drug compliance: reduced risk of MI and mortality in depressed patients'. American Journal of Medicine ,**124**: 318–24.

Schmitt, A., Rujescu, D., Gawlik, M., Hasan, A., Hashimoto, K., Iceta, S., Jarema, M., Kambeitz, J., Kasper, S., Keeser, D., Kornhuber, J., Koutsouleris, N., Lanzenberger, R., Malchow, B. Saoud, M., Spies, M., Stöber, G., Thibaut, F., Riederer, P., and **Falkai, P.** (2016a). 'Consensus paper of the WFSBP Task Force on Biological Markers: Criteria for biomarkers and endophenotypes of schizophrenia part II: Cognition, neuroimaging and genetics'. World Journal of Biological Psychiatry, **17**: 406–28.

Schmitt, A., Martins-de-Souza, D., Akbarian, S., Cassoli, J.S., Ehrenreich, H., Fischer, A., Fonteh, A., Gattaz, W.F., Gawlik, M., Gerlach, M., and **Grünblatt, E.** (2016b). 'Consensus paper of the WFSBP Task Force on Biological Markers: Criteria for biomarkers and endophenotypes of schizophrenia, part III: Molecular mechanisms'. World Journal of Biological Psychiatry, **18**: 330–56.

Schoenberg V.J. and **Rosamond W.D.** (2000). 'Understanding the fundamentals of epidemiology: An evolving text'. Available at: <http://www.epidemiolog.net/>.

Schou, M. (1997). 'Forty years of lithium treatment'. Archives of General Psychiatry, **54**: 9–13.

Schwartz, M.A. and **Wiggins O.P.** (1987a). 'Diagnosis and ideal types: A contribution to psychiatric classification'. Comprehensive Psychiatry, **28**: 277–91.

Schou, M., Sæther, S.G., Borowski, K., Teegen, B., Kondziella, D., Stoecker, W., Vaaler, A., and **Reitan, S.K.** (2016). 'Prevalence of serum anti-neuronal autoantibodies in patients admitted to acute psychiatric care'. Psychological Medicine, **46**: 3303–13.

Schwartz, M.A. and **Wiggins O.P.** (1987b). 'Typifications the first step for clinical diagnosis in psychiatry'. Journal of Nervous and Mental Disease, **175**: 65–77.

Scott, S., **Pfohl, B.**, **Battaglia, M.**, and **Bellodi, L.** (1998). 'The cooccurrence of DSM-III-R personality disorders'. Journal of Personality Disorders, **12**: 302–15.

Sedgwick, P. (2014). 'Statistical question relative risks versus odds ratios'. British Medical Journal, **348**: g1407.

Seeman, P. and **Tallerico, T.**, 1998. Antipsychotic drugs which elicit little or no parkinsonism bind more loosely than dopamine to brain D2 receptors, yet occupy high levels of these receptors. Molecular Psychiatry, **3**(2): 123–4.

Sekar, A., **Bialas, A.R.**, **de Rivera, H.**, **Davis, A.**, **Hammond, T.R.**, **Kamitaki, N.**, **Tooley, K.**, **Presumey, J.**, **Baum, M.**, **Van Doren, V.**, and **Genovese, G.** (2016). 'Schizophrenia risk from complex variation of complement component 4'. Nature, **530**: 177–83.

Selinger, C.P. (2009). 'The right to consent: Is it absolute?' British Journal of Medical Practitioners, **2**: 50–4.

Semkovska, M. and **McLoughlin, D.M.** (2010). 'Objective cognitive performance associated with electroconvulsive therapy for depression: A systematic review and meta-analysis'. Biological Psychiatry, **68**: 568–77.

Sen, S., **Duman, R.**, and **Sanacora, G.** (2008). 'Serum brain-derived neurotrophic factor, depression, and antidepressant medications: Meta-analyses and implications'. Biological Psychiatry, **64**: 527–32.

Severus, E., **Taylor, M.J.**, **Sauer, C.**, **Pfennig, A.**, **Ritter, P.**, **Bauer, M.**, and **Geddes, J.R.** (2014). 'Lithium for prevention of mood episodes in bipolar disorders: Systematic review and meta-analysis'. International Journal of Bipolar Disorders, **2**: 15.

Shah, A.S., **Griffiths, M.**, **Lee, K.K.**, **McAllister, D.A.**, **Hunter, A.L.**, **Ferry, A.V.**, **Cruikshank, A.**, **Reid, A.**, **Stoddart, M.**, **Strachan, F.**, and **Walker, S.** (2015). 'High sensitivity cardiac troponin and the under-diagnosis of myocardial infarction in women: prospective cohort study'. British Medical Journal, **350**: 7873–80.

Shah, P. and **Mountain, D.** (2007). 'The medical model is dead: Long live the medical model'. British Journal of Psychiatry, **191**: 375–7.

Shakoor, S., **Zavos, H.M.**, **Haworth, C.M.**, **McGuire, P.**, **Cardno, A.G.**, **Freeman, D.**, and **Ronald, A.** (2016). 'Association between stressful life events and psychotic experiences in adolescence: evidence for gene–environment correlations'. British Journal of Psychiatry, **208**: 532–53.

Shalev, I., **Heim, C.M.**, and **Noll, J.G.** (2016). 'Child maltreatment as a root cause of mortality disparities: A call for rigorous science to mobilize public investment in prevention and treatment'. JAMA Psychiatry, **73**: 897–8.

Sharma, T., **Guski, L.S.**, **Freund, N.**, and **Gøtzsche, P.C.** (2016). 'Suicidality and aggression during antidepressant treatment: Systematic review and meta-analyses based on clinical study reports'. British Medical Journal, **352**: i65.

Shaw, C.M., **Creed, F.H.**, **Tomenson, B.M.**, **Riste, L.**, and **Cruikshank J.K.** (1999). 'Prevalence of anxiety and depressive illness and help seeking behaviour in African Caribbeans and white Europeans: Two phase general population survey'. British Medical Journal, **318**: 302–6.

Shedler, J., **Beck, A.**, **Fonagy, P.**, **Gabbard, G.O.**, **Gunderson, J.**, **Kernberg, O.**, **Michels, R.**, and **Westen, D.** (2010). 'Personality disorders in DSM-5'. American Journal of Psychiatry, **167**: 1026–28.

Shepherd, M. and Zangwill. O.L. (eds) (1983). *Handbook of Psychiatry 1: General Psychopathology*. Cambridge: Cambridge University Press.

Shine, B., McKnight, R.F., Leaver, L., and **Geddes, J.R.** (2015). 'Long-term effects of lithium on renal, thyroid, and parathyroid function: A retrospective analysis of laboratory data'. Lancet, **386**: 461–8.

Shorter, E. (2014). 'The 25th anniversary of the launch of Prozac gives pause for thought: Where did we go wrong?' British Journal of Psychiatry, **204**: 331–2.

Shrout P.E, Spitzer R.L., and **Fleiss J.L.** (1987). 'Quantification of agreement in psychiatric diagnosis revisited'. Archives of General Psychiatry, **44**: 172–7.

Sibelli, A., Chalder, T., Everitt, H., Workman, P., Windgassen, S., and **Moss-Morris, R.** (2016). 'A systematic review with meta-analysis of the role of anxiety and depression in irritable bowel syndrome onset'. Psychological Medicine, **46**: 3065–80.

Siebert, S., Lyall, D.M., Mackay, D.F., Porter, D., McInnes, I.B., Sattar, N., and **Pell, J.P.** (2016). 'Characteristics of rheumatoid arthritis and its association with major comorbid conditions: Cross-sectional study of 502 649 UK Biobank participants'. RMD Open, **2**: e000267.

Sievers M.L. (1961). 'The second "great imitator"—tuberculosis'. Journal of the American Medical Association, **17**: 809–10.

Silver H.K. and **Finkelstein M.** (1967). 'Deprivation dwarfism'. Journal of Pediatrics, **70**: 317–24.

Silbersweig, D. and **Loscalzo, J.** (2017). 'Precision psychiatry meets network medicine: Network psychiatry'. JAMA Psychiatry, **74**: 665–6.

Sim, K., Lau, W.K., Sim, J., Sum, M.Y., and **Baldessarini, R.J.** (2016). 'Prevention of relapse and recurrence in adults with major depressive disorder: Systematic review and meta-analyses of controlled trials'. International Journal of Neuropsychopharmacology, **19**: pyv076.

Singer, M., Bulled, N., Ostrach, B., and **Mendenhall, E.** (2017). 'Syndemics and the biosocial conception of health'. Lancet, **389**: 941–50.

Singh, G.M., Danaei, G., Farzadfar, F., Stevens, G.A., Woodward, M., Wormser, D., Kaptoge, S., Whitlock, G., Qiao, Q., Lewington, S., and **Di Angelantonio, E.** (2013). 'The age-specific quantitative effects of metabolic risk factors on cardiovascular diseases and diabetes: A pooled analysis'. PloS One, **8**: e65174.

Singh, H., Meyer, A.N., and **Thomas, E.J.** (2014). 'The frequency of diagnostic errors in outpatient care: Estimations from three large observational studies involving US adult populations'. BMJ Quality and Safety, **23**: 727–31.

Singleton N., Bumpstead R., O'Brien M., Lee A., and **Meltzer H.** (2001). 'Psychiatric morbidity among adults living in private households, 2000'. London: Her Majesty's Stationery Office.

Skapinakis, P., Weich, S., Lewis, G., Singleton, N., and **Araya, R.** (2006). 'Socio-economic position and common mental disorders: Longitudinal study in the general population in the UK'. British Journal of Psychiatry, **189**: 109–17.

Skilleter, A.J., Weickert, C.S., Vercammen, A., Lenroot, R., and **Weickert, T.W.** (2015). 'Peripheral BDNF: A candidate biomarker of healthy neural activity during learning is disrupted in schizophrenia'. Psychological Medicine, **45**: 841–54.

Skodol, A.E., Oldham, J.M., Bender, D.S., Dyck, I.R., Stout, R.L., Morey, L.C., Shea, M.T., Zanarini, M.C., Sanislow, C.A., Grilo, C.M., and **McGlashan, T.H.** (2005). 'Dimensional representations of DSM-IV personality disorders: Relationships to functional impairment'. American Journal of Psychiatry, **162**: 1919–25.

Skodol, A.E., Morey, L.C., Bender, D.S., and **Oldham, J.M.** (2015). 'The alternative DSM-5 model for personality disorders: A clinical application'. American Journal of Psychiatry, **172**: 606–13.

Smilowitz, N.R., Pirmohamed A., and **Weisz, G.** (2016). 'Published articles reporting studies by industry employees on interventional cardiology devices: Scope and association with study outcomes'. JAMA Internal Medicine. Published online 28 March 2016. doi:10.1001/jamainternmed.2016.0367.

Smith, D.J., Escott-Price, V., Davies, G., Bailey, M.E., Colodro-Conde, L., Ward, J., Vedernikov, A., Marioni, R., Cullen, B., Lyall, D., and **Hagenaars, S.P.** (2016). 'Genome-wide analysis of over 106 000 individuals identifies 9 neuroticism-associated loci'. Molecular Psychiatry, **21**: 749–57.

Smith, K. (2017). 'The best drug treatment for psychotic depression: antidepressants, antipsychotics or both combined?' British Journal of Psychiatric Advances, **23**: 3–8.

Smith, L.A., Cornelius, V., Warnock, A., Tacchi, M.J., and **Taylor, D.** (2007). 'Pharmacological interventions for acute bipolar mania: A systematic review of randomized placebo-controlled trials'. Bipolar Disorders, **9**: 551–60.

Smith, M.L. and **Glass, G.V.** (1977). 'Meta-analysis of psychotherapyoutcome studies'. American Psychologist, **32**: 752–60.

Sokal R.R. (1974). 'Classification: Purposes, principles, progress, prospects'. Science, **185**: 1115–23.

Sommer, I.E. (2010). 'The continuum hypothesis of psychosis: David's criticisms are timely'. Psychological Medicine, **40**: 195961.

Son, J.M., de la Foz, V.O., Martinez-Garcia, O., Moreno, T., Parrilla-Escobar, M., Valdizan, E.M., and **Crespo-Facorro, B.** (2016). 'Clinical outcome after antipsychotic treatment discontinuation in functionally recovered first-episode nonaffective psychosis individuals: A 3-year naturalistic follow-up study'. Journal of Clinical Psychiatry, **77**: 492–500.

Song, J., Bergen, S.E., Kuja-Halkola, R., Larsson, H., Landén, M., and **Lichtenstein, P.** (2015). 'Bipolar disorder and its relation to major psychiatric disorders: A family-based study in the Swedish population'. Bipolar Disorders, **17**: 184–93.

Song, J., Bergen, S.E., Di Florio, A., Karlsson, R., Charney, A., Ruderfer, D.M., Stahl, E.A., Chambert, K.D., Moran, J.L., Gordon-Smith, K., and **Forty, L.** (2016). 'Genome-wide association study identifies SESTD1 as a novel risk gene for lithium-responsive bipolar disorder'. Molecular Psychiatry, **21**: 1290–7.

Spiteri, M.A., Cook, D.G., and **Clarke, S.W.** (1988). 'Reliability of eliciting physical signs in examination of the chest'. Lancet, **331**: 873–5.

Spitzer R.L., Cohen J., Fleiss J.L., and **Endicott J.** (1967). 'Quantification of agreement in psychiatric diagnosis'. Archives of General Psychiatry, **17**: 83–7.

Spitzer, R.L. and **Fleiss, J.L.** (1974). 'A re-analysis of the reliability of psychiatric diagnosis'. British Journal of Psychiatry, **125**: 341–7.

Spitzer R.L, Endicott J., and **Robbins E.** (1978). 'Research diagnostic criteria: rationale and reliability'. Archives of General Psychiatry, **35**: 773–82.

Stanghellini, G., Langer, Á.I., Ambrosini, A., and **Cangas, A.J.** (2012). 'Quality of hallucinatory experiences: Differences between a clinical and a non-clinical sample'. World Psychiatry, **11**: 110–13.

Stanghellini G. and Fuchs T. (eds) (2013). *One Century of Karl Jaspers' General Psychopathology*. Oxford: Oxford University Press.

Starfield, B. (2000). 'Is US health really the best in the world?' Journal of the American Medical Association, **284**: 483–5.

Stausberg, J., Lehmann, N., Kaczmarek, D., and **Stein, M.** (2008). 'Reliability of diagnoses coding with ICD-10'. International Journal of Medical Informatics, **77**: 50–7.

Steel, Z., Chey, T., Silove, D., Marnane, C., Bryant, R.A., and **Van Ommeren, M.** (2009). 'Association of torture and other potentially traumatic events with mental health outcomes among populations exposed to mass conflict and displacement: A systematic review and meta-analysis'. Journal of the American Medical Association, **302**: 537–49.

Stein, D.J. (2015). 'Antidepressant-placebo differences: Is the glass half full or half empty?' World Psychiatry, **14**: 257–8.

Steinbrecher, N., Koerber, S., Frieser, D. and **Hiller, W.** (2011). 'The prevalence of medically unexplained symptoms in primary care'. Psychosomatics, **52**: 263–71.

Stengel E. (1959). 'Classification of mental disorders'. Bulletin of World Health Organisation, **21**: 601–63.

Stewart, R. (2002). 'Vascular dementia: a diagnosis running out of time'. British Journal of Psychiatry, **180**: 152–6.

Stochl, J., Khandaker, G.M., Lewis, G., Perez, J., Goodyer, I.M., Zammit, S., Sullivan, S., Croudace, T.J., and **Jones, P.B** (2015). 'Mood, anxiety and psychotic phenomena measure a common psychopathological factor'. Psychological Medicine, **45**: 1483–93.

Stoltenborgh, M., van IJzendoorn, M.H., Euser, E.M., and **Bakermans-Kranenburg, M.J.** (2011). 'A global perspective on child sexual abuse: meta-analysis of prevalence around the world'. Child Maltreatment, **16**: 79–101.

Stone, J., Wojcik, W., Durrance, D., and **Carson, A.** (2002). 'What should we say to patients with symptoms unexplained by disease? "The number needed to offend"'. British Medical Journal, **325**: 1449–50.

Stovell, D, Wearden A, Morrison A.P., and **Hutton A.** (2016). 'Service users' experiences of the treatment decision-making process in psychosis: A phenomenological analysis'. Psychosis, **8**: 1–13.

Strauss, J.S. and **Carpenter, W.T.** (1972). 'The prediction of outcome in schizophrenia: I. Characteristics of outcome'. Archives of General Psychiatry, **27**: 739–46.

Sugarman, P.A. and Craufurd, D., 1994. 'Schizophrenia in the Afro-Caribbean community'. The British Journal of Psychiatry, **164**(4): 474–80.

Suliman, S., Hemmings, S.M.and Seedat, S. (2013). 'Brain-Derived Neurotrophic Factor (BDNF) protein levels in anxiety disorders: Systematic review and meta-regression analysis'. Frontiers in Integrative Neuroscience, 7 article 55.

Sullivan, P.F., Kendler, K.S., and **Neale, M.C.** (2003). 'Schizophrenia as a complex trait: Evidence from a meta-analysis of twin studies'. Archives of General Psychiatry, **60**: 1187–92.

Sullivan, P.F., Daly, M.J., and **O'Donovan, M.** (2012). 'Genetic architectures of psychiatric disorders: The emerging picture and its implications'. Nature Reviews Genetics, **13**: 537–51.

Suppes, T., Badessarini, R. J., Faedda, G. L., and **Tohen M.** (1991). 'Risk of recurrence following discontinuation of lithium treatment in bipolar disorder'. Archives of General Psychiatry, **48**: 1082–8.

Susser, M. (1991). 'What is a cause and how DO we know one? A grammar for pragmatic epidemiology'. American Journal of Epidemiology, **133**: 633–48.

Susser, M. (1998). Falsification,verification and causal inference in epidemiology: reconsideration in the light of Sir Karl Popper's philosophy In: K.J. Rothman (ed.). *Causal Inference*. Chestnut Hill, MA: Epidemiology Resources, Inc., pp. 33–58.

Sutterland, A.L., Fond, G., Kuin, A., Koeter, M.W.J., Lutter, R., Gool, T., Yolken, R., Szoke, A., Leboyer, M., and **Haan, L.** (2015). 'Beyond the association. Toxoplasma gondii in schizophrenia, bipolar disorder, and addiction: Systematic review and meta-analysis'. Acta Psychiatrica Scandinavica, **132**: 161–79.

Szasz T. (1960). 'The myth of mental illness'. American Psychologist, **15**: 113–18.

Szatmari, P. (2011). 'New recommendations on autism spectrum disorder'. British Medical Journal, **342**: d2456.

Tajika, A., Ogawa, Y., Takeshima, N., Hayasaka, Y., and **Furukawa, T.A.** (2015). 'Replication and contradiction of highly cited research papers in psychiatry: 10-year follow-up'. British Journal of Psychiatry, **207**: 357–62.

Takeuchi, H., Kantor, N., Sanches, M., Fervaha, G., Agid, O., and **Remington, G.** (2017). 'One-year symptom trajectories in patients with stable schizophrenia maintained on antipsychotics versus placebo: Meta-analysis'. British Journal of Psychiatry, **211**: 137–43.

Takwoingi, Y., Riley, R.D., and **Deeks, J.J.** (2015). 'Meta-analysis of diagnostic accuracy studies in mental health'. Evidence Based Mental Health, **18**: 103–9.

Tambs, K., Czajkowsky, N., Røysamb, E., Neale, M.C., Reichborn-Kjennerud, T., Aggen, S.H., Harris, J.R., Ørstavik, R.E., and **Kendler, K.S.** (2009). 'Structure of genetic and environmental risk factors for dimensional representations of DSM-IV anxiety disorders'. British Journal of Psychiatry, **195**: 301–7.

Tamminga, C.A., Ivleva, E.I., Keshavan, M.S., Pearlson, G.D., Clementz, B.A., Witte, B., Morris, D.W., Bishop, J., Thaker, G.K., and **Sweeney, J.A.** (2013). 'Clinical phenotypes of psychosis in the Bipolar-Schizophrenia Network on Intermediate Phenotypes (B-SNIP)'. American Journal of Psychiatry, **170**: 1263–74.

Tamminga, C.A., Pearlson, G., Keshavan, M., Sweeney, J., Clementz, B., and **Thaker, G.** (2014). 'Bipolar and schizophrenia network for intermediate phenotypes: Outcomes across the psychosis continuum'. Schizophrenia Bulletin, **40**(Suppl 2): S131–S137.

Tansella, M. (2002). 'The scientific evaluation of mental health treatments: an historical perspective'. Evidence Based Mental Health, **5**: 4–5.

Tarricone, I., Stivanello, E., Poggi, F., Castorini, V., Marseglia, M.V., Fantini, M.P., and **Berardi, D.** (2012). 'Ethnic variation in the prevalence of depression and anxiety in primary care: A systematic review and meta-analysis'. Psychiatry Research, **195**: 91–106.

Taylor A.E. and **Munafo M.R.** (2016). 'Triangulating meta-analyses: the example of the serotonin transporter gene, stressful life events and major depression'. BMC Psychology, 4: 23–31.

Taylor, D. (2015). 'The straw man of prescribing in psychiatry: Commentary on . . . drug-centred psychopharmacology'. British Journal of Psychiatric Advances, **21**: 237–9.

Taylor, M.A. and **Abrams, R.** (1975). 'A critique of the St. Louis psychiatric research criteria for schizophrenia'. American Journal of Psychiatry, **132**: 1276–80.

Taylor, M.A., Shorter, E., Vaidya, N.A., and **Fink, M.** (2010). 'The failure of the schizophrenia concept and the argument for its replacement by hebephrenia: applying the medical model for disease recognition'. Acta Psychiatrica Scandinavica, **122**: 173–83.

Taylor M.A. (2013). *Hippocrates Cried. The Decline of American Psychiatry*. Oxford: Oxford University Press.

Teasdale, G. and **Jennett, B.** (1974). 'Assessment of coma and impaired consciousness: A practical scale'. Lancet, **304**: 81–4.

Teasdale, G. and **Jennett, B.** (1976). 'Assessment and prognosis of coma after head injury'. Acta Neurochirurgica, **34**: 45–55.

Teicher, M.H. and **Samson, J.A.** (2013). 'Childhood maltreatment and psychopathology: A case for ecophenotypic variants as clinically and neurobiologically distinct subtypes'. American Journal of Psychiatry, **170**: 1114–33.

Tenback, D.E., **Van Harten, P.N.**, **Slooff, C.J.**, and **Van Os, J.** (2010). 'Incidence and persistence of tardive dyskinesia and extrapyramidal symptoms in schizophrenia'. Journal of Psychopharmacology, **24**: 1031–5.

Tennant N. and **Thompson I.E.** (1980). 'Causes and logic in epidemiological psychiatry 2: Causal models and logical inference'. British Journal of Psychiatry, **137**: 579–82.

Tesli, M., **Wirgenes, K.V.**, **Hughes, T.**, **Bettella, F.**, **Athanasiu, L.**, **Hoseth, E.S.**, **Nerhus, M.**, **Lagerberg, T.V.**, **Steen, N.E.**, **Agartz, I.**, and **Melle, I.** (2016). 'VRK2 gene expression in schizophrenia, bipolar disorder and healthy controls'. British Journal of Psychiatry, **209**: 114–20.

Thibaut, F., **Boutros, N.N.**, **Jarema, M.**, **Oranje, B.**, **Hasan, A.**, **Daskalakis, Z.J.**, **Wichniak, A.**, **Schmitt, A.**, **Riederer, P.**, and **Falkai, P.** (2015). 'Consensus paper of the WFSBP Task Force on Biological Markers: Criteria for biomarkers and endophenotypes of schizophrenia part I: Neurophysiology'. World Journal of Biological Psychiatry, **16**: 280–90.

Thomas, C.S., **Stone, K.**, **Osborn, M.**, **Thomas, P.F.** and **Fisher, M.** (1993). 'Psychiatric morbidity and compulsory admission among UK-born Europeans, Afro-Caribbeans and Asians in central Manchester'. British Journal of Psychiatry ,**163**: 91–9.

Thornton T (2015). 'Against explanatory minimalism in psychiatry'. Frontiers in Psychiatry, **6**: 171. doi:10.3389/fpsyt.2015.00171.

Tiihonen, J., **Lönnqvist, J.**, **Wahlbeck, K.**, **Klaukka, T.**, **Niskanen, L.**, **Tanskanen, A.**, and **Haukka, J.** (2009). '11-year follow-up of mortality in patients with schizophrenia: A population-based cohort study (FIN11 study)'. Lancet, **374**: 620–7.

Tiihonen, J., **Mittendorfer-Rutz, E.**, **Torniainen, M.**, **Alexanderson, K.**, and **Tanskanen, A.** (2016). 'Mortality and cumulative exposure to antipsychotics, antidepressants, and benzodiazepines in patients with schizophrenia: An observational follow-up study'. American Journal of Psychiatry, **173**: 600–6.

Tikkinen, K.A., **Leinonen, J.S.**, **Guyatt, G.H.**, **Ebrahim, S.**, and **Järvinen, T.L.** (2012). 'What is a disease? Perspectives of the public, health professionals and legislators'. BMJ Open, **2**: e001632.

Timmis, A. (2015). 'Acute coronary syndromes'. British Medical Journal, **351**: h5153.

Tolin, D.F. (2010). 'Is cognitive–behavioral therapy more effective than other therapies?: A meta-analytic review'. Clinical Psychology Review, **30**: 710–20.

Tolin, D.F., **Gilliam, C.**, **Wootton, B.M.**, **Bowe, W.**, **Bragdon, L.B.**, **Davis, E.**, **Hannan, S.E.**, **Steinman, S.A.**, **Worden, B.**, and **Hallion, L.S.** (2016). 'Psychometric properties of a structured diagnostic interview for DSM-5 anxiety, mood, and obsessive-compulsive and related disorders'. Assessment, **25**(1): 3–13.

Tononi, G. and **Koch, C.** (2015). 'Consciousness: here, there and everywhere?' Philosophical Transactions of the Royal Society Biological Sciences, **370**: p. 20140167.

Torniainen, M., **Mittendorfer-Rutz, E.**, **Tanskanen, A.**, **Björkenstam, C.**, **Suvisaari, J.**, **Alexanderson, K.**, and **Tiihonen, J.** (2014). 'Antipsychotic treatment and mortality in schizophrenia'. Schizophrenia Bulletin, **41**: 656–63.

Torrey, E.F., **Bartko, J.J.**, and **Yolken, R.H.** (2012). 'Toxoplasma gondii and other risk factors for schizophrenia: An update'. Schizophrenia Bulletin, **38**: 642–7.

Tortelli, A., **Errazuriz, A.**, **Croudace, T.**, **Morgan, C.**, **Murray, R.M.**, **Jones, P.B.**, **Szoke, A.**, and **Kirkbride, J.B.** (2015). 'Schizophrenia and other psychotic disorders in Caribbean-born migrants and their descendants in England: Systematic review and meta-analysis of incidence rates, 1950–2013'. Social Psychiatry and Psychiatric Epidemiology, **50**: 1039–55.

Treadwell, J. and **McCartney, M.** (2016). 'Overdiagnosis and overtreatment: generalists—it's time for a grassroots revolution'. British Journal of General Practice, **66**: 116–17.

Tsuang, M.T., **Woolson, R.F.**, and **Fleming, J.A.** (1979). 'Long-term outcome of major psychoses: I. Schizophrenia and affective disorders compared with psychiatrically symptom-free surgical conditions'. Archives of General Psychiatry, **36**: 1295–301.

Tsuang, M.T. and **Dempsey, G.M.** (1979). 'Long-term outcome of major psychoses: II. Schizoaffective disorder compared with schizophrenia, affective disorders, and a surgical control group'. Archives of General Psychiatry, **36**: 1302–04.

Turkheimer, E., **Pettersson, E.**, and **Horn, E.E.** (2014). 'A phenotypic null hypothesis for the genetics of personality'. Annual Review of Psychology, **65**: 515–40.

Turner, D. T., **van der Gaag, M.**, **Karyotaki, E.**, and **Cuijpers, P.** (2014). 'Psychological interventions for psychosis: A meta-analysis of comparative outcome studies'. American Journal of Psychiatry, **171**: 523–38.

Turner, E.H., **Matthews, A.M.**, **Linardatos, E.**, **Tell, R.A.**, and **Rosenthal, R.** (2008). 'Selective publication of antidepressant trials and its influence on apparent efficacy'. New England Journal of Medicine, **358**: 252–60.

Turner, E.H., **Knoepflmacher, D.**, and **Shapley, L.** (2012). 'Publication bias in antipsychotic trials: an analysis of efficacy comparing the published literature to the US Food and Drug Administration database'. PLoS Medicine, **9**: e1001189.

Tye, K.M., **Prakash, R.**, **Kim, S.Y.**, **Fenno, L.E.**, **Grosenick, L.**, **Zarabi, H.**, **Thompson, K.R.**, **Gradinaru, V.**, **Ramakrishnan, C.**, and **Deisseroth, K.** (2011). 'Amygdala circuitry mediating reversible and bidirectional control of anxiety'. Nature, **471**: 358–62.

Tyrer P., **Al Muderis O.**, and **Gulbrandsen G.** (2001). 'Distribution of case-load in community mental health teams'. Psychiatric Bulletin, **25**: 10–12.

Tyrer, P., **Crawford, M.**, **Mulder, R.** and **ICD-11 Working Group for the Revision of Classification of Personality Disorders** (2011). 'Reclassifying personality disorders'. Lancet, **377**: 1814–15.

Tyrer, P., **Reed, G.M.**, and **Crawford, M.J.** (2015). 'Classification, assessment, prevalence, and effect of personality disorder', Lancet, **385**: 717–26.

Tyrer, P. (2017). 'Comorbidity, consanguinity and co-occurrence'. British Journal of Psychiatric Advances, **23**: 167–8.

UK ECT Review Goup (2003). 'Efficacy and safety of electroconvulsive therapy in depressive disorders: A systematic review and meta-analysis'. Lancet, **361**: 799–808.

US Department of Health and Human Services (2014). 'The health consequences of smoking—50 years of progress: a report of the Surgeon General'. Atlanta, GA. Available at: <https://www.surgeongeneral.gov/library/reports/50-years-of-progress/full-report.pdf>.

Vachon, D.D., **Krueger, R.F.**, **Rogosch, F.A.**, and **Cicchetti, D.** (2015). 'Assessment of the harmful psychiatric and behavioral effects of different forms of child maltreatment'. JAMA Psychiatry, **72**: 1135–42.

Valenti, E., **Banks, C.**, **Calcedo-Barba, A.**, **Bensimon, C.M.**, **Hoffmann, K.M.**, **Pelto-Piri, V.**, **Jurin, T.**, **Mendoza, O.M.**, **Mundt, A.P.**, **Rugkåsa, J.**, and **Tubini, J.** (2015). 'Informal coercion in psychiatry: A focus group study of attitudes and experiences of mental health professionals in ten countries'. Social Psychiatry and Psychiatric Epidemiology, **50**: 1297–308.

van der Gaag, M., **Cuijpers, A.**, **Hoffman, T.**, **Remijsen, M.**, **Hijman, R.**, **de Haan, L.**, **van Meijel, B.**, **van Harten, P.N.**, **Valmaggia, L.**, **De Hert, M.**, and **Wiersma, D.** (2006a). 'The five-factor model of the Positive and Negative Syndrome Scale I: Confirmatory factor analysis fails to confirm 25 published five-factor solutions'. Schizophrenia Research, **85**: 273–9.

Van den Hout M. (2014). 'Psychiatric symptoms as pathogens'. Clinical Neuropsychiatry, **11**: 153–9.

Van der Gaag, M., **Hoffman, T.**, **Remijsen, M.**, **Hijman, R.**, **de Haan, L.**, **van Meijel, B.**, **van Harten, P.N.**, **Valmaggia, L.**, **De Hert, M.**, **Cuijpers, A.** and **Wiersma, D.** (2006b). 'The five-factor model of the Positive and Negative Syndrome Scale II: a ten-fold cross-validation of a revised model'. Schizophrenia Research, **85**: 280–7.

van Nierop, M., **Viechtbauer, W.**, **Gunther, N.**, **Van Zelst, C.**, **De Graaf, R.**, **Ten Have, M.**, **Van Dorsselaer, S.**, **Bak, M.**, and **van Winkel, R.** (2015). 'Childhood trauma is associated with a specific admixture of affective, anxiety, and psychosis symptoms cutting across traditional diagnostic boundaries'. Psychological Medicine, **45**: 1277–88.

Van Os, J., **Fahy, T.A.**, **Jones, P.**, **Harvey, I.**, **Sham, P.**, **Lewis, S.**, **Bebbington, P.**, **Toone, B.**, **Williams, M.** and **Murray, R.** (1996). 'Psychopathological syndromes in the functional psychoses: Associations with course and outcome'. Psychological Medicine, **26**: 161–76.

Van Os, J., **Gilvarry, C.**, **Bale, R.**, **Van Horn, E.**, **Tattan, T.**, and **White, I.** (1999). 'A comparison of the utility of dimensional and categorical representations of psychosis'. Psychological Medicine, **29**: 595–606.

Van Os, J., **Bak, M.**, **Hanssen, M.**, **Bijl, R.V.**, **De Graaf, R.**, and **Verdoux, H.** (2002). 'Cannabis use and psychosis: a longitudinal population-based study'. American Journal of Epidemiology, **156**: 319–27.

Van Os, J. (2015). 'The transdiagnostic dimension of psychosis: implications for psychiatric nosology and research'. Shanghai Archives of Psychiatry, **27**: 82–6.

Van Os, J. and **Reininghaus, U.** (2016). 'Psychosis as a transdiagnostic and extended phenotype in the general population'. World Psychiatry, **15**: 118–24.

Van Praag, H. (1992). 'Reconquest of the subjective. Against the waning of the psychiatric diagnosis'. British Journal of Psychiatry, **160**: 266–72.

Vancampfort, D., **Correll, C.U.**, **Galling, B.**, **Probst, M.**, **De Hert, M.**, **Ward, P.B.**, **Rosenbaum, S.**, **Gaughran, F.**, **Lally, J.**, and **Stubbs, B.** (2016). 'Diabetes mellitus in people with schizophrenia, bipolar disorder and major depressive disorder: A systematic review and large scale meta-analysis'. World Psychiatry, **15**: 166–74.

Varese, F., **Smeets, F.**, **Drukker, M.**, **Lieverse, R.**, **Lataster, T.**, **Viechtbauer, W.**, **Read, J.**, **van Os, J.**, and **Bentall, R.P.** (2012). 'Childhood adversities increase the risk of psychosis: A meta-analysis of patient-control, prospective-and cross-sectional cohort studies'. Schizophrenia Bulletin, **38**: 661–71.

Vassos, E., **Pedersen, C.B.**, **Murray, R.M.**, **Collier, D.A.**, and **Lewis, C.M.** (2012). 'Meta-analysis of the association of urbanicity with schizophrenia'. Schizophrenia Bulletin, **38**: 1118–23.

Vassos, E., **Agerbo, E.**, **Mors, O.**, and **Pedersen, C.B.** (2016). 'Urban–rural differences in incidence rates of psychiatric disorders in Denmark'. British Journal of Psychiatry, **208**: 435–80.

Vaughan, B., **Goldstein, M.H.**, **Alikakos, M.**, **Cohen, L.J.**, and **Serby, M.J.** (2014). 'Frequency of reporting of adverse events in randomized controlled trials of psychotherapy vs. psychopharmacotherapy'. Comprehensive Psychiatry, **55**: 849–55.

Viera A.J. and **Garrett J.M.** (2005). 'Understanding interobserver agreement: The Kappa statistic'. Family Medicine, **37**: 360–3.

Viera, A.J. (2017). 'Whatever happened to the polypill?' British Medical Journal, **356**: j1474.

Vita, A., **De Peri, L.**, **Deste, G.**, **Barlati, S.**, and **Sacchetti, E.** (2015). 'The effect of antipsychotic treatment on cortical gray matter changes in schizophrenia: Does the class matter? A meta-analysis and meta-regression of longitudinal magnetic resonance imaging studies'. Biological Psychiatry, **78**: 403–12.

Vobecky M., **Leduc P.D.**, **Devroede G.**, and **Madarnas P.** (1989). 'The reliability of routine pathologic diagnosis of colorectal adenocarcinoma'. Cancer, **64**: 1261–5.

Vos, T., **Barber, R.M.**, and **Bell, B.** (2015). 'Global Burden of Disease Study 2013 Collaborators. Global, regional, and national incidence, prevalence, and years lived with disability for 301 acute and chronic diseases and injuries in 188 countries, 1990–2013: A systematic analysis for the Global Burden of Disease Study 2013'. Lancet, **386**: 743–800.

Vreeker, A., **Boks, M.P.M.**, **Abramovic, L.**, **Verkooijen, S.**, **Van Bergen, A.H.**, **Hillegers, M.H.J.**, **Spijker, A.T.**, **Hoencamp, E.**, **Regeer, E.J.**, **Riemersma-Van der Lek, R.F.**, and **Stevens, A.W.M.M.** (2016). 'High educational performance is a distinctive feature of bipolar disorder: A study on cognition in bipolar disorder, schizophrenia patients, relatives and controls'. Psychological Medicine, **46**: 807–18.

Wakefield, J.C. (1992). 'The concept of mental disorder: On the boundary between biological facts and social values'. American Psychologist, **47**: 373–88.

Wakefield, J.C. (2014). 'Wittgenstein's nightmare: Why the RDoC grid needs a conceptual dimension'. World Psychiatry, **13**: 38–40.

Walker B.R., **Colledge N.R.**, **Ralston S.H.**, and **Penman I.** *Davidson's Principles and Practice of Medicine*, 22nd edn. (2014). Edinburgh: Churchill Livingstone (Elsevier).

Walker, E.R., **McGee, R.E.**, and **Druss, B.G.** (2015a). 'Mortality in mental disorders and global disease burden implications: A systematic review and meta-analysis'. JAMA Psychiatry, **72**: 334–41.

Walker, Z., **Possin, K.L.**, **Boeve, B.F.**, and **Aarsland, D.** (2015b). 'Lewy body dementias'. Lancet, **386**: 1683–97.

Wallace, D.E., **McGreal, G.T.**, **O'Toole, G.**, **Holloway, P.**, **Wallace, M.**, **McDermott, E.W.** and **Blake, J.** (2000). 'The influence of experience and specialisation on the reliability of a common clinical sign'. Annals of the Royal College of Surgeons of England, **82**: 336–8.

Wallace, S., **Nazroo, J.**, and **Bécares, L.** (2016). 'Cumulative effect of racial discrimination on the mental health of ethnic minorities in the United Kingdom'. American Journal of Public Health, **106**: 1294–300.

Walsh, B.T., **Seidman, S.N.**, **Sysko, R.**, and **Gould, M.** (2002). 'Placebo response in studies of major depression: Variable, substantial, and growing'. Journal of the American Medical Association, **287**: 1840–7.

Wampold, B.E., **Minami, T.**, **Baskin, T.W.**, and **Tierney, S.C.** (2002). 'A meta-(re) analysis of the effects of cognitive therapy versus "other therapies" for depression'. Journal of Affective Disorders, **68**: 159–65.

Wampold, B.E. (2015). 'How important are the common factors in psychotherapy? An update'. World Psychiatry, **14**: 270–7.

Wampold, B.E., Flückiger, C., Del Re, A.C., Yulish, N.E., Frost, N.D., Pace, B.T., Goldberg, S.B., Miller, S.D., Baardseth, T.P., Laska, K.M., and **Hilsenroth, M.J.** (2017). 'In pursuit of truth: A critical examination of meta-analyses of cognitive behavior therapy'. Psychotherapy Research, **27**: 14–32.

Wang, K., Merin, A., Rendina, H.J. and **Pachankis, J.E.** (2016a). 'Genital herpes stigma: Toward the measurement and validation of a highly prevalent yet hidden public health problem'. Stigma and Health, **3**(1): 27–34.

Wang Y., Xia J., Helfer B., Li C., and **Leucht S.** (2016b). 'Valproate for schizophrenia'. Cochrane Database of Systematic Reviews, **11**: CD004028.

Wartolowska, K., Judge, A., Hopewell, S., Collins, G.S., Dean, B.J., Rombach, I., Brindley, D., Savulescu, J., Beard, D.J., and **Carr, A.J.** (2014). 'Use of placebo controls in the evaluation of surgery: Systematic review'. British Medical Journal, **348**: g3253.

Waszczuk, M.A., Coulson, A.E., Gregory, A.M., and **Eley, T.C.** (2016). 'A longitudinal twin and sibling study of the hopelessness theory of depression in adolescence and young adulthood'. Psychological Medicine, **46**: 1935–49.

Weed (1998). Causal criteria and Popperian refutation. In: K.J. Rothman (ed.). *Causal Inference*. Chestnut Hill, MA: Epidemiology Resources, Inc., pp. 15–32.

Weidow, J., Cederlund, C.G., Ranstam, J. and **Kärrholm, J.** (2006). 'Ahlbäck grading of osteoarthritis of the knee: Poor reproducibility and validity based on visual inspection of the joint'. Acta Orthopaedica, 77: 262–6.

Welch, G., Schwartz, L., and **Woloshin, S.** (2011). *Overdiagnosed: Making People Sick in Pursuit of Health*. Boston, MA: Beacon Press.

Weiler-Ravell, D., Leventhal, A., Coker, R.J., and **Chemtob, D.** (2004). 'Compulsory detention of recalcitrant tuberculosis patients in the context of a new tuberculosis control programme in Israel'. Public Health, **118**: 323–32.

Weiss, A.J., Elixhauser, A., Bae, J., and **Encinosa, W.** (2013). 'Origin of adverse drug events in US hospitals, 2011'. HCUP Statistical Brief, **158.**

Wells A. (1997). *Cognitive Therapy of Anxiety Disorders: A Practice Manual and Conceptual Guide*. Chichester: Wiley.

Wester, K., Jönsson, A.K., Spigset, O., Druid, H., and **Hägg, S.** (2008). 'Incidence of fatal adverse drug reactions: A population based study'. British Journal of Clinical Pharmacology, **65**: 573–9.

White, L.R., Edland, S.D., Hemmy, L.S., Montine, K.S., Zarow, C., Sonnen, J.A., Uyehara-Lock, J.H., Gelber, R.P., Ross, G.W., Petrovitch, H., and **Masaki, K.H.** (2016). 'Neuropathologic comorbidity and cognitive impairment in the Nun and Honolulu-Asia Aging Studies'. Neurology, **86**: 1000–8.

WHO World Health Organization (1992). 'The ICD-10 classification of mental and behavioural disorders: clinical descriptions and diagnostic guidelines'. Geneva: World Health Organization.

Widom, C.S., Czaja, S.J., Bentley, T., and **Johnson, M.S.** (2012). 'A prospective investigation of physical health outcomes in abused and neglected children: New findings from a 30-year follow-up'. American Journal of Public Health, **102**: 1135–44.

Widiger, T.A., and **Samuel, D.B.** (2005). 'Diagnostic categories or dimensions? A question for the Diagnostic and Statistical Manual of Mental Disorders'. Journal of Abnormal Psychology, **114**: 494–504.

Widiger, T.A., and **Simonsen, E.** (2005). 'Alternative dimensional models of personality: Finding a common ground'. Journal of Personality Disorder, **19**: 110–30.**Wiersma, D.**, **Nienhuis, F.J.**, **Slooff, C.J.**, and **Giel, R.** (1998). 'Natural course of schizophrenic disorders: A 15-year followup of a Dutch incidence cohort'. Schizophrenia Bulletin, **24**: 75–85.

Wijkstra, J., **Lijmer, J.**, **Burger, H.**, **Cipriani, A.**, **Geddes, J.** aand **Nolen, W.A.** (2017). 'Pharmacological treatment for psychotic depression'. British Journal of Psychiatric Advances, **23**: 2.

Wileman, L., **May, C.**, and **Chew-Graham, C.A.** (2002). 'Medically unexplained symptoms and the problem of power in the primary care consultation: A qualitative study'. Family Practice, **19**: 178–82.

Wilkinson, R. and **Pickett, K.** (2010). *The Spirit Level: Why Equality is Better for Everyone.* London: Penguin.

Williams, E.D., **Tillin, T.**, **Richards, M.**, **Tuson, C.**, **Chaturvedi, N.**, **Hughes, A.D.**, and **Stewart, R.** (2015). 'Depressive symptoms are doubled in older British South Asian and Black Caribbean people compared with Europeans: Associations with excess co-morbidity and socioeconomic disadvantage'. Psychological Medicine, **45**: 1861–71.

Williams, J.B., **Gibbon, M.**, **First, M.B.**, **Spitzer, R.L.**, **Davies, M.**, **Borus, J.**, **Howes, M.J.**, **Kane, J.**, **Pope, H.G.**, **Rounsaville, B.**, and **Wittchen, H.U.** (1992). 'The structured clinical interview for DSM-III-R (SCID): II. Multisite test-retest reliability'. Archives of General Psychiatry, **49**: 630–6.

Williams, P.V. and **McGlashan, T.H.** (1987). 'Schizoaffective psychosis: I. Comparative long-term outcome'. Archives of General Psychiatry, **44**: 130–7.

Wilshire, C.E. and **Ward, T.** (2016). 'Psychogenic explanations of physical illness: Time to examine the evidence'. Perspectives on Psychological Science, **11**: 606–31.

Wing, J.K., **Beevor, A.S.**, **Curtis, R.H.**, **Park, S.B.**, **Hadden, S.** and **Burns, A.** (1998). 'Health of the Nation Outcome Scales (HoNOS). Research and development'. British Journal of Psychiatry, **172**: 11–18.

Winokur, G. (1990). 'The concept of secondary depression and its relationship to comorbidity'. Psychiatric Clinics of North America, **13**(4), 567–83.

Winsper, C., **Marwaha, S.**, **Lereya, S.T.**, **Thompson, A.**, **Eyden, J.** and **Singh, S.P.** (2016). 'A systematic review of the neurobiological underpinnings of borderline personality disorder (BPD) in childhood and adolescence'. Reviews in the Neurosciences, **27**: 827–47.

Woods, S.W., **Morgenstern, H.**, **Saksa, J.R.**, **Walsh, B.C.**, **Sullivan, M.C.**, **Money, R.**, **Hawkins, K.A.**, **Gueorguieva, R.V.**, and **Glazer, W.M.** (2010). 'Incidence of tardive dyskinesia with atypical and conventional antipsychotic medications: Prospective cohort study'. Journal of Clinical Psychiatry, **71**: 463–74.

Wray, N.R. and **Sullivan, P.F.** (2017). 'Genome-wide association analyses identify 44 risk variants and refine the genetic architecture of major depression'. bioRxiv: 167577.

Wright, A.G., **Krueger, R.F.**, **Hobbs, M.J.**, **Markon, K.E.**, **Eaton, N.R.**, and **Slade, T.** (2013). 'The structure of psychopathology: Toward an expanded quantitative empirical model'. Journal of Abnormal Psychology, **122**: 281–94.

Wu EQ, Birnbaum HG, Shi L, Ball DE, Kessler RC, Moulis M, Aggarwal J. (2005). 'The economic burden of schizophrenia in the United States in 2002'. Journal of Clinical Psychiatry, **66**: 1–478.

Wunderink, L., **Nienhuis, F.J.**, **Sytema, S.**, **Slooff, C.J.**, **Knegtering, R.**, and **Wiersma, D.** (2007). 'Guided discontinuation versus maintenance treatment in remitted first-episode psychosis: Relapse rates and functional outcome'. Journal of Clinical Psychiatry, **68**: 654–61.

Wunderink, L., **Nieboer, R.M.**, **Wiersma, D.**, **Sytema, S.**, and **Nienhuis, F.J.** (2013). 'Recovery in remitted first-episode psychosis at 7 years of follow-up of an early dose reduction/discontinuation or maintenance treatment strategy: Long-term follow-up of a 2-year randomized clinical trial'. JAMA Psychiatry, **70**: 913–20.

Wulff, H.R. (1999). 'The concept of disease: from Newton back to Aristotle'. Lancet, **354**: SIV50.

Yeomans D, **Moncrieff J** and **Huws R.** (2015). 'Drug-centred psychopharmacology: A non-diagnostic framework for drug treatment'. (2015). British Journal of Psychiatric Advances, **21**: 229–36.

Wykes, T., **Huddy, V.**, **Cellard, C.**, **McGurk, S.R.**, and **Czobor, P.** (2011). 'A meta-analysis of cognitive remediation for schizophrenia: Methodology and effect sizes'. American Journal of Psychiatry, **168**: 472–85.

Xian, Y., **O'Brien, E.C.**, **Fonarow, G.C.**, **Olson, D.M.**, **Schwamm, L.H.**, **Hannah, D.**, **Lindholm, B.**, **Maisch, L.**, **Lytle, B.L.**, **Greiner, M.A.**, and **Wu, J.** (2015). 'Patient-Centered Research into Outcomes Stroke Patients Prefer and Effectiveness Research: Implementing the patient-driven research paradigm to aid decision making in stroke care'. American Heart Journal, **170**: 36–45.

Yates, D. (2013). 'Neuronal circuits: Piecing together anxiety'. Nature Reviews Neuroscience, **14**: 305.

Yildiz, A., **Nikodem, M.**, **Vieta, E.**, **Correll, C.U.**, and **Baldessarini, R.J.** (2015). 'A network meta-analysis on comparative efficacy and all-cause discontinuation of antimanic treatments in acute bipolar mania'. Psychological Medicine, **45**: 299–317.

Young, J. and **Inouye, S.K.** (2007). 'Delirium in older people'. British Medical Journal, **334**: 842–6.

Yung, A.R. and **Lin, A.** (2016). 'Psychotic experiences and their significance'. World Psychiatry, **15**: 130–1.

Zachar P. and **Kendler K.S.** (2007). 'Psychiatric disorders: A conceptual taxonomy'. American Journal of Psychiatry, **164**: 557–65.

Zachar, P., Stoyanov, D.S., Aragona, M., and Jablensky, A. (eds) (2015). *Alternative Perspectives on Psychiatric Validation—DSM, ICD, RDoC, and Beyond*. Oxford: Oxford University Press.

Zachar, P. (2015). 'Psychiatric disorders: natural kinds made by the world or practical kinds made by us?' World Psychiatry, **14**: 288–90.

Zachar, P., **Krueger, R.F.**, and **Kendler, K.S.** (2016). 'Personality disorder in DSM-5: an oral history'. Psychological Medicine, **46**: 1–10.

Zanarini, M.C., 2000. 'Childhood experiences associated with the development of borderline personality disorder'. Psychiatric Clinics of North America, **23**(1): 89–101.

Zandi, T., **Havenaar, J.M.**, **Laan, W.**, **Kahn, R.S.**, and **van den Brink, W.** (2016). 'Effects of a culturally sensitive assessment on symptom profiles in native Dutch and Moroccan patients with a first psychosis referral'. Transcultural Psychiatry, **53**: 45–59.

Zavodnick, A.D. and **Ali, R.** (2012). Lamotrigine in the treatment of unipolar depression with and without comorbidities: A literature review. Psychiatric Quarterly, **83**(3): 371–83.

Zavos, H.M., **Freeman, D.**, **Haworth, C.M.**, **McGuire, P.**, **Plomin, R.**, **Cardno, A.G.**, and **Ronald, A.** (2014). 'Consistent etiology of severe, frequent psychotic experiences and milder, less frequent manifestations: A twin study of specific psychotic experiences in adolescence'. JAMA Psychiatry, **71**: 1049–57.

Zhang, W., **Deng, W.**, **Yao, L.**, **Xiao, Y.**, **Li, F.**, **Liu, J.**, **Sweeney, J.A.**, **Lui, S.** **Gong, Q.** (2015). 'Brain structural abnormalities in a group of never-medicated patients with long-term schizophrenia'. American Journal of Psychiatry, **172**: 995–1003.

Zhu, X., **Need, A.C.**, **Petrovski, S.**, and **Goldstein, D.B.** (2014). 'One gene, many neuropsychiatric disorders: lessons from Mendelian diseases'. Nature Neuroscience, **17**: 773–81.

Zimmerman, M., **Chelminski, I.**, **Young, D.**, **Dalrymple, K.**, and **Martinez, J.** (2013). 'Is dimensional scoring of borderline personality disorder important only for subthreshold levels of severity?' Journal of Personality Disorders, **27**: 244–51.

Zimmerman, M., **Clark, H.L.**, **Multach, M.D.**, **Walsh, E.**, **Rosenstein, L.K.** and **Gazarian, D.** (2015). 'Have treatment studies of depression become even less generalizable? A review of the inclusion and exclusion criteria used in placebo-controlled antidepressant efficacy trials published during the past 20 years'. Mayo Clinic Proceedings, **90**: 1180–6.

Zimmerman, M., **Multach, M.D.**, **Dalrymple, K.**, and **Chelminski, I.** (2017). 'Clinically useful screen for borderline personality disorder in psychiatric out-patients'. British Journal of Psychiatry, **210**: 165–6.

Zipursky, R.B., **Reilly, T.J.**, and **Murray, R.M.** (2013). 'The myth of schizophrenia as a progressive brain disease'. Schizophrenia Bulletin, **39**: 1363–72.

Zipursky, R.B. and **Agid, O.** (2015). 'Recovery, not progressive deterioration, should be the expectation in schizophrenia'. World Psychiatry, **14**: 94–6.

Index

Tables and figures are indicated by an italic *t* and *f* following the page number.